Women with

A Practical Management Handbook

Women with Epilepsy

A Practical Management Handbook

Edited by

Esther Bui, MD, FRCPC
Staff Neurologist and Lecturer,
Division of Neurology and Division of Obstetrical Medicine, Department of Medicine,
Sunnybrook Health Sciences Centre, University of Toronto, ON, Canada

Autumn Klein, MD, PhD
Formerly of the Department of Neurology,
UPMC Presbyterian/Magee Women's Hospital, Pittsburgh, PA, USA

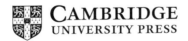

CAMBRIDGE
UNIVERSITY PRESS

University Printing House, Cambridge CB2 8BS, United Kingdom

Cambridge University Press is part of the University of Cambridge.

It furthers the University's mission by disseminating knowledge in the
pursuit of education, learning and research at the highest international
levels of excellence.

www.cambridge.org
Information on this title: www.cambridge.org/9781107659889

© Cambridge University Press 2014

First published 2014

Printed and bound in the United Kingdom by Clays Ltd, St Ives plc

*A catalogue record for this publication is available from the British
Library*

Library of Congress Cataloging-in-Publication Data
Women with epilepsy (2014)
Women with epilepsy : a practical management handbook / edited by
Esther Bui, Autumn Klein.
   p. ; cm.
Includes bibliographical references and index.
ISBN 978-1-107-65988-9 (Paperback)
I. Bui, Esther, editor of compilation.   II. Klein, Autumn, editor of
compilation.   III. Title.
[DNLM: 1. Epilepsy.   2. Women's Health. WL 385]
RC372.3
616.85′30082–dc23   2013041804

ISBN 978-1-107-65988-9 Paperback

Contents

List of contributors   vii

Preface   xi

1   **Epidemiology of women with epilepsy**   1
Kristi A. McIntosh and Nathalie Jette

2   **Psychiatric comorbidities of epilepsy in women**   20
Sherese Ali

3   **Sleep-related comorbidities in women with epilepsy**   34
Carin Dove and Brian J. Murray

4   **Hormonal influences in women with epilepsy**   50
Alberto Verrotti, Marianna Sebastiani, Alessandra Scaparrotta, and Carla Verrotti

5   **Antiepileptic drugs and hormones**   65
Pavel Klein and Jaromir Janousek

6   **Genetic causes of epilepsies in women**   80
Danielle Molinari Andrade

7   **Epilepsy in girls during childhood and adolescence**   92
Cristina Y. Go and O. Carter Snead, III

8   **Catamenial epilepsy**   101
Sima Indubhai Patel and Nancy Foldvary-Schaefer

9   **Fertility in women with epilepsy**   113
Mark Quigg

10   **Selecting contraception for women with epilepsy**   127
Page B. Pennell and Anne Davis

11   **Preconception counseling for women with epilepsy**   141
Elizabeth E. Gerard

12   **Teratogenicity and antiepileptic drugs**   157
Georgia Montouris

13   **Seizure management in pregnancy**   170
A. Gabriela Lizama and Pamela Crawford

14   **Obstetric and fetal monitoring in women with epilepsy**   182
Dini Hui and Ori Nevo

15   **Pregnancy and epilepsy: neuroimaging**   189
Kalliopi A. Petropoulou

16   **Obstetrical anesthesia and the pregnant epileptic patient**   206
Fatima Zahir and Jonathan H. Waters

17   **Seizure management in the postpartum period**   215
Elinor Ben-Menachem

18   **Breastfeeding and use of antiepileptics**   223
Weerawadee Chandranipapongse and Shinya Ito

19 **Postpartum safety issues for women with epilepsy** 242
Diane T. Sundstrom and Patricia Osborne Shafer

20 **Management of the neonate: clinical examination and surveillance** 251
Eugene Ng

21 **Menopause and HRT in women with epilepsy** 260
Cynthia L. Harden

22 **Bone health in adolescent girls and postmenopausal women with epilepsy** 264
Alison M. Pack

Index 275

Contributors

Sherese Ali, MD
Assistant Professor, University of Toronto,
Staff Psychiatrist, Neuropsychiatry,
Psychosomatic Medicine and Global Mental
Health, Toronto Western Hospital, University
Health Network, Toronto, ON, Canada

Danielle Molinari Andrade, MD, MSc
Director, Epilepsy Genetics Program,
Associate Professor, Neurology, University
of Toronto, Krembil Neuroscience Centre,
Toronto Western Hospital, Toronto, ON,
Canada

Elinor Ben-Menachem
Department of Neurology, Sahlgren
University Hospital, Göteborg, Sweden

Weerawadee Chandranipapongse, MD
Clinical Fellow, Division of Clinical
Pharmacology and Toxicology,
Department of Paediatrics, The Hospital
for Sick Children, University of Toronto,
Toronto, ON, Canada

Pamela Crawford, MB, ChB, MD, FRCP
Consultant Neurologist, Visiting Professor
in Community Neurological Studies, York
Hospital, York, UK

Anne Davis, MD, MPH
Associate Professor of Clinical Obstetrics
and Gynecology, Department of Obstetrics
and Gynecology, Columbia University
Medical Center, New York, NY, USA

Carin Dove, MD
Department of Neurology, Sunnybrook
Health Sciences Centre, Toronto, ON,
Canada

Nancy Foldvary-Schaefer, DO, MS
Professor of Medicine, Cleveland Clinic
Lerner College of Medicine, Cleveland

Clinic Neurological Institute, Cleveland,
OH, USA

Elizabeth E. Gerard, MD
Assistant Professor of Neurology, Director,
Women's Neurology Center, Northwestern
University, Department of Neurology,
Chicago, IL, USA

Cristina Y. Go, MD
Assistant Professor of Paediatrics
(Neurology), The Hospital for Sick Children,
University of Toronto, Toronto, ON, Canada

Cynthia L. Harden, MD
Professor of Neurology, Hofstra North
Shore-LIJ School of Medicine, Chief, Division
of Epilepsy and Electroencephalography,
North Shore-Long Island Jewish Health
System, Great Neck, NY, USA

Dini Hui, MD, FRCSC
Division of Maternal Fetal Medicine,
Department of Obstetrics and
Gynaecology, Sunnybrook Health Sciences
Centre, University of Toronto, Toronto,
ON, Canada

Shinya Ito, MD, FRCPC
Professor and Head, Division of Clinical
Pharmacology and Toxicology,
Department of Paediatrics, The Hospital
for Sick Children, University of Toronto,
Toronto, ON, Canada

Jaromir Janousek, MD
Research Associate, Mid-Atlantic
Epilepsy and Sleep Center, Bethesda, MD,
USA

Nathalie Jette, MD, MSc, FRCPC
Associate Professor of Neurology,
Department of Clinical Neurosciences and
Hotchkiss Brain Institute, Department of

Community Health Sciences and Institute for Public Health, University of Calgary, AB, Canada

Pavel Klein, MB, BChir
Director, Epilepsy Center, Director, Mid-Atlantic Epilepsy and Sleep Center, Bethesda, MD, and Associate Professor, Department of Neurology, The George Washington University, Washington, DC, USA

A. Gabriela Lizama, MD
Clinical Fellow, Department of Neurology, Yale University, New Haven, CT, USA

Kristi A. McIntosh, MPH
PhD Candidate, School of Population & Public Health, The University of British Columbia, Vancouver, BC, Canada

Georgia Montouris, MD
Clinical Associate Professor of Neurology, Boston University School of Medicine, Director of Epilepsy Services, Boston Medical Center, Boston, MA, USA

Brian J. Murray, MD, FRCPC D,ABSM
Associate Professor of Neurology, Sunnybrook Health Sciences Centre, University of Toronto, Toronto, ON, Canada

Ori Nevo, MD
Division of Maternal Fetal Medicine, Department of Obstetrics and Gynaecology, Sunnybrook Health Sciences Centre, University of Toronto, Toronto, ON, Canada

Eugene Ng, MD, FRCPC, FAAP
Assistant Professor of Paediatrics, Chief, Newborn and Developmental Paediatrics, Sunnybrook Health Sciences Centre, University of Toronto, Toronto, ON, Canada

Alison M. Pack, MD, MPH
Associate Professor of Neurology, Columbia University Medical Center, New York, NY, USA

Sima Indubhai Patel, MD
University of Minnesota Physicians/MINCEP Epilepsy Care, Assistant Professor of Clinical Neurology, University of Minnesota, MN, USA

Page B. Pennell, MD
Associate Professor of Neurology, Harvard Medical School, Director of Research, Division of Epilepsy, Division of Women's Health, Brigham and Women's Hospital, Boston, MA, USA

Kalliopi A. Petropoulou, MD
Neuroradiologist Assistant Professor, SUNY Upstate University Hospital Radiology Department, Syracuse, NY, USA

Mark Quigg, MD, MSc, FANA
Professor of Neurology, Medical Director, Clinical EEG/EP/Epilepsy Monitoring, University of Virginia, Charlottesville, VA, USA

Alessandra Scaparrotta, MD
Department of Pediatrics, University Hospital G. d'Annunzio of Chieti, Chieti, Italy

Marianna Sebastiani, MD
Department of Pediatrics, University of Chieti, Chieti, Italy

Patricia Osborne Shafer, RN, MN
Beth Israel Deaconess Medical Center, Department of Neurology and Comprehensive Epilepsy Center, Boston, MA, USA

O. Carter Snead, III, MD
Head, Division of Neurology (Pediatrics), The Hospital for Sick Children, Toronto, ON, Canada

Diane T. Sundstrom, RN, BSN
Beth Israel Deaconess Medical
Center, Department of Neurology
and Comprehensive Epilepsy Center,
Boston, MA, USA

Alberto Verrotti
Department of Pediatrics, University
Hospital G. d'Annunzio of Chieti, Chieti,
Italy

Carla Verrotti, MD, PhD
Professor of Gynecology and Obstetrics,
Department of Gynecologic, Obstetric and
Neonatal Sciences, Unit of Obstetrics and
Gynecology, University Hospital of Parma,
Parma, Italy

Jonathan H. Waters, MD
Professor of Anesthesiology and
Bioengineering, University of Pittsburgh,
Chief of Anesthesiology, Magee Womens
Hospital of UPMC, Pittsburgh, PA, USA

Fatima Zahir, MD
Obstetric Anesthesia Fellow, Magee
Womens Hospital of UPMC, Magee
Womens Hospital, Pittsburgh, PA, USA

Preface

This book began with a simple desire to create a practical, portable tool to help busy practitioners care for women with epilepsy. It was developed for neurologists, internists, obstetricians and gynecologists, family physicians, anesthetists, midwives, nurses, social workers, pharmacists, neonatologists, and all those who care for women with epilepsy. The diversity of our audience reflects the inherent multidisciplinary nature of this practice. Caring for women with epilepsy, especially during pregnancy, has challenges that many of us frequently feel ill-equipped to manage. Questions such as:

- How do hormones influence seizures, and how is this best managed?
- What is the teratogenicity of newer drugs such as topiramate or levetiracetam?
- What is the best form of birth control to use in women with epilepsy?
- How do I give my patient the best chance of seizure freedom during pregnancy?
- What factors can predict seizures in pregnancy?
- How do I manage seizures or status epilepticus in pregnancy especially during labor and delivery?
- Do hormone replacement therapies pose a risk for seizure exacerbation?

I still recall the many sleepless nights ruminating over whether I was providing the best possible care for these women. This culminated when a young pregnant patient of mine with epilepsy deteriorated into status epilepticus. The challenges of this, and many other cases, have catalyzed for me a strong desire to summarize key and critical concepts in the care of these women. I am grateful to have worked with world experts on these topics. They have successfully distilled key practice points and provided comprehensive basic science data, pregnancy registry data, and expert opinion to further enrich our understanding and ability to counsel patients. This book is designed as a quick, accessible, everyday, easy-to-use manual that puts the essentials of caring for women with epilepsy at one's fingertips.

On a very personal note, it is with a heavy heart that I conclude this preface with a tribute to Autumn Klein my co-editor. Autumn was a force to be reckoned with, one in a million, a unique person who had a remarkable ability to be on the leading edge of her own field and yet simultaneously filled with humility and a curiosity that easily engaged others to learn with her. Autumn and I mutually viewed this book to be a labor of love on a topic that we both were passionate about. We worked closely together over the past 2 years to bring this book to life. Autumn died in the Spring of 2013, before she could see the completion of this work. I know with certainty that she would have wanted to, as I do, dedicate this book to our daughters. To Cianna, know that despite all the awards, accolades, and tributes that your mother received, you were her greatest prize. To my own daughter Madelaine, this work and all others to follow would be meaningless without you. You are my own greatest life achievement. I want to thank my husband Carlo, who has tirelessly championed my hopes and dreams, my parents John and Ruth, who gave up their own dreams to allow me to follow mine, my brothers San, Mark, and Luke who lead a blazing trail for me to follow, and Nick Dunton at Cambridge University Press who recognized the potential in me.

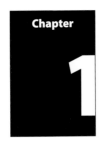

Epidemiology of women with epilepsy

Kristi A. McIntosh and Nathalie Jette

Key points:

- Gender differences are observed in specific epilepsy syndromes
- Women with epilepsy (WWE) are at increased risk for depression, anxiety, sexual dysfunction, and infertility
- WWE of childbearing age encounter challenges associated with contraceptive therapy, pregnancy, and anticonvulsant use
- WWE during menopause face unique concerns related to hormone replacement therapy and osteoporosis

Introduction

Epilepsy is one of the most common neurological conditions affecting men and women of all ages. In this chapter, we review the epidemiology of the epilepsies along with the epidemiology of comorbidity and special issues WWE encounter throughout their life.

Epidemiology of epilepsy

Fifty million individuals worldwide are estimated to have epilepsy at any given time [1]. Prevalence of epilepsy is defined as the number of persons with epilepsy in a specific population at one point in time, divided by the number of persons in that population and time. Incidence of epilepsy is defined as the number of new cases of epilepsy over a specified time period [1]. The reported incidence and prevalence of epilepsy varies widely between studies. Reasons for these estimated differences may include variations in the case ascertainment methods, the lack of accepted diagnostic criteria, the variations in the study location, and possible underreporting due to the stigma associated with epilepsy.

The overall prevalence of epilepsy is estimated to be between 5 and 10 cases per 1,000 persons, excluding febrile convulsions, single seizures, and inactive epilepsy [2–6], but the median lifetime prevalence of epilepsy has been reported to be as high as 15.4 per 1,000 (4.8–49.6) in rural areas and 10.3 per 1,000 (2.8–37.7) in urban areas of developing countries [3]. The prevalence of epilepsy is slightly higher in males than females in many door-to-door studies and record-review studies. Still, the difference in prevalence between the genders is very slight and usually not significant [1, 7]. However, some studies do report a gender difference in the epilepsy prevalence. For example, in a Danish study

Women with Epilepsy, ed. Esther Bui and Autumn Klein. Published by Cambridge University Press.

A

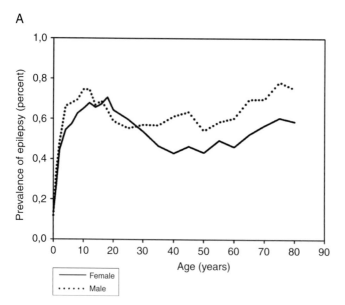

Figure 1.1: A: 5-year prevalence of epilepsy in Denmark. Estimates were based on 4,977,482 persons born in Denmark and resident in Denmark on December 31, 1999, including 28,303 diagnosed with epilepsy between 1995 and 1999. B: Age- and gender-specific incidence of epilepsy in Denmark. Estimates were based on 5,491,652 people born in Denmark followed up for development of epilepsy between 1995 and 2002, including 33,140 who developed epilepsy. The incidence measures the number of new cases per 100,000 person-years at risk. Reproduced with permission from Christensen et al. [2]

B

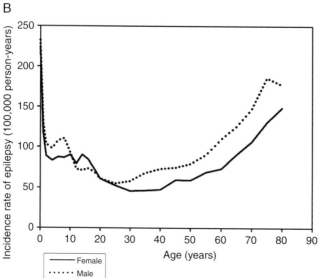

using population-based data from a national registry (Figure 1.1, A), the prevalence of epilepsy was higher in men compared to women for most age groups, except for the 16–25 year age group [2, 8]. In this study, men were also found to have higher incidence rates than women in all age categories with the exception of the 10–20 year age category (Figure 1.1, B) [2].

The overall incidence of epilepsy is usually reported to be about 40–70 cases per 100,000 person-years in developed countries, and about 100–190 cases per 100,000 person-years in developing countries [3, 7]. In a recent systematic review and meta-analysis, the median incidence of epilepsy was reported to be 45.0/100,000 person-years for high-income

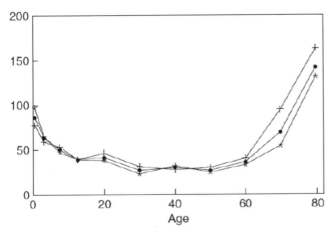

Figure 1.2: Age- and gender-specific incidence/100,000 of epilepsy in Rochester, Minnesota, 1935–1984. Total (solid circles), male (plus signs), female (stars). Reproduced with permission from Hauser et al. [10].

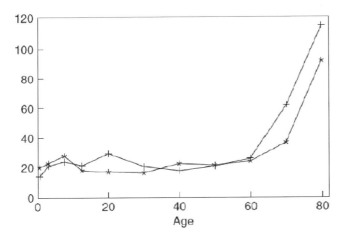

Figure 1.3: Age- and gender-specific incidence/100,000 of partial epilepsy in Rochester, Minnesota, 1935–1984. Male (plus signs), female (stars). Reproduced with permission from Hauser et al. [10].

countries and 81.7/100,000 person-years for low- and middle-income countries [9]. The incidence of epilepsy is often reported to have a bimodal distribution (Figure 1.2). It is highest in early childhood, lowest in early adult years, and then increases again after age 55 with the highest reported incidence in those over 75 years of age [10]. A similar pattern is described in both males and females.

The lifetime risk is the probability that a person will develop epilepsy over his or her lifetime. Based on calculations in a recent population-based study, 1 in 26 people will develop epilepsy during their lifetime, and men have a higher risk of developing epilepsy (1 of every 21 males) than women (1 of every 28 females) [11].

The causes behind these gender differences have not been elucidated. One hypothesis as to why epilepsy may be more common in men than in women is that men have a higher incidence of trauma-related disease, which in turn is associated with epilepsy. Focal epilepsy has also been found to occur more frequently among men than women (Figure 1.3). This higher incidence in men relative to women has not been reported in adolescents. This may be due to the higher incidence of primary generalized epilepsy (PGE) in

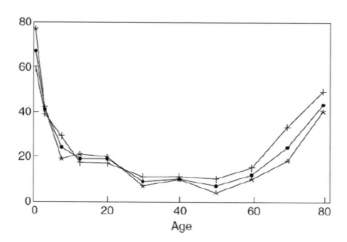

Figure 1.4: Age- and gender-specific incidence/100,000 of generalized onset epilepsy in Rochester, Minnesota, 1935–1984. Total (solid circles), male (plus signs), female (stars). Reproduced with permission from Hauser et al. [10].

women between the ages of 12 and 20 years (Figure 1.4). This increased incidence of generalized epilepsy in women relative to men in adolescence could be attributed to hormonal factors [8]. It has been hypothesized that sex hormones may contribute to the development of idiopathic generalized epilepsy in women, in which case this difference would be more obvious before menopause and decline with age, as demonstrated in the Danish study discussed above [8]. Furthermore, it has been suggested that higher reported estimates in males compared to females in many studies may be due to concealment of symptoms by women in certain cultures where women are considered "unmarriageable" if they have epilepsy [1].

Comorbidities

A number of mental health conditions are increased in persons with epilepsy compared to those without epilepsy [12]. Having epilepsy is also associated with a higher prevalence of somatic comorbidities compared to the general population [6, 13]. Here, we discuss gender differences in the epidemiology of mood and anxiety as well as sleep disorders in epilepsy. This is discussed in greater detail in Chapters 2 and 3.

Psychiatry
Mood disorders in epilepsy

Mood disorders are prevalent in those with epilepsy, with major depression being the most common mood disorder [14]. Recently, studies have shown that a history of major depression is associated with an increased risk for developing seizures and vice versa [15]. This two-way relationship suggests a possible shared pathogenetic origin [15].

Female gender is found to be associated with depression in those with or without epilepsy [14, 16]. Among women without epilepsy (WWoE), the prevalence of depressive mood disorders has been reported to be approximately two times higher in women than in men. In a nationally representative Canadian health survey using structured interviews for the assessment of major depressive disorder, depression was identified in 13% of those with epilepsy compared to 7% of those without epilepsy [14]. WWE were 2.6 times more

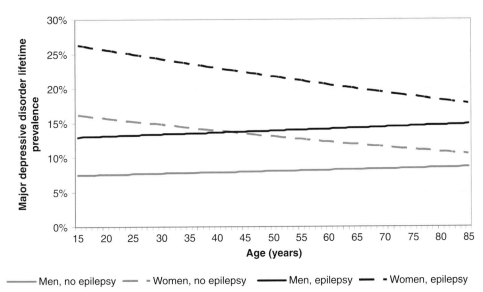

Figure 1.5: Logistic regression (fitted) models predicting the lifetime prevalence (proportion in percentage) of major depression disorder (on the y-axis) based on age (on the x-axis) and gender. Reproduced with permission from Tellez-Zenteno et al. [12].

likely (95% confidence intervals (CI), 1.6–4.3) to be depressed than men with epilepsy [14]. In another large Canadian population-based study using similar methodology, the odds of lifetime major depression was found to be higher in people with epilepsy compared to those without epilepsy [12]. The lifetime prevalence of major depressive disorder in those with epilepsy was 17.4% (95% CI, 10.0–24.9), compared to 10.7% (95% CI, 10.2–11.2) in those without epilepsy, with an odds ratio (OR) of 1.8 (95% CI, 1.0–3.1). In other population-based studies lifetime prevalence has been estimated to be as high as 30% [80]. Furthermore, the lifetime prevalence of major depressive disorders, while still increased for those with epilepsy has been shown to decline with age in women while remaining relatively stable in men (Figure 1.5) [12].

While no population-based studies have examined the incidence of postpartum depression (PPD) in WWE, smaller studies have reported an increased frequency of PPD in WWE compared to WWoE. For example, an Italian study of 55 postpartum women with and without epilepsy found that PPD occurred in 39% of WWE compared to 12% of WWoE (p<0.05) [17]. No specific causative factor, however, has been identified to explain this disparity.

Anxiety disorders

Whereas much is known about the association between epilepsy and depression, less is known about the epidemiology of anxiety disorders in those with epilepsy.

In a cross-sectional, population-based study from the UK using diagnoses from primary care records, anxiety disorders were reported in 11% of people with epilepsy (n = 5,834), compared to 5.6% of those without epilepsy (n = 831,163) [18]. The risk of anxiety was higher in both men and WWE compared to control, but higher in WWE overall. In the female 16–64 year age group, anxiety was reported in 14.2% of 2,338 WWE compared to 7.5% of 410,851 WWoE (RR, 1.95; 95% CI, 1.8–2.2). In the 64 year and older age group, 9.0% of 642 WWE had anxiety compared to 7.8% of 118,516 WWoE (RR, 1.2; 95% CI, 0.9–1.5).

In a population-based Canadian health survey using structured interviews based on DSM-IV, those with epilepsy were more likely than those without epilepsy to report lifetime anxiety disorders with an OR of 2.4 (95% CI, 1.5–3.8). Of those with epilepsy, 12.8% (95% CI, 6.0–19.7) reported an anxiety disorder in the past 12 months compared to 4.6% (95% CI, 4.3–4.9) in the group without epilepsy. Similarly, 22.8% (95% CI, 14.8– 30.9) of those with epilepsy compared to 11.2% (95% CI, 10.8–11.7) of those without epilepsy reported a lifetime anxiety disorder. In both women and men with epilepsy, panic disorder and agoraphobia became more prevalent with age (and was found to be higher in women compared to men with epilepsy) but this was not found to occur in the general population [12].

Sleep

Sleep disturbances are reported more frequently in adults with epilepsy than in adults without epilepsy. Increasing evidence suggests that obstructive sleep apnea (OSA), excessive daytime sleepiness (EDS), and sleep maintenance insomnia (difficulty staying asleep) are more commonly found in adults with epilepsy than in those without [19–21]. However, population-based studies on sleep disturbances in patients with epilepsy are lacking. Furthermore, there has been little attention to gender differences in existing smaller studies.

In a mail survey of 1,183 Dutch outpatients, the 6-month prevalence of sleep disturbances in people with focal epilepsy was more than two times greater than that of healthy controls (38.6% vs. 18.0%) [22]. This was felt not to be due to any one particular type of sleep disturbance but rather all sleep disturbances were significantly more prevalent in the patients with epilepsy. A prospective Swiss study of 100 adult epilepsy patients found sleep complaints were three times as likely (30% vs. 10%) in a population of people with epilepsy compared with controls [21]. Of those with epilepsy, 52% were found to have sleep maintenance insomnia compared to 38% of controls [21]. In small case series, OSA has been reported in 10% of adults with epilepsy, 20% of children with epilepsy, and approaching 30% in drug-resistant epilepsy patients [19]. Furthermore, OSA is more likely to occur in those who are older, male, overweight, with drug-resistant or late onset epilepsy [19, 20].

More sleep problems are encountered by children with epilepsy than their healthy siblings and other healthy controls [20]. Gender does not appear to contribute to the frequency of problems with sleep in children [20].

Epilepsy in childhood and adolescence
Inheritance and genetics

Several factors have been found to be associated with a predisposition to epilepsy, particularly in families where one member is already affected. Affected children have a greater risk of being born to a mother with epilepsy (2.8–8.7%) compared to a father with epilepsy (1.0 to 3.6%) [23]. How early a parent developed epilepsy also predicts the likelihood of a child developing epilepsy [23]. A parent who develops epilepsy before age 20 has a 2.3–6% risk of their children developing epilepsy, while a parent who develops epilepsy after age 20 has a 1.0–3.6% risk of their children developing epilepsy [23]. Furthermore, in families who have both an affected parent and child, the risk of epilepsy for other siblings increases

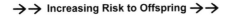

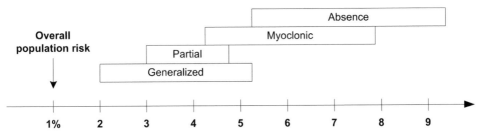

Figure 1.6: Percent of offspring affected with epilepsy. Reproduced with permission from Winawer and Shinnar [23].

from approximately 3% to 8% [23]. The epilepsy syndrome or seizure type also contributes to the likelihood of epilepsy developing in relatives. Occurrence of epilepsy in relatives is increased when the proband has idiopathic epilepsy with seizures such as myoclonic or absence seizures. In those with myoclonic seizures, a 4–8% risk of any epilepsy in offspring is seen, while in those with absence seizures, a 5–9% risk of any epilepsy is observed. The risk of epilepsy in those related to individuals with generalized epilepsy is greater than in those related to individuals with partial epilepsy in some studies; however this has not been observed in all studies (Figure 1.6) [23].

Epilepsy in girls and female adolescents

Gender differences have been identified in various epilepsy syndromes. Idiopathic generalized epilepsy, which accounts for 15–20% of the epilepsies, can be found more frequently in females than in males [24]. Childhood absence epilepsy (CAE) was reported in 2.5% of boys compared to 11.4% of girls in a Norwegian population-based study [25]. Juvenile absence epilepsy (JAE) and juvenile myoclonic epilepsy (JME) were found to be more common among females than males using data from 2,488 individuals with epilepsy from a Danish outpatient epilepsy clinic and the Danish Twin Registry [8]. JAE was 3 times more common in females than males (76% vs. 24%), whereas JME was 1.5 times more common in females than males (61% vs. 39%) [8]. However, there has been less agreement as to whether gender differences exist in localization-related epilepsies (LRE). While one prospective study of 996 patients with suspected seizures conducted over a 4-year period in Australia reported an equal gender distribution of hippocampal sclerosis (81% in men vs. 79% in women) [26], another retrospective study of 153 patients presenting for pre-surgical evaluation in Germany found that the expression of focal epilepsy due to mesial temporal sclerosis is not the same in females and in males [27]. Females were more likely to experience isolated auras than males (OR, 2.1; 95% CI, 1.1–4.2), and less likely to have secondary generalized seizures (OR, 0.44, 95% CI, 0.21–0.92). Furthermore, they also found that electrographic findings were more likely to be on the same side of hippocampal sclerosis in females compared to males (98% vs. 84%). Finally, specific hereditary epilepsy syndromes such as Rett syndrome, Aicardi syndrome, subcortical band heterotopia and epilepsy and mental retardation limited to females (EFMR) are seen primarily in females due to mutations identified in the X chromosome. These syndromes are discussed in detail in Chapter 6.

Catamenial epilepsy

Catamenial epilepsy is defined as a doubling in daily seizure frequency during specific phases of the menstrual cycle [28]. Three categories of catamenial seizure patterns have been described: perimenstrual (C1 pattern), periovulatory (C2 pattern), and entire second half of the cycle (Figure 8.1) in anovulatory cycles (C3 pattern) [28]. Population-based studies exploring the prevalence of catamenial epilepsy are lacking. However, a catamenial pattern was found in 39% of women with LRE in a prospective study of 87 women [29] and 31% of adolescent females in a prospective study of 42 WWE from an Egyptian pediatric neurology clinic [30]. Furthermore, the laterality and focality of epilepsy may play an important role in the ability for reproductive hormones to affect the seizure pattern during the monthly cycle [31].

Epilepsy in childbearing
Fertility and epilepsy
Sexual dysfunction

Population-based studies examining sexual dysfunction in WWE are lacking. However, smaller series have found that WWE are more likely to suffer from sexual dysfunction than WWoE. The epilepsy syndrome and its localization influence sexual function. An American study explored sexual dysfunction in 57 reproductive-aged women on antiepileptic drug (AED) monotherapy recruited from tertiary epilepsy centers compared to 17 WWoE. Lower scores for sexual dysfunction were found in women with primary generalized epilepsy (20.0%) and localization-related epilepsy (20.7%) compared to controls (9%) [32]. Furthermore, sexual dysfunction is seen more frequently in right than left temporal lobe epilepsy (TLE) in both men and women [33].

Another controlled prospective American study of 36 women with TLE recruited from a neurology outpatient service, and 12 controls recruited from the community, examined whether changes in sexual function were found more frequently in women with unilateral TLE [33]. Indeed, sexual function scores were substantially worse with right TLE than left TLE. Additionally, 50.0% of women with right TLE and 30.0% of women with left TLE had sexual dysfunction as compared with 8.3% of WWoE. However, these differences were only significant for those with right TLE [33]. Some AEDs, particularly older, enzyme-inducing AEDs, contribute to sexual dysfunction due to potential influences on the hypothalamic-pituitary-gonadal axis resulting in changes in the levels of hormones supporting sexual behavior (Chapter 9). Enzyme-inducing AEDs are believed to increase sex hormone-binding globulin and thereby decrease bioavailable testosterone which contributes to the emergence of sexual dysfunction [33]. While not statistically significant, 40.7% of WWE receiving AEDs reported increased sexual dysfunction compared to 33.3% of those not receiving AEDs in this same study [33].

Reproductive dysfunction

In WWE, menstrual cycle irregularities, increased risk of infertility, or signs of polycystic ovary syndrome (PCOS) are frequently encountered. Both seizures and AEDs have been causally implicated [34]. Some of the greatest challenges in comparing the results from studies looking at menstrual disorders in WWE are the lack of menstrual disorder definitions, and of population-based studies. Most published studies report data from highly selected, biased populations (e.g., women referred to a neuroendocrine clinic).

In a retrospective, questionnaire-based study of 265 WWE and 142 matched WWoE from three different Norwegian hospitals, menstrual disorders were significantly higher in WWE (48.0%) than in controls (30.7%) [35]. In another retrospective American analysis of 100 women with LRE, menstrual disorders were identified by 32% [36]. In a case-control study, 12/36 (33.3%) of WWE compared to 14/100 (14%) community-based WWoE (p = 0.02) had menstrual disorders (defined as "abnormal cycle interval, oligomenorrhea, polymenorrhea, increased variability of cycle interval or menometrorrhagia") [37].

Menstrual cycle irregularities, anovulation, higher androgen levels, carbohydrate intolerance with obesity, and polycystic-appearing ovaries are characteristics of PCOS. A lack of a standardized definition of PCOS could explain the varying reported rates in both women with and without epilepsy [38]. Once again, however, there is a lack of population-based studies examining the epidemiology of PCOS in WWE.

In a recent Finnish study examining reproductive endocrine function in 148 WWE, PCOS was found to occur in 28% of WWE, 52% of WWE on valproate (VPA), and 11% of controls. WWE on VPA were 5.46 times more likely to have PCOS when compared to controls (95% CI, 2.23–13.03) [39]. In a recent meta-analysis including 556 WWE treated with VPA, 593 women treated with other AEDs, 120 untreated WWE, and 329 healthy controls, the likelihood of developing PCOS was 1.95 times greater in VPA-treated WWE compared to other AED-treated women [38]. The possibility of developing features of PCOS in those treated with VPA seems to depend on the age at which the female was first treated with VPA [40]. In a prospective American study of 225 WWE taking VPA compared to 222 WWE taking lamotrigine (LTG), the occurrence of PCOS symptoms occurred more frequently in women started on VPA rather than LTG before the age of 26 years compared to WWE in whom VPA was started at the age of 26 years or older [40].

Another pattern of reproductive dysfunction described in patients with epilepsy is hypothalamic amenorrhea. This is one of the more severe yet common patterns of hypo-gonadotropic hypogonadism. In one study, 50 women with TLE referred for neurologic evaluation were studied, with 8 (16%) found to have amenorrhea. This is much higher than the expected frequency of 1.5% in the general population [41]. Furthermore, it has been found to occur more commonly in RTLE than LTLE [37, 42]. However, population-based estimates of amenorrhea in WWE have not yet been published.

There are, however, population-based data examining fertility rates in WWE between 1991 and 1995 compared to the 1993 population fertility rates for England and Wales [43]. The fertility rate in WWE aged 15–44 was 47.1 live births per 1,000 women per year (95% CI, 42.3–52.2), compared with a national rate of 62.6. The most significant decrease in fertility rates was among the WWE in the 25–39 year age group (p<0·001). In a more recent, prospective cohort of 375 WWE enrolled in an epilepsy and pregnancy registry in India, 38% failed to conceive, with the most important predictors of infertility being multiple AEDs, older age, and lower education [44].

Lower birth rates may be due to lower marriage rates, reproductive dysfunction, fear of birth defects, and concern for an increased risk of epilepsy in the offspring [45]. In a population-based study of 19 American states, 55.5% (95% CI, 51.3–59.7) of those with epilepsy were married or in a common-law relationship compared to 64.1% (95% CI, 63.6–64.7) of those without epilepsy. Of those with epilepsy, 22.9% (95% CI, 20.0–26.2) were formerly married compared to 18.0% (95% CI, 17.6–18.3) of those without epilepsy. Finally, 21.5% (95% CI, 17.7–26.0) of those with epilepsy were never married compared to 17.9% (95% CI, 17.4–18.4) of those without epilepsy [6]. Similar findings have been reported in an Indian study of 300 epilepsy patients. Of those with epilepsy (n = 300), 44.6% of women were never married compared to 22.3% of women in the general population (n = 4,687). Of those with epilepsy, 51.1% of women were married compared to 75.7% of women in the general population. Finally, 4.3% of WWE were divorced compared to 2% of women in the general population [46]. Fertility in WWE is discussed in further detail in Chapter 9.

Contraception and epilepsy

It is estimated that nearly half of all pregnancies among WWE are unplanned, similar to the frequency seen in the general population [79]. Contraceptive management in WWE is paramount, due to the possible maternal and fetal complications if contraception fails. Furthermore, the use of enzyme-inducing AEDs can result in birth control failure and contribute to the relatively high number of unplanned pregnancies in WWE [47, 48]. Therefore, preconception counseling to all WWE of childbearing age is necessary.

The prevalence of contraceptive use in 1,630 Dutch women of childbearing age on AEDs was calculated in a study using a population-based pharmaceutical dispensing database [49]. The authors found that only 34.3% of AED users were prescribed highly effective contraceptives compared with 41.2% of the general population of women of childbearing age (p<.001). They also found that of WWE who used enzyme-inducing AEDs in combination with a highly effective contraceptive method, 43.5% of them were on an oral contraceptive (OC) containing less than the recommended 50 μg of estrogen. These findings are consistent with a large, population-based study of childbearing WWE on AEDs in the UK. This latter study found that 16.7% of WWE were on OC, and of those on both an enzyme-inducing AED and an OC, 56% were on OC with an estrogen content less than 50 μg [50].

Despite the well-known effects of estrogen on lowering seizure threshold, an association between estrogen-containing OC and seizure exacerbation in WWE has not been seen. A large UK cohort study of 17,032 WWE followed for up to 26 years examined whether there was a relationship between OC use and an increase in the incidence of epilepsy or seizures [51]. No association was found between OC use and the development of epilepsy in WWoE or between OC use and seizure frequency in WWE.

Preconception counseling

There are no studies examining how common preconception counseling is for WWE. However, the use of preconception folic acid by WWE was reviewed by a committee assembled by the American Academy of Neurology (AAN) and American Epilepsy Society (AES) and is discussed below [52]. A prospective study of 970 pregnancies and 979 offspring in WWE reported a significant correlation between serum folic acid concentrations <4.4 nmol/L and malformations in newborns (adjusted OR, 5.8; 95% CI, 1.3–27) [53]. However, several other studies reviewed did not show a relationship between folic acid and major congenital malformations (MCMs), but were insufficiently powered to exclude a significant risk reduction from folic acid supplementation. Prevention of MCMs in offspring of WWE taking AEDs may occur with preconception folic acid supplementation.

The effectiveness of preconception folic acid supplementation was examined in a recent prospective, observational study by looking at the rate of MCMs in a group of women on AED monotherapy in the UK [54]. In the 1,935 cases that received preconception folic acid, 76 MCMs (3.9%; 95% CI, 3.1–4.9) and 8 neural tube defects (NTDs) (0.4%; 95% CI, 0.2–0.8) were observed. There were 53 occurrences of a MCM (2.2%; 95% CI, 1.7–2.9) and 8 NTDs (0.34%; 95% CI, 0.2–0.7) in the 2,375 women who obtained folic acid but did not start taking it until later in the pregnancy (n = 1,825) or not at all (n = 550). Folic acid supplementation in this population of WWE was not associated with a reduction in the frequency of MCMs or NTDs. This study suggests that extrapolating findings from population-based studies of all pregnant women that took folate to groups of selected WWE enrolled in registries may be inappropriate. The higher risk of MCMs in WWE may be multifactorial and may also be explained by mechanisms other than those directly related to folic acid metabolism.

The evidence regarding the effectiveness of preconception counseling for WWE, calculated by a decrease in adverse pregnancy outcomes was recently published as a Cochrane review [55]. No studies met all study eligibility criteria. There is thus no strong evidence regarding the effectiveness of preconception counseling in decreasing adverse pregnancy outcomes for WWE and their offspring [56]. More population-based studies looking at folic acid intake in WWE and its benefits are required.

The prophylactic effect of folic acid supplementation on the likelihood of spontaneous abortion and pre-term delivery was examined prospectively in pregnant WWE on AEDs. These WWE were all registered in EURAP (an International Registry of AEDs and Pregnancy) at a single center, with 388 pregnancies in 244 patients investigated [57]. WWE that did not supplement with folic acid were more likely to have a spontaneous abortion than those who did supplement (OR, 2.6; 95% CI, 1.2–5.6). Consequently, pregnancies with folic acid supplementation were associated with a significant reduction of spontaneous abortion.

AEDs and fetal effects

The occurrence of fetal malformations is associated with the use of AEDs in pregnancy. Different AEDs are associated with different types of malformations in the offspring. Epilepsy and pregnancy registries exist to collect such information, as randomized clinical trials are difficult to conduct in pregnancy. Registries are found in many countries and differ in methodology and outcomes. Pharmaceutical companies may collect pregnancy data related to their product while other registries are driven by independent research groups who may collect and publish data on more than one AED for comparison [58]. Here, we primarily discuss population-based studies reporting on AEDs and the risk of MCMs. This is discussed further in Chapter 12.

One population-based retrospective study of WWE from Finland using data from the National Medical Birth Registry showed a higher risk of MCMs in the newborns of WWE exposed to any in utero AED (OR, 1.7; 95% CI, 1.1–2.8) compared to the newborns of WWE not exposed to AEDs. The likelihood of MCMs in infants exposed to in utero VPA monotherapy (OR, 4.2; 95% CI, 2.3–7.6) or polytherapy (OR, 3.5; 95% CI, 1.4–8.1) was also increased [59].

A systematic review and meta-analysis of international published registries examined the incidence of MCMs and other pregnancy outcomes after in utero AED exposure [60]. Fifty-nine studies involving 65,533 pregnancies in WWE and 1,817,024 in WWoE were included. The incidence of MCMs in offspring born to WWE was greater (7.1%; 95% CI, 5.6–8.5) compared to offspring born to WWoE (2.3%; 95% CI, 1.5–3.1). Incidence was greatest for AED polytherapy (16.8%; 95% CI, 0.5–33.1). The highest MCMs' incidence rate belonged to VPA, at 10.7% (95% CI, 8.2–13.3) for monotherapy. VPA monotherapy and polytherapy drugs that included phenobarbital (PB), PHT, or VPA significantly increased the risk of MCMs in offspring exposed in utero.

A population-based cohort study of 837,795 infants born in Denmark investigated the relationship between in utero exposure to newer generation AEDs during the first trimester of pregnancy and the likelihood of developing MCMs [61]. Of the 1,532 infants exposed to LTG, oxcarbazepine (OXC), topiramate (TPM), gabapentin (GBP), or levetiracetam (LEV) during the first trimester, 3.2% were diagnosed with a MCM compared with 2.4% who were not exposed to an AED, with an adjusted OR of 1.0 (95% CI, 0.7–1.4). Of 1,019 AED-exposed newborns, a MCM was discovered in 38 (3.7%) exposed to LTG during the first trimester (OR, 1.2; 95% CI, 0.8–1.7), in 11 of 393 newborns (2.8%) exposed to OXC (OR, 0.9; 95% CI, 0.5–1.6), and in 5 of 108 newborns (4.6%) exposed to TPM (OR, 1.4; 95% CI, 0.6–3.6). Only 1 (1.7%) infant exposed to GBP (n = 59) and no infants exposed to LEV (n = 58) were diagnosed with MCMs, but the use of these AEDs is still less common in pregnancy.

There have also been studies examining the association between AED use and cognitive outcomes in children. A prospective, observational (non-population-based) study from epilepsy centers in the USA and the UK examined the cognitive effects of fetal exposure to AEDs in 309 children at 3 years of age [62]. Pregnant WWE were enrolled who were taking AED monotherapy (carbamazepine (CBZ), LTG, PHT, or VPA). Significantly lower IQ scores were found in 3-year-old children who had been exposed in utero to VPA compared to those children exposed to any other AEDs. After adjustment for maternal IQ, standardized AED dose in the mother, age of mother at delivery, gestational age of the neonate at delivery, and preconception folate supplementation, the mean IQ was 101 for children exposed to LTG, 99 for those exposed to PHT, 98 for those exposed to CBZ, and 92 for those exposed to VPA. A dose-dependent relationship between VPA use and IQ was noted.

An observational (non-population-based) study of WWE and their children was conducted through the Australian Pregnancy Register for WWE and Allied Disorders [63]. Researchers looked at the language skills of 102 school-aged children exposed prenatally to AEDs. With regards to mean language scores, children exposed to VPA monotherapy or polytherapy were significantly below normal, while children exposed to CBZ or LTG monotherapy, or polytherapy without VPA, were not. Additionally, first-trimester VPA usage resulted in a decrease in language scores.

Pregnancy and epilepsy

WWE have been found to have a higher risk of pregnancy and delivery complications. However, it is not clear if this is due to more severe epilepsy or the use of AEDs during pregnancy. A recent population-based study investigated whether pregnant WWE had a greater likelihood of complications during pregnancy and also explored the effects of AED use using databases on all births in Norway from 1999–2005 [64]. Main outcomes included pre-eclampsia, gestational hypertension, eclampsia, vaginal bleeding, and prematurity. WWE were more likely to have mild pre-eclampsia (OR, 1.3; 95% CI, 1.1–1.5) and delivery before week 34 (OR, 1.2; 95% CI, 1.0–1.5). WWE on AEDs were more likely to develop mild pre-eclampsia (OR, 1.8; 95% CI, 1.3–2.4), gestational hypertension (OR, 1.5; 95% CI, 1.0–2.2), vaginal bleeding late in pregnancy (OR, 1.9; 95% CI, 1.1–3.2), and delivery before 34 weeks of gestation (OR, 1.5; 95% CI, 1.1–2.0) when compared to WWoE. However, these increased risks of complications were not seen in WWE not using AED.

A population-based study using the same databases as above including all births in Norway looked at whether WWE have a greater likelihood of complications during labor, and investigated the impact of AEDs [65]. Outcomes included induction, cesarean section, use of forceps and vacuum, abnormal presentation, placental abruption, mechanical disproportion, postpartum hemorrhage, atony, and decreased Apgar scores after 5 minutes. An elevated risk of induction (OR, 1.3; 95% CI, 1.1–1.4), cesarean section (OR, 1.4; 95% CI, 1.3–1.6), and postpartum hemorrhage (OR, 1.2; 95% CI, 1.1–1.4) were seen in WWE (on or off AEDs) compared with WWoE. However, even higher estimates were obtained in WWE on AEDs with ORs (95% CIs) of 1.6 (1.4–1.9), 1.6 (1.4–1.9), and 1.5 (1.3–1.9), respectively. The likelihood of an Apgar score less than 7 was higher in WWE on AEDs (OR, 1.6; 95% CI, 1.1–2.4) compared to WWoE. Only a mildly increased likelihood of cesarean delivery was found among WWE without AED compared to WWoE (OR, 1.3; 95% CI, 1.2–1.5). This is discussed further in Chapter 14.

Another recent population-based study investigated pregnancy, delivery, and MCM outcomes in WWE using data also collected from the compulsory Medical Birth Registry of Norway [66]. A surprising 66% of WWE did not use AEDs during pregnancy. AED-exposed infants were more frequently found to be pre-term (OR, 1.3; 95% CI, 1.1–1.6), and to have birth weight <2.500 g (OR, 1.7; 95% CI, 1.4–2.3), head circumference <2.5 percentile (OR, 2.0; 95% CI, 1.4–2.7), and low Apgar scores (OR, 1.6; 95% CI, 1.1–2.3) compared to WWoE. Small for gestational age (SGA) infants (<10 percentile) were more often born to WWE in both AED-exposed (OR, 1.2; 95% CI, 1.0–1.5) and unexposed (OR, 1.2; 95% CI, 1.0–1.4) groups. Increased MCMs were only found after in utero exposure to VPA (5.6%; OR, 2.3; 95% CI, 1.3–4.2) and AED polytherapy including VPA (6.1%; OR, 2.5; 95% CI, 1.2–5.1). Cesarean sections were performed more frequently in pregnant WWE regardless of their AED-exposure.

A group assembled by the AAN and the AES reviewed the evidence associated with the care of WWE during pregnancy which included adverse perinatal outcomes [67]. They reported on a prospective community-based study from Finland which found that WWE on AEDs during pregnancy (n = 127) are twice as likely to have SGA infants compared to WWoE (n = 24,778) (OR, 2.16; 95% CI, 1.34–3.47; absolute risk 17.3%) [68]. There was no difference in the rate of SGA in WWE not taking AEDs compared to controls. One-minute Apgar scores of less than 7 occurred more frequently in WWE taking AEDs (n = 127) compared to controls (OR, 2.29; 95% CI, 1.29–4.05) [68]. This outcome did not occur more frequently in the neonates of WWE not taking AEDs.

Seizure control during pregnancy

No population-based studies have examined seizure control during pregnancy. However some of the pregnancy registries have studied this in selected WWE. EURAP (an International Registry of AEDs and Pregnancy) reported prospectively documented seizure control and treatment in 1,956 pregnancies of 1,882 WWE [69]. Fifty-eight percent of all pregnant WWE were seizure-free throughout pregnancy. LRE (OR, 2.5; 95% CI, 1.7–3.9), polytherapy (OR, 9.0; 95% CI, 5.6–14.8), and OXC monotherapy (for tonic-clonic seizures only) (OR, 5.4; 95% CI, 1.6–17.1) predicted the occurrence of seizures. Seizure control stayed constant during pregnancy in 63.6% of WWE pregnancies. Of those, 92.7% remained seizure-free during the complete pregnancy. There was an increase in the frequency of seizures in 17.3% of pregnant WWE and 15.9% of pregnant WWE had a decrease. The same AED treatment continued in 62.7% of the pregnancies.

The likelihood of seizing during pregnancy has been reported to be significantly decreased if there have been no seizures for a year before pregnancy according to an Australian registry-based study of 841 AED-treated pregnancies [70]. Of all AED-treated WWE, 49.7% had seizures while pregnant. The risk of having seizures during pregnancy was 24.9% with a minimum of 1 year seizure freedom before pregnancy, 22.8% with a minimum of 2 years of seizure freedom, 20.5% with a minimum of 3 years of seizure freedom and 20% with 4 years or greater of seizure freedom. The association between the length of time of seizure freedom prior to becoming pregnant and the chances of being seizure-free during and after pregnancy was the most relevant finding of this study. With 1 year of seizure freedom before pregnancy, the likelihood of seizures in pregnancy was decreased by 50–70% [70]. This is discussed further in Chapter 13.

Postpartum monitoring
Lactation
Population-based studies of breastfeeding WWE have yet to be conducted. However, pregnant WWE who were taking a single AED (CBZ, LTG, PHT, and VPA) were enrolled between 1999 and 2004 in an observational, prospective study from epilepsy centers in the USA and the UK. The implications of breastfeeding during AED therapy on cognitive outcomes in 3-year-old children were investigated in this study [71]. Of the 199 children studied, 42% were breastfed. There were no differences in IQs for breastfed children compared to non-breastfed children for all AEDs combined and for each of the four individual AED groups. Mean-adjusted IQ scores (95% CIs), across all AEDs, for children who were breastfed was 99 (96–103) while non-breastfed was 98 (95–101). This investigation does not show adverse effects of breastfeeding during AED therapy on cognitive outcomes in children exposed in utero to four common AEDs. Implications of AED use in the breastfed neonate are discussed in Chapter 18.

Epilepsy in menopause
Menopause, hormone replacement therapy
Treatment of epilepsy may disrupt the effects of hormone replacement therapy (HRT) and conversely HRT may influence the occurrence of seizures. During menopause, catamenial seizures may increase in frequency due to hyperestrogenism and then decrease afterwards. Sexual dysfunction may be exacerbated due to the lack of estrogen in menopause and epilepsy itself [72, 73]. Menopause tends to occur about 3 years earlier with a history of one or more seizures per month for much of the duration of epilepsy and lifetime use of multiple enzyme-inducing AEDs [74]. Premature ovarian failure (POF) in WWE has been noted in some studies but no predisposing factors such as epilepsy duration, seizure severity, or use of enzyme-inducing AEDs have been identified [42, 75]. As of yet, no population-based studies of menopause in WWE have been conducted. Menopause in WWE is further discussed in Chapter 21.

Bone health

Osteoporosis is associated with both menopause and the use of AEDs. The occurrence of menopause and the use of AEDs in WWE concurrently may combine to exacerbate this risk. Osteoporosis and fractures may increase in menopausal WWE because of hypoestrogenism in menopause and the use of cytochrome P450-inducing AEDs [72].

A Danish, population-based case-control study investigated fracture risk associated with various AEDs (124,655 fracture cases and 373,962 controls) using the National Hospital Discharge Register and the National Pharmacological Database [76]. After adjustment, a significant association was found between CBZ (OR, 1.18; 95% CI, 1.10–1.26), OXC (OR, 1.14; 95% CI 1.03–1.26), clonazepam (CLZ) (OR, 1.27; 95% CI 1.15–1.41), PB (OR, 1.79; 95% CI, 1.64–1.95), and VPA (OR, 1.15; 95% CI, 1.05–1.26) and the likelihood of fracture. This association was not seen in ethosuximide (ETX), LTG, PHT, primidone (PR), tiagabine (TGB), TPM, and vigabatrin (VGB). Age and gender did not affect the risk of fracture [76].

A Canadian, retrospective, cohort study of 15,792 patients with nontraumatic fractures matched with up to 3 controls (n = 47,289) investigated the relationship between AED use and nontraumatic fractures in those aged 50 years and older [77]. Pharmacy data determined current and prior AED usage. Fracture risk was significantly higher for most of the AEDs being investigated (CBZ, CLZ, GBP, PB, and PHT). The likelihood of developing a fracture ranged from an adjusted OR of 1.2 (95% CI, 1.1–1.5) for CLZ to 1.9 (95% CI, 1.6–2.3) for PHT. VPA was the only AED not associated with a greater fracture risk (adjusted OR, 1.1; 95% CI, 0.7–1.7), which persisted after adjusting for sociodemographic variables, comorbidities, and use of home care services. The risk however was not stratified by sex as both the AED exposed group and the control groups were matched for age and sex.

WWE of reproductive age are also at risk of experiencing bone loss while on AED, as shown in a prospective American study of WWE in taking AED monotherapy (CBZ, LTG, PHT, or VPA) [78]. Of note, no control group of WWoE was included for comparison. In the PHT group, a significant decrease (2.6%) was found at the femoral neck over 1 year unlike those treated with CBZ, LTG, and VPA, who did not have evidence of bone turnover or decreased bone mineral density.

References

1. Banerjee PN, Filippi D and Allen Hauser W. The descriptive epidemiology of epilepsy – a review. *Epilepsy Res* 2009; 85 (1):31–45.

2. Christensen J, Vestergaard M, Pederson MG, et al. Incidence and prevalence of epilepsy in Denmark. *Epilepsy Res* 2007; 76(1):60–5.

3. Ngugi AK, Bottomley C, Kleinschmidt I, et al. Estimation of the burden of active and life-time epilepsy: a meta-analytic approach. *Epilepsia* 2010; 51(5):883–90.

4. Forsgren L, Beghi E, Oun A, et al. The epidemiology of epilepsy in Europe – a systematic review. *Eur J Neurol* 2005; 12(4):245–53.

5. Tellez-Zenteno JF, Pondal-Sordo M, Matijevic S, et al. National and regional prevalence of self-reported epilepsy in Canada. *Epilepsia* 2004; 45(12):1623–9.

6. Kobau R, Zahran H, Thurman DJ, et al. Epilepsy surveillance among adults – 19 states, behavioral risk factor surveillance system, 2005. *MMWR Surveill Summ* 2008; 57(6):1–20.

7. Kotsopoulos IA, van Merode T, Kessels FG, et al. Systematic review and meta-analysis of incidence studies of epilepsy and unprovoked seizures. *Epilepsia* 2002; 43(11):1402–9.

8. Christensen J, Kieldsen MJ, Anderson H, et al. Gender differences in epilepsy. *Epilepsia* 2005; 46(6):956–60.

9. Ngugi AK, Kariuki SM, Bottomley C, et al. Incidence of epilepsy: a systematic review and meta-analysis. *Neurology* 2011; 77(10):1005–12.

10. Hauser WA, Annegers JF and Kurland LT. Incidence of epilepsy and unprovoked seizures in Rochester, Minnesota: 1935–1984. *Epilepsia* 1993; 34(3):453–68.

11. Hesdorffer DC, Logroscino G, Benn EK, et al. Estimating risk for developing epilepsy: a population-based study in Rochester, Minnesota. *Neurology* 2010; 76(1):23–7.

12. Tellez-Zenteno JF, Patten SB, Jette N, et al. Psychiatric comorbidity in epilepsy: a population-based analysis. *Epilepsia* 2007; 48(12):2336–44.

13. Tellez-Zenteno JF, Matijevic S and Wiebe S. Somatic comorbidity of epilepsy in the general population in Canada. *Epilepsia* 2005; 46(12):1955–62.

14. Fuller-Thomson E and Brennenstuhl S. The association between depression and epilepsy in a nationally representative sample. *Epilepsia* 2009; 50(5):1051–8.

15. Hesdorffer DC, Hauser WA, Olafsson E, et al. Depression and suicide attempt as risk factors for incident unprovoked seizures. *Ann Neurol* 2006; 59(1):35–41.

16. Kanner AM. Depression in epilepsy: prevalence, clinical semiology, pathogenic mechanisms, and treatment. *Biol Psychiatry* 2003; 54(3):388–98.

17. Turner K, Piazzini A, Franza A, et al. Epilepsy and postpartum depression. *Epilepsia* 2009; 50:24–7.

18. Gaitatzis A, Carroll K, Majeed A, et al. The epidemiology of the comorbidity of epilepsy in the general population. *Epilepsia* 2004; 45(12):1613–22.

19. Manni R and Terzaghi M. Comorbidity between epilepsy and sleep disorders. *Epilepsy Res* 2010; 90(3):171–7.

20. van Golde EGA, Gutter T and de Weerd AW. Sleep disturbances in people with epilepsy: prevalence, impact and treatment. *Sleep Med Rev* 2011; 15(6):357–68.

21. Khatami R, Zutter D, Siegel A, et al. Sleep-wake habits and disorders in a series of 100 adult epilepsy patients – a prospective study. *Seizure* 2006; 15(5):299–306.

22. de Weerd A, de Haas S, Otte A, et al. Subjective sleep disturbance in patients with partial epilepsy: a questionnaire-based study on prevalence and impact on quality of life. *Epilepsia* 2004; 45 (11):1397–1404.

23. Winawer MR and Shinnar S. Genetic epidemiology of epilepsy or what do we tell families? *Epilepsia* 2005; 46(Suppl 10):24–30.

24. McHugh JC and Delanty N. Chapter 2 epidemiology and classification of epilepsy. *Int Rev of Neurobiol* 2008; 83:11–26.

25. Waaler PE, Blom BH, Skeidsvoll H, et al. Prevalence, classification, and severity of epilepsy in children in western Norway. *Epilepsia* 2000; 41(7):802–10.

26. Briellmann RS, Jackson GD, Mitchell LA, et al. Occurrence of hippocampal sclerosis: is one hemisphere or gender more vulnerable? *Epilepsia* 1999; 40(12):1816–20.

27. Janszky J. Medial temporal lobe epilepsy: gender differences. *J Neurol Neurosurg Psychiatry* 2004; 75(5):773–5.

28. Herzog AG. Catamenial epilepsy: definition, prevalence pathophysiology and treatment. *Seizure* 2008; 17(2):151–9.

29. Herzog AG, Harden CL, Liporace J, et al. Frequency of catamenial seizure exacerbation in women with localization-related epilepsy. *Ann Neurol* 2004; 56 (3):431–4.

30. El-Khayat HA, Oliman NA, Tomoum HY, et al. Reproductive hormonal changes and catamenial pattern in adolescent females with epilepsy. *Epilepsia* 2008; 49(9):1619–26.

31. Quigg M, Smithson SD, Fowler KM, et al. Laterality and location influence catamenial seizure expression in women with partial epilepsy. *Neurology* 2009; 73(3):223–7.

32. Morrell MJ, Flynn KL, Done S, et al. Sexual dysfunction, sex steroid hormone abnormalities, and depression in women

with epilepsy treated with antiepileptic drugs. *Epilepsy Behav* 2005; 6(3):360–5.

33. Herzog AG, Coleman AE, Jacobs AR, et al. Relationship of sexual dysfunction to epilepsy laterality and reproductive hormone levels in women. *Epilepsy Behav* 2003; 4(4):407–13.

34. Pack AM. Implications of hormonal and neuroendocrine changes associated with seizures and antiepileptic drugs: a clinical perspective. *Epilepsia* 2010; 51:150–53.

35. Svalheim S, Taubøll E, Bjørnenak T, et al. Do women with epilepsy have increased frequency of menstrual disturbances? *Seizure* 2003; 12(8):529–33.

36. Herzog AG and Friedman MN. Menstrual cycle interval and ovulation in women with localization-related epilepsy. *Neurology* 2001; 57(11):2133–5.

37. Herzog AG, Coleman AE, Jacobs AR, et al. Interictal EEG discharges, reproductive hormones, and menstrual disorders in epilepsy. *Ann Neurol* 2003; 54(5):625–37.

38. Hu X, Wang J, Dong W, et al. A meta-analysis of polycystic ovary syndrome in women taking valproate for epilepsy. *Epilepsy Res* 2011; 97(1–2):73–82.

39. Lofgren E, Mikkonen K, Tolonen U, et al. Reproductive endocrine function in women with epilepsy: the role of epilepsy type and medication. *Epilepsy Behav* 2007; 10(1):77–83.

40. Morrell, MJ, Hayes FJ, Sluss PM, et al. Hyperandrogenism, ovulatory dysfunction, and polycystic ovary syndrome with valproate versus lamotrigine. *Ann Neurol* 2008; 64(2):200–211.

41. Herzog AG, Seibel MM, Schomer DL, et al. Reproductive endocrine disorders in men with partial seizures of temporal lobe origin. *Arch Neurol* 1986; 43(4):347–50.

42. Herzog AG, Seibel MM, Schomer DL, et al. Reproductive endocrine disorders in women with partial seizures of temporal lobe origin. *Arch Neurol* 1986; 43(4):341–6.

43. Wallace H, Shorvon S and Tallis R. Age-specific incidence and prevalence rates of treated epilepsy in an unselected population of 2 052 922 and age-specific fertility rates of women with epilepsy. *Lancet* 1998; 352(9145):1970–73.

44. Sukumaran SC, Sarma PS and Thomas SV. Polytherapy increases the risk of infertility in women with epilepsy. *Neurology* 2010; 75(15):1351–5.

45. Pack AM. Infertility in women with epilepsy: what's the risk and why? *Neurology* 2010; 75(15):1316–7.

46. Gopinath M, Sarma PS and Thomas SV. Gender-specific psychosocial outcome for women with epilepsy. *Epilepsy Behav* 2011; 20(1):44–7.

47. Pack AM, Davis AR, Kritzer J, et al. Antiepileptic drugs: are women aware of interactions with oral contraceptives and potential teratogenicity? *Epilepsy Behav* 2009; 14(4):640–4.

48. Pennell PB. Hormonal aspects of epilepsy. *Neurol Clin* 2009; 27(4):941–65.

49. Wang H, Bos JH and de Jong-van den Berg LT. Co-prescription of antiepileptic drugs and contraceptives. *Contraception* 2012; 85(1):28–31.

50. Shorvon SD, Tallis RC and Wallace HK. Antiepileptic drugs: coprescription of proconvulsant drugs and oral contraceptives: a national study of antiepileptic drug prescribing practice. *J Neurol Neurosurg Psychiatry* 2002; 72(1):114–5.

51. Vessey M, Painter R and Yeates D. Oral contraception and epilepsy: findings in a large cohort study. *Contraception* 2002; 66(2):77–9.

52. Harden CL, Pennell PB, Koppel BS, et al. Management issues for women with epilepsy–focus on pregnancy (an evidence-based review): III. Vitamin K, folic acid, blood levels, and breast-feeding: Report of the Quality Standards Subcommittee and Therapeutics and Technology Assessment Subcommittee of the American Academy of Neurology and the American Epilepsy Society. *Epilepsia* 2009; 50(5):1247–55.

53. Kaaja E, Kaaja R and Hiilesmaa V. Major malformations in offspring of women with epilepsy. *Neurology* 2003; 60(4):575–9.

54. Morrow JI, Hunt SJ, Russell AJ, et al. Folic acid use and major congenital malformations in offspring of women with epilepsy: a prospective study from the UK Epilepsy and Pregnancy Register. *J Neurol Neurosurg Psychiatry* 2009; 80(5): 506–11.

55. Winterbottom JB, Smyth RM, Jacoby A, et al. Preconception counselling for women with epilepsy to reduce adverse pregnancy outcome. *Cochrane Database Syst Rev* 2008; (3):CD006645.

56. Winterbottom J, Smyth R, Jacoby A, et al. The effectiveness of preconception counseling to reduce adverse pregnancy outcome in women with epilepsy: what's the evidence? *Epilepsy Behav* 2009; 14(2):273–9.

57. Pittschieler S, Brezinka C, Jahn B, et al. Spontaneous abortion and the prophylactic effect of folic acid supplementation in epileptic women undergoing antiepileptic therapy. *J Neurol* 2008; 255(12): 1926–31.

58. Tomson T, Battino D, French J, et al. Antiepileptic drug exposure and major congenital malformations: the role of pregnancy registries. *Epilepsy Behav* 2007; 11(3):277–82.

59. Artama M, Auvinen A, Raudaskoski T, et al. Antiepileptic drug use of women with epilepsy and congenital malformations in offspring. *Neurology* 2005; 64(11):1874–8.

60. Meador K, Reynolds MW, Crean S, et al. Pregnancy outcomes in women with epilepsy: a systematic review and meta-analysis of published pregnancy registries and cohorts. *Epilepsy Res* 2008; 81(1):1–13.

61. Molgaard-Nielsen D and Hviid A. Newer-generation antiepileptic drugs and the risk of major birth defects. *JAMA* 2011; 305(19):1996–2002.

62. Meador KJ, Baker GA, Browning N, et al. Cognitive function at 3 years of age after fetal exposure to antiepileptic drugs. *N Engl J Med* 2009; 360(16):1597–605.

63. Nadebaum C, Anderson VA, Vajda F, et al. Language skills of school-aged children prenatally exposed to antiepileptic drugs. *Neurology* 2011; 76(8):719–26.

64. Borthen I, Eide MG, Veiby G, et al. Complications during pregnancy in women with epilepsy: population-based cohort study. *BJOG: An International Journal of Obstetrics & Gynaecology* 2009; 116 (13):1736–42.

65. Borthen I, Eide MG, Daltveit AK, et al. Delivery outcome of women with epilepsy: a population-based cohort study. *BJOG* 2010; 117(12):1537–43.

66. Veiby G, Daltveit AK, Engelson BA, et al. Pregnancy, delivery, and outcome for the child in maternal epilepsy. *Epilepsia* 2009; 50(9):2130–39.

67. Harden CL, Pennell PB, Koppel BS, et al. Management issues for women with epilepsy – focus on pregnancy (an evidence-based review): II. Teratogenesis and perinatal outcomes. *Epilepsia* 2009; 50(5):1237–46.

68. Viinikainen K, Heinonen S, Eriksson K, et al. Community-based, prospective, controlled study of obstetric and neonatal outcome of 179 pregnancies in women with epilepsy. *Epilepsia* 2006; 47(1): 186–92.

69. Seizure control and treatment in pregnancy: observations from the EURAP Epilepsy Pregnancy Registry. *Neurology* 2006; 66(3):354–60.

70. Vajda FJ, Hitchcock A, Graham J, et al. Seizure control in antiepileptic drug-treated pregnancy. *Epilepsia* 2008; 49(1):172–6.

71. Meador KJ, Baker GA, Browning N, et al. Effects of breastfeeding in children of women taking antiepileptic drugs. *Neurology* 2010; 75(22):1954–60.

72. Erel T and Guralp O. Epilepsy and menopause. *Arch Gynecol Obstet* 2011; 284(3):749–55.

73. Harden CL, Pulver MC, Ravdin L, et al. The effect of menopause and perimenopause on the course of epilepsy. *Epilepsia* 1999; 40(10):1402–7.

74. Harden CL, Koppel BS, Herzog AG, et al. Seizure frequency is associated with age at

menopause in women with epilepsy. *Neurology* 2003; 61(4):451–5.

75. Klein P, Serje A and Pezzullo JC. Premature ovarian failure in women with epilepsy. *Epilepsia* 2001; 42(12):1584–9.

76. Vestergaard P, Rejnmark L and Mosekilde L. Fracture risk associated with use of antiepileptic drugs. *Epilepsia* 2004; 45(11):1330–7.

77. Jette N, Lix LM, Metge CJ, et al. Association of antiepileptic drugs with nontraumatic fractures: a population-based analysis. *Arch Neurol* 2011; 68(1):107–12.

78. Pack AM, Morrell MJ, Randall A, et al. Bone health in young women with epilepsy after one year of antiepileptic drug monotherapy. *Neurology* 2008; 70(18):1586–93.

79. Davis AR, Pack AM, Kritzer J, et al. Reproductive history, sexual behavior and use of contraception in women with epilepsy. *Contraception* 2008; 77(6):405–9.

80. Kanner AM. Depression in epilepsy: prevalence, clinical semiology, pathogenic mechanisms, and treatment. *Biol Psychiatry* 2003; 54:388–98.

Psychiatric comorbidities of epilepsy in women

Sherese Ali

Key points:

- Up to one in three women with epilepsy (WWE) have a lifetime risk of depression
- Depression can be seen in association with preictal, ictal, postictal, and interictal states
- WWE have an increased risk of anxiety and postpartum depression
- Unlike the general population, WWE are equally likely to have completed suicide compared to men with epilepsy
- Psychotropic drugs have significant drug-drug interactions with anticonvulsants, influences on seizure threshold, and teratogenicity

Introduction

The prevalence of psychiatric comorbidity in epilepsy is higher than that of other medical disorders, with an estimated prevalence of 25–50% [1]. A complex neurobiological relationship between epilepsy and psychiatric disorders has been purported, accounting in part for this comorbidity, which extends beyond coping with a chronic medical illness and its psychosocial impact. Community-based epidemiological studies consistently demonstrate that depression is the most common comorbidity of any medical or psychiatric disorder with an estimated prevalence rate of 30% versus 15% in the general population [1–3]. There are less reliable estimates of prevalence of anxiety disorders, which are themselves highly comorbid with depression [3]. The prevalence of bipolar disorder and schizophrenia in patients with epilepsy is estimated at 10% versus 1% and 0.3–0.7%, respectively, in the general population [2].

Affective disorders
Depression

Affective disorders include depression, anxiety, and bipolar disorder. The lifetime prevalence of depression is estimated at 10% in males and 25% in females in the general population. The lifetime prevalence of depression in patients with epilepsy is estimated to be as high as 30% in population-based studies and up to 50% in tertiary care centers, with a noticeable lack of gender difference, although some studies still report a small gender bias towards women [4].

Women with Epilepsy, ed. Esther Bui and Autumn Klein. Published by Cambridge University Press.
© Cambridge University Press 2014.

A neurobiological and bidirectional relationship between the two disorders has long been suggested since Hippocrates first suggested it six centuries ago. Studies show a 4-fold increase in depression in newly diagnosed epilepsy patients, and up to 17-fold if the seizures were partial. Investigations into common pathogenic mechanisms implicate decreased serotonin (5-HT) and noradrenaline (NE), which both form the basis of depression pharmacotherapy and have been shown to facilitate kindling and exacerbate seizure frequency in rats [4]. Indeed several antiepileptic drugs (AEDs) (carbamazepine (CBZ), lamotrigine (LMT), zonisamide (ZNM), valproate (VPA), and vigabatrin (VGB)) are presynaptic 5-HT receptor agonists [4].

The duration of depressive symptoms and temporal relationship to seizure activity give rise to the terms periictal (preictal and postictal), ictal (directly part of the seizure), and interictal depression.

Preictal, ictal, and postictal depression

Preictal depression is considered part of the prodromal dysphoria preceding seizure(s) often by hours to days, ictal depression as part of the seizure, and postictal depression as part of the recovery phase. The prevalence of preictal and ictal depressive symptoms is not known but it is considered uncommon to rare. No gender difference has been identified. Postictal depression might be the most common, with a recent review suggesting that it can be identified in up to 50% of patients with medically refractory epilepsy and has a median duration of 24 hours, with a range of several hours to 5 days [6]. It may represent an exacerbation of chronic depression. The available data suggest a slight gender bias towards women, 62% of 100 patients [7].

A rare component of seizure semiology, ictal depression is a sudden onset of dysphoria more commonly seen in temporal lobe epilepsy [5]. There is, however, limited population-based data to further characterize this rare phenomenon. No association with epilepsy variables, such as hemispheric lateralization, or demographic factors such as gender has been reported. There are a few case reports of its occurrence with psychotic symptoms and impulsive suicidal behavior during nonconvulsive status epilepticus [5].

Interictal depression (interictal dysphoric disorder)

Interictal depression, also known as interictal dysphoric disorder (IDD) is defined by DSM-IV criteria as depression that is more pervasive and unrelated temporally to seizure activity. It is the most common type of depressive disorder in epilepsy, with prevalence estimates of 25–70% with no gender difference [4]. In addition to the biopsychosocial risk factors usually associated with depression (for example family history and adverse life events), additional biological risk factors include side effects of AEDs and mesial versus neocortical temporal lobe epilepsy [8]. Its occurrence seems to be independent of successful seizure control [4].

Although DSM-IV is used to diagnose interictal depression, there are some qualitative differences in the symptoms. These include more complaints of cognitive impairment, fatigue, anergia, pain, anxiety, and medication side effects, rather than of depressed mood or endogenous symptoms such as guilt [8]. Perhaps the most prominent difference is in the quality of the mood, with low mood and intermittent, episodic irritability and euphoric moods often raising suspicion for a bipolar spectrum disorder. The duration of the mood disturbance may not meet the minimum 2-week duration criteria for a depressive episode as they follow a more chronic and intermittent course, relapsing and remitting within several days [8]. There is, therefore, a risk of underdiagnosis.

Depressive behaviors, such as poor medication compliance, poor sleep, lack of daily structure, irregular eating, have a negative impact on epilepsy, including poorer seizure control and poorer response to medical and surgical treatment. Depression is the strongest predictor of decreased quality of life compared to any other epilepsy variable, including seizure control. It is associated with an increase in suicidal ideation, behavior, and completion, increased health care utilization for non-psychiatric problems, and increased health care costs [3].

Cognitive behavior therapy (CBT) and interpersonal therapy are approved psychological treatments for depression. Other adjunctive psychotherapies include psycho-education, supportive therapy, and assistance with coping. Pharmacotherapies include use of selective serotonin reuptake inhibitor (SSRI), serotonin and norepinephrine reuptake inhibitor (SNRIs), or tricyclic antidepressants (TCAs). Electroconvulsive therapy has been used safely in select patients with epilepsy. Repetitive transcranial magnetic stimulation and deep brain stimulation are currently in their infancy and being studied for depression and epilepsy. Vagal nerve stimulation has been studied and used in selected cases of refractory epilepsy with noticeable positive mood effects. This has stimulated considerable interest in its potential use for depression in epilepsy since it can have beneficial effects on both disorders.

Postpartum blues and postpartum depression

Postpartum blues affects 25–75% of mothers. It is defined as symptoms of tearfulness, fatigue, mild sleep disturbance, maintenance of insight, absence of psychotic symptoms, and maintained desire to bond with the baby, with an onset within 2 days after parturition and resolves over the course of 1 week postpartum. It is not considered pathological, is not associated with a risk of harm to self or baby, and is thought to be an emotional consequence of rapid changes in hormone levels after birth.

In contrast, postpartum depression (PPD) occurs in 10–15% of women and has an onset within the postpartum period, defined as 1 month after parturition. Only three studies examined prevalence rates in women with epilepsy and found an increased rate of 25–39% [9–11]. There were no associated epilepsy or demographic variables, except multiparity and AED polytherapy for treatment-resistant epilepsy in one study, however this study lacked a control group [11]. To date, no specific risk factors have been identified to account for the increased prevalence of PPD in women with epilepsy.

In PPD, symptoms meet DSM-IV symptom criteria for a major depressive episode, but have additional distinct symptoms of mood lability, anxiety, fear of not being a good mother, fear that the baby does not like or want them, disinterest in the baby, less affection and less responsiveness towards the baby, initial insomnia rather than early-morning awakening, panic attacks, psychomotor agitation, and spontaneous crying. It carries an increased risk of suicide. Babies of mothers with postpartum depression tend to be more irritable, show less social behaviors such as vocalizations and cooing, and make fewer positive facial expressions [9].

PPD can be classified as mild, moderate, or severe. In DSM-IV terms PPD is a Major Depressive Episode, Mild/Moderate/Severe without Psychosis, with Postpartum Onset. When it is severe *with* psychosis, it refers to postpartum psychosis (PPP). In postpartum psychosis, fears develop into delusions, such as believing they are bad mothers, or that the baby is evil. It carries both an increased risk of suicide and a risk of infanticide and is considered a psychiatric emergency. Its prevalence in the population is rare and there are no estimates specifically in the epilepsy population. PPP may be a harbinger of a later diagnosis of bipolar disorder.

The treatment for postpartum depression in women with epilepsy is the same as in those without epilepsy, with special consideration being given to effect on seizure threshold, safety during lactation and drug interactions with AEDs (discussed later in this chapter and shown in Tables 2.3 and 2.6). The Canadian Network for Mood and Anxiety Treatment (CANMAT) Clinical Guidelines [12] indicate that there is level 3 evidence that citalopram, nortriptyline, sertraline, and paroxetine can be used as first line antidepressants in lactating mothers due to low to undetectable levels in breast fed babies. Empirical data provided strong support for the efficacy of psychotherapy alone, such as counseling and CBT, in the treatment of PPD [9, 12]. Studies reporting steroid hormone-associated deficiency in central nervous system gamma-aminobutyric acid A (GABA-A) regulation leading to postpartum depression and increased neuronal excitability, raise ideas about the use of benzodiazepines in women with epilepsy comorbid with postpartum depression [13].

Premenstrual dysphoric disorder (PMDD)

The prevalence of PMDD is estimated at 3–6% of premenopausal women [14]. Estrogen is thought to have regulatory effects on serotonin, GABA, and dopamine, resulting in the negative mood effects and physical symptoms of PMDD [14]. The DSM-IV diagnostic criteria for PMDD are shown in Table 2.1.

In addition to the direct hormonal effects of the menstrual cycle on seizure exacerbation in catamenial epilepsy, the monthly mood fluctuations in PMDD can contribute to increased seizure frequency.

Table 2.1: DSM-IV diagnostic criteria for PMDD

At least five symptoms, at least one being a cardinal symptom, present in most menstrual cycles over the past year in at least two consecutive cycles, with symptoms beginning in the luteal phase and beginning to remit within a few days of onset of the follicular phase, being absent in the week post-menses.

Cardinal symptoms:
1) markedly depressed mood, hopelessness, or self-deprecating thoughts
2) marked tension, feeling "keyed up" or "on edge"
3) marked affective lability (e.g., feeling suddenly sad or tearful, or increased rejection sensitivity)
4) persistent and marked anger or irritability, or increased interpersonal conflicts

Associated symptoms:
5) decreased interest
6) difficulty concentrating
7) lethargy
8) overeating or food cravings
9) hypersomnia or insomnia
10) feeling overwhelmed or out of control

Symptoms are severe enough to affect socio-occupational function and not better accounted for by another psychiatric condition or comorbidity

SSRIs are first line pharmacotherapy for PMDD. Fluoxetine, paroxetine, and sertraline either in intermittent dosing or continuous treatment are FDA-approved for PMDD [14]. Non-pharmacologic measures include regular sleep, exercise, and small, frequent, nutritionally balanced meals. Vitamin B6, vitamin E, calcium, magnesium, and tryptophan have also been reported to be helpful [14]. Stress reduction techniques, anger management, cognitive behavior therapy, and psycho-education can all be beneficial. The use of hormone therapy has been studied but is not FDA-approved for PMDD. There is no data on whether treatment of PMDD with SSRIs or psychotherapy is effective in catamenial epilepsy, and this remains an area of future research. Often then, women with catamenial epilepsy and PMDD may end up on additional intermittent-dosing AED treatment concomitant with intermittent- or continuous-dosing SSRI treatment.

Anxiety

The prevalence of anxiety in the general population is 9% for men and 16% for women, while the prevalence of interictal anxiety disorders has been estimated at 10–25% [15]. One study estimated the lifetime prevalence of anxiety in epilepsy at 39%, with epileptic patients being 2.4 times more likely to report any type of anxiety in their lifetime [1].

Comorbid anxiety disorders reported in epilepsy include generalized anxiety disorder (GAD), panic disorder, agoraphobia, and social phobia, with GAD being the most common [15]. The phobic anxieties are thought to be linked to poor seizure control, and concerns about unpredictably having seizures in public [15]. Ictal fear and panic is a fairly common manifestation of anxiety in temporal lobe seizures [15]. It is distinguishable from panic attacks by its short duration of only a few seconds and confinement to the ictus with complete recovery postictally.

Anxiety disorders are often highly comorbid with depression and this holds true in patients with epilepsy, with one study showing 73% of 199 patients with epilepsy and depression meeting DSM-IV criteria for an anxiety disorder using the Mini International Neuropsychiatric Interview [3].

SSRIs and SNRIs are used to treat both anxiety and depression. Due to transient side effects of insomnia, irritability, and worsening anxiety in the first 2 weeks of SSRI use, some patients may require a benzodiazepine during those first 2 weeks of treatment. Psychotherapeutic interventions such as cognitive behavior therapy are approved for the treatment of anxiety and depression. Other methods include mindfulness-based stress reduction, breathing exercises, and progressive muscular relaxation.

Bipolar disorder

Bipolar symptoms are frequently observed in patients with epilepsy but are thought to more likely represent the affective instability of interictal dysphoric disorder (IDD) [16]. The phenotype of bipolar disorder in patients with epilepsy is thought to be modified by the use of AEDs, such that there is decreased symptom amplitude with a more rapid-cycling pattern, as in IDD. Although the estimated prevalence is 10–12% with no gender preference, epidemiological studies are difficult to interpret as studies may be detecting IDD rather than true bipolar disorder [16]. True mania in epilepsy is considered rare, with the exception of postictal mania and post-epilepsy surgery mania [8].

Postictal mania

In a review study, one author examining the semiology of interictal versus postictal psychoses found that manic symptoms were more closely associated with postictal psychosis than with interictal psychosis [8]. Three factors were also more closely associated with postictal (manic-like) than interictal (schizophreniform) psychosis: temporal lobe epilepsy, 87% versus 59%, respectively; complex partial seizures, 82% versus 67%, respectively; and structural abnormalities of the temporal lobe on MRI, 35% versus 20%, respectively.

Post-epilepsy surgery mania

The available data suggest that de novo manic episodes occur in about 10% of patients after temporal lobectomy, especially right-sided lobectomies or if there are bilateral abnormalities. The manic episodes tend to have an onset within several days to a few weeks postoperatively and have a short course with spontaneous remission. While they are thought to be associated with poor postoperative seizure outcome, they are thus far considered psychiatrically benign, but long-term psychiatric follow-up studies are lacking [8].

Since both these conditions are self-limited, treatment with psychotropics is often not necessary. In cases of protracted postictal mania, short-term antipsychotics with anti-manic efficacy, such as risperidone, olanzapine, or quetiapine, or high potency D2 antagonists, such as haloperidol, or benzodiazepines, such as lorazepam, may be used as adjunctive therapy to the AEDs to speed recovery.

Psychotic disorders
Psychoses of epilepsy
Periictal and ictal psychosis

Preictal psychotic symptoms may include visual, olfactory, or gustatory hallucinations. Ictal psychosis is rare and may be experienced as auditory or visual illusions or hallucinations, depersonalization, derealization, or a sense of "someone behind." Symptoms are very short-lived, several seconds to <1 minute and are rarely recalled as psychotic. Differentiating this from a primary ictal phenomenon can be difficult. Because of how rare these are, there is not enough data to determine gender ratios.

Postictal psychosis (PIP) is the most common of the three, with a prevalence estimate of up to 18%, and accounts for an estimated 25% of cases of psychosis in epilepsy [17]. It may be more likely to occur when there is more than one independent epileptic focus, such as in patients with multiple cavernomas or tuberous sclerosis. There are more reports of males than females with PIP in the literature. It is often a missed diagnosis because of a classic clinical feature of the syndrome: a mentally lucid interval of about 3 days between seizures and the onset of psychosis, resulting in dismissal of a relationship between the two. It typically occurs after a cluster of seizures, usually in patients with complex partial seizures often with secondary generalization. Mean duration of symptoms is 3.0–14.3 days with a range of 1–90 days [17]. Symptoms include visual and auditory hallucinations, delusions of any type (religious, somatic, paranoid, grandiose) but mostly religious, mild changes in levels of consciousness and behavior suggestive of encephalopathy, and affective disturbance that can include hypomanic symptoms. In the latter case, especially when accompanied by grandiose delusions, the diagnosis is often postictal mania, rather than psychosis. EEG may show minimal diffuse slowing compatible with encephalopathy, but may otherwise be normal during the psychotic stage.

Some patients respond well to benzodiazepines, which may be the first choice of therapy, with antipsychotics such as risperidone being used in cases of worsening psychosis [17]. Though antipsychotics associated with an increased risk of seizures, such as clozapine, loxapine, and chlorpromazine, should be considered carefully, most people with epilepsy on AEDs could be safely treated with either a first or second generation antipsychotic [29–31]. Postictal psychosis is most often a self-limiting syndrome, which can be managed conservatively with observation and supportive care, including constant supervision where necessary for safety. It may develop into a chronic interictal psychosis in up to 25% of cases, particularly if it is recurrent [18].

A history of PIP is not considered an absolute contraindication to epilepsy surgery, especially if the chance of becoming seizure-free with surgery is considered high [17]. Only one study recorded outcome of surgery and found postoperative mood disorders in 8/38 patients with preoperative PIP [17]. Careful postoperative psychiatric monitoring is therefore considered essential.

Interictal psychosis

Interictal psychosis is a chronic psychosis temporally *unrelated* to seizure activity. It features symptoms more reminiscent of schizophrenia, in contrast to PIP, which has a strong affective component resembling bipolar disorder. It occurs insidiously in about 5% of patients [18]. No data is available on gender bias, but anecdotal reports more often feature males than females. Religious themes and persecutory auditory hallucinations are prominent. There is a higher incidence of negative symptoms than in PIP, first rank symptoms of schizophrenia are virtually absent [18]. Treatment is similar to that of schizophrenia, including pharmacotherapy and psychosocial rehabilitation.

Forced normalization (or alternative psychosis)

First described by Landolt in 1953, this concept is still controversial and no reliable epidemiological data exist. It refers to emergence of psychotic symptoms after obtaining acute seizure control in patients with chronic uncontrolled epilepsy. It is considered uncommon and little is known about its actual mechanism [32].

Post-epilepsy surgery psychosis

De novo psychosis following temporal lobectomy occurs at an average rate of 7% [18]. It usually occurs within the first 6 months after temporal lobectomy and is considered transient. After 6 months, its incidence approaches that of the baseline rate in patients with medically refractory epilepsy [18]. From the limited data, potential risk factors are operative age over 30, family history of psychosis, and preoperative psychosis. No gender predisposition is known.

Suicide

Several studies document a 3-fold higher risk of death by suicide in patients with well-controlled epilepsy than in controls, in the absence of psychiatric disorder. A review of 21 studies found a mean rate of 11.5% of suicide as cause of death in patients with epilepsy. The rate is considered higher in patients with temporal lobe epilepsy and is also elevated

Table 2.2: Mini International Neuropsychiatric Interview

In the past month did you:	Points for answering "YES"
1. Think that you would be better off dead or wish that you were dead?	1
2. Want to harm yourself?	2
3. Think about suicide?	6
4. Have a suicide plan?	10
5. Attempt suicide?	10
6. Have you ever in your lifetime made a suicide attempt?	4
Low Risk	1–5 points
Moderate Risk	6–9 points
High Risk	>9 points

after epilepsy surgery. No gender difference in suicide attempt versus completion has been found in patients with epilepsy. In the general population, women are nine times more likely than men to attempt by non-lethal means rather than complete suicide. In patients with epilepsy however, this gender bias does not exist. In several studies, only depression and a previous suicide attempt, no other demographic or epilepsy variables, were identified as risk factors in patients with epilepsy [19, 20].

In 2008, the FDA issued a safety warning on the risk of suicidality associated with 11 AEDs. It was based on a meta-analysis of 199 randomized clinical trials, which has since been shown to have had several methodological flaws, including lack of standardization of the definition of "suicidality," lack of statistically significant findings except for two AEDs, topiramate and lamotrigine, not accounting for polytherapy or psychiatric comorbidity, and large ranges in the odds ratio of suicide in the various studies [21]. A retrospective study of levetiracetam use in epilepsy identified out of 517 patients, 0.4% experienced suicidal ideation [33]. There have since been several studies that have shown that AEDs in patients with epilepsy do not confer additional risk of suicide or have produced mixed results due to significant methodological flaws [22–24].

Psychiatric monitoring is recommended in both male and female patients with comorbid depression and/or a previous lifetime history of suicide attempt. The MINI suicide risk assessment shown in Table 2.2 is a quick and easily administered tool for routine monitoring of suicidal risk.

Psychogenic non-epileptic seizures (PNES)

PNES is not an uncommon comorbidity with epilepsy, occurring in about 15–25% of admissions to epilepsy monitoring units and in up to 50% of "medically refractory" patients, with a male:female ratio of 1:3 [25]. PNES are episodes resembling epileptic seizures that are not associated with epileptiform EEG changes and are judged to have an underlying psychological cause. According to DSM-IV, it is categorized as Conversion Disorder, one of the five somatoform disorders. By definition, it is therefore unconsciously produced without evidence of secondary gain. However, it can become secondarily reinforced by the attention that patients may gain from family or medical professionals. It can complicate the picture of underlying epilepsy. The video-EEG is considered the gold standard for diagnosis.

PNES is typically associated with a history of chronic family dysfunction which may include non-sexual trauma and sexual abuse. Alexithymia is a prominent characteristic, whereby patients have difficulty reading, acknowledging or discussing emotions, and become very focused on physical and somatic symptoms. Attention is often unduly focused on finding a physical cause for the symptoms and lack of insight into the psychological nature of the events is a poor prognostic factor for recovery. A high incidence of borderline personality disorder (25–40%) in patients with PNES further complicates recovery [29].

The first phase of treatment consists of sensitive and effective presentation of the diagnosis and psycho-education, leading to significant reduction in PNES frequency before any further intervention even starts. Further treatment is primarily psychotherapeutic and the best evidence exists for cognitive behavior therapy or behavior therapy where there are cognitive limitations. Symptoms of Axis I disorders, most commonly depression and post-traumatic stress disorder (PTSD), may eventually emerge and appropriate psychiatric treatment for these disorders can then ensue. Many underlying psychiatric disorders including borderline personality disorder, depression, and PTSD are over-represented in females. Furthermore, female gender is considered a poor prognostic factor in patients with PNES.

Effect of psychotropic medications on seizure threshold

Seizures have been reported with almost all antidepressant classes and compounds, although causation has not been reliably established and controlled studies are lacking. Available evidence from clinical studies suggests that in the absence of overdose, the risk is relatively low for SSRIs and atypical antipsychotics. Table 2.3 shows the risk stratification of various psychotropic medications derived from the available data. In general, all the low- and intermediate-risk psychotropics are considered safe in therapeutic doses with concomitant appropriate AED coverage. High-risk psychotropics have a dose-dependent increase in risk but absolute risk quotes per dose are not available except for clozapine. High-risk psychotropics are best avoided except in rare select cases of severe refractory comorbid psychiatric disorders with very close monitoring and AED coverage.

Neuropsychiatric effects of antiepileptic drugs

Some AEDs have positive psychiatric effects and Table 2.4 shows those that are approved for use in psychiatric disorders. Although all AEDs are capable of producing some neuro-psychiatric side effects of varying degrees, e.g., cognitive slowing and sedation, some that carry more specific negative psychiatric side effects are shown in Table 2.5, with incidences in percent where data is available.

Psychotropic drugs in pregnancy and lactation

Table 2.6 shows a summary of the available data on the safety of psychotropic medications during pregnancy and lactation. Note that lithium should be avoided in patients with epilepsy where possible. In the rare circumstance that it is being used, the following is the recommended monitoring for lithium during pregnancy:

- Observe infant for sedation, withdrawal, and toxicity.
- Monitor cord blood lithium levels during pregnancy.

Table 2.3: Psychotropic medications and seizure risk [4, 5]

High risk (dose-dependent increases in risk)	Intermediate risk	Low risk
Chlorpromazine >1g/day	Haloperidol	Fluphenazine
Clozapine (dose-dependent): • 0.7% per 100 mg • <300 mg/day – 1% • 300–600 mg/day – 2.7% • 600–900 mg/day – 4.4% • Myoclonic > GTC > partial		Trifluoperazine
Thioridazine	Venlafaxine	Risperidone
Bupropion (especially >450 mg/day)	Duloxetine	†Paliperidone
Clomipramine	Imipramine	‡Iloperidone
Maprotiline		Quetiapine
Amoxapine		Olanzapine
*Mianserin		Aripiprazole
Lithium		Ziprasidone
		‡Asenapine
		Paroxetine
		Sertraline
		Fluoxetine
		Fluvoxamine
		Citalopram
		Escitalopram
		Amitriptyline
		Trazodone
		Monoamine Oxidase Inhibitors
		Methylphenidate (20 mg/day)

- Low risk – relative risk not statistically significant from risk of de novo seizure in the general population
- Intermediate risk – some but not all uncontrolled studies, retrospective case reports and series suggesting some increase in seizure frequency
- High risk – sufficient data to provide consensus on statistically significant elevation of seizure risk

* Tetracyclic antidepressant, no longer available in the USA
† Paliperidone – no reports of seizures since introduction in 2006
‡ Iloperidone and asenapine – no reports of seizures since recent introduction in 2009, considered to have the lowest risk

Table 2.4: AEDs currently approved or being used in psychiatric conditions [26]

AED	Approved indications in psychiatry	Other uses in psychiatry
Benzodiazepines	• Generalized anxiety disorder • Panic disorder • Insomnia • Alcohol benzodiazepine withdrawal	• Catatonia • Aggression • Adjunctive therapy in BAD
Carbamazepine (<1% incidence of depression)	• 2nd line agent for maintenance in bipolar disorder and acute mania	• Anger/irritability/mood swings • Impulsivity, aggression
Valproate (<1% incidence of depression)	• 1st line agent for bipolar disorder, maintenance, acute mania, mixed episode, rapid cycling	
Lamotrigine	• 1st line agent for bipolar disorder, maintenance, bipolar depression	
Pregabalin	• Generalized anxiety disorder	
Phenytoin		• 3rd line, adjunctive agent in bipolar disorder
Topiramate		• 3rd line, adjunctive agent in bipolar disorder • Weight loss, binge-eating
Oxcarbazepine		• 3rd line, adjunctive agent in bipolar disorder
Gabapentin		• 3rd line, adjunctive agent in bipolar disorder • Anxiety (social anxiety disorder)

- Monitor maternal serum lithium levels during pregnancy, especially during third trimester, due to significant physiological changes leading to changes in drug metabolism and clearance.
- At birth, check neonatal thyroid function, urea, and electrolytes.

Psychotropic-antiepileptic drug interactions [28]

There are only a few clinically significant drug interactions between psychotropic medications and AEDs. The most significant are enzyme-inducing anticonvulsants, such as carbamazepine and phenytoin, due to liver-inducing effects of most drugs, including induction of its own metabolism. Carbamazepine and phenytoin have caused clinically significant

Table 2.5: AEDs associated with significant psychiatric side effects [26]

AED	Psychiatric side effects
Barbiturates (phenobarbital, primidone)	Depression 10%
Vigabatrin	Depression 10%, psychosis 1%
Topiramate	Depression 10%, mania, psychosis
High-dose zonisamide	Depression 7%, mania
Leviteracetam	Depression 4%, anger, aggression, agitation
Tiagibine	Depression 4%, nervousness, anxiety
Felbamate	Depression 4%
Rufinamide	Depression
Ethosuximide	Depression <1%
Phenytoin	Depression <1%
Oxcarbazepine	Depression <1%
Gabapentin	Depression <1%

Table 2.6: Safety of psychotropic medications during pregnancy and lactation [12, 27]

Drug/Drug class	Data on teratogenecity	Data on lactation
SSRIs	*Paroxetine*: cardiac malformations, not recommended for use during pregnancy Minor anomalies, but no increased risk of major malformations with other SSRIs	*Fluoxetine*: Adverse effects reported in 4/190 infants, (3: colic; 1: seizure-like activity at 3 weeks, and unresponsive episodes at 4 months) No reports of adverse effects with other SSRIs, which have undetectable levels in serum of breastfed babies
SNRIs	No teratogenic effects known	No published adverse events to date
Bupropion	No teratogenic effects known	No published adverse events to date
Trazodone	No teratogenic effects known	No published adverse events to date
Mirtazapine	No teratogenic effects known	No published adverse events to date
TCAs	No teratogenic effects known, neonatal anticholinergic side effects	No published adverse events to date
Haloperidol	Sparse data available, avoid in 1st trimester, minimize use as much as possible	No reliable reports of harm
Atypical antipsychotics	Sparse data available, avoid in 1st trimester, minimize use as much as possible	No published adverse events to date

Table 2.6: (cont.)

Drug/Drug class	Data on teratogenecity	Data on lactation
Carbamazepine	2.9% NTDs, anencephaly, craniofacial defects, IUGR, cardiac abnormalities	Safe, monitor CBC and liver function
Valproate	8.7% NTDs and major malformations	Safe, monitor CBC and liver function
Lamotrigine	2.7% major malformations	No published adverse events to date
Lithium	Ebstein's anomaly of the heart 0.05-.01% vs. 0.005% in general population; RR = 2–10 More commonly it causes "floppy baby" syndrome with cyanosis and hypotonicity; reports of neonatal hypothyroidism and nephrogenic diabetes insipidus	Lithium levels recorded at 10–50% of maternal levels in 1st week, then 33%; fetal renal clearance is decreased in first 5 months of age; lithium effects: hypotonicity, cyanosis, thyroid dysfunction, abnormal ECG; best avoided, at least during first 5 months of breastfeeding
Benzodiazepines	0.07% cleft lip/cleft palate	

CBC – complete blood count
IUGR – intrauterine growth retardation
NTDs – neural tube defects
SNRI – serotonin and norepinephrine reuptake inhibitor
SSRI – selective serotonin reuptake inhibitor

reductions in levels of haloperidol and atypical antipsychotics. Discontinuation of cytochrome p450 (CYP 450) enzyme-inducing agents may result in increased antipsychotic concentrations with associated risk of toxicity. Fluvoxamine can lead to carbamazepine toxicity via CYP3A4 inhibition. Valproate has an inhibitory effect on liver metabolism and tends to increase levels of most drugs. Topiramate, oxcarbazepine, and felbamate have only very mild liver-inducing effects. Lamotrigine is metabolized by hepatic uridine glucuronosyl transferease (UGT) microsomal enzymes UGT1A3 and UGT1A4, and therefore has no drug interactions with psychotropic drugs, which are largely metabolized via the CYP 450 system. Gabapentin, pregabalin, leviteracetam, and lacosamide have no demonstrable effect on CYP 450 enzymes. In general, carefully administered psychotropics are safe for use in epilepsy.

References

1. Karouni M, Arulthas S, Larsson PG, et al. Psychiatric comorbidity in patients with epilepsy: a population-based study. *Eur J Clin Pharmacol* 2010; 66:1151–60.

2. Ottman R, Lipton RB, Ettinger AB, et al. Comorbidities of epilepsy: results from the epilepsy comorbidities and health (EPIC) survey. *Epilepsia* 2011; 52(2):308–15.

3. Kanner AM. Psychiatric issues in epilepsy: the complex relation of mood, anxiety disorders and epilepsy. *Epilepsy Behav* 2009; 15:83–7.

4. Kanner AM. Depression in epilepsy: prevalence, clinical semiology, pathogenic mechanisms, and treatment. *Biol Psychiatry* 2003; 54:388–98.

5. Prueter C and Norra C. Mood disorders and their treatment in patients with epilepsy. *J Neuropsychiatry Clin Neurosci* 2005; 17(1):20–8.

6. Kanner AM, Trimble M and Schmitz B. Postictal affective episodes. *Epilepsy Behav* 2010; 19(2):156–8.

7. Kanner AM, Soto A and Gross-Kanner H. Prevalence and clinical characteristics of

postictal psychiatric symptoms in partial epilepsy. *Neurology* 2004; 62:708–13.

8. Schmitz B. Depression and mania in patients with epilepsy. *Epilepsia* 2005; 46 (Suppl 4):45–9.

9. Turner K, Piazzini A, Franza A, et al. Postpartum depression in women with epilepsy versus women without epilepsy. *Epilepsy Behav* 2006; 9:293–7.

10. Turner K, Piazzini A, Franza A, et al. Epilepsy and postpartum depression. *Epilepsia* 2009; 50(Suppl 1):24–7.

11. Galanti M, Newport DJ, Pennell PB, et al. Postpartum depression in women with epilepsy: influence of antiepileptic drugs in a prospective study. *Epilepsy Behav* 2009; 16:426–30.

12. Lam RW, Kennedy SH, Grigoriadis S, et al. Canadian network for mood and anxiety treatments (CANMAT) clinical guidelines for the management of depressive disorder in adults. III Pharmacotherapy. *J Affect Disord* 2009; 117:S26–S43.

13. Maguire J and Mody I. Steroid hormone fluctuations and GABA$_A$R plasticity. *Psychoneuroendocrinology* 2009; 34S:S84–S90.

14. Pinkerton JV, Guico-Pabia CJ and Taylor HS. Menstrual cycle-related exacerbation of disease. *Am J Obstet Gynecol* 2010; 202 (3):221–31.

15. Jackson MJ and Turkington D. Depression and anxiety in epilepsy. *J Neurol Neurosurg Psychiatry* 2012; 76(Suppl I):i45–7.

16. Lau C, Ettinger EB and Hamberger S. Do mood instability symptoms in epilepsy represent formal bipolar disorder? *Epilepsia* 2012; 53(2):e37–42.

17. Trimble M, Kanner AB and Schmitz B. Postictal psychosis. *Epilepsy Behav* 2010; 19:159–61.

18. Nadkarni S, Arnedo V and Devinsky O. Psychosis in epilepsy patients. *Epilepsia* 2007; 48(Suppl 9):17–9.

19. Hećimović H, Salpekar J, Kanner AM, et al. Suicidality and epilepsy: a neuropsychological perspective. *Epilepsy Behav* 2011; 22:77–84.

20. Jones JE, Hermann BP, Barry JJ, et al. Rates and risk factors for suicide, suicidal ideation, and suicide attempts in chronic epilepsy. *Epilepsy Behav* 2003; 4:S31–S38.

21. Kanner AM. Depression and epilepsy: a review of multiple facets of their close relation. *Neurol Clin* 2009; 27:865–80.

22. Arana A, Wentworth CE and Ayuso-Mateos JL. Suicide-related events in patients treated with antiepileptic drugs. *Eng J Med* 2010; 363:542–51.

23. Bagary M. Epilepsy, antiepileptic drugs and suicidality. *Curr Opin Neurol* 2011; 24:177–82.

24. Mula M, Hesdorffer DC. Suicidal behavior and antiepileptic drugs in epilepsy: analysis of the emerging evidence. *Drug Healthc Patient Saf* 2011; 3:15–20.

25. Reuber M. Psychogenic nonepileptic seizures: answers and questions. *Epilepsy Behav* 2008; 12(4):622–35.

26. Kaufman KR. Antiepileptic drugs in the treatment of psychiatric disorders. *Epilepsy Behav* 2011; 21:1–11.

27. Galbally M, Roberts M and Buist A. Mood stabilizers in pregnancy: a systematic review. *Aust N Ze J Psychiatry* 2010; 44: 967–77.

28. Spina E and Perucca E. Clinial significance of pharmacokinetic interactions between antiepileptic and psychotropic durgs. *Epilepsia* 2002; 43(Suppl 2):37–44.

29. Whitworth AB and Fleischhacker WW. Adverse effects of antipsychotic drugs. *Int Clin Psychopharmacol* 1995; 9(Suppl 5):21–7.

30. Toth P and Frankenburg FR. Clozapine and seizures: a review. *Can J Psychiatry* 1994; 39:236.

31. Adachi N, Kanemoto K, de Toffol B, et al. Basic treatment principles for psychotic disorders in patients with epilepsy. *Epilepsia* 2013; 54 (Suppl 1):19–33.

32. Landolt H. Some clinical EEG correlations in epileptic psychoses (twilight states). *EEG Clin Neurophysiol* 1953; 5:121.

33. Mula M and Sander JW. Suicidal ideation in epilepsy and levetiracetam therapy. *Epilepsy Behav* 2007; 11:130–2.

Chapter 3

Sleep-related comorbidities in women with epilepsy

Carin Dove and Brian J. Murray

Key points:

- Seizures can aggravate sleep quality, and poor quality sleep can aggravate seizure disorders
- Antiepileptic medications can alter sleep architecture, and aggravate daytime sleepiness; timing of therapy can have significant effects on this profile
- Hormonal, reproductive, and life cycle events alter sleep and consequently have effects on sleep disorders that may be present in women
- Sleep disorders such as insufficient sleep, sleep disordered breathing, and restless legs syndrome are common in women
- Simple sleep interventions can often have significant impact on seizure management and quality of life for women

Introduction

The interactions between sleep and epilepsy are numerous, yet much remains to be elucidated. Comparatively, little is known about the combination of epilepsy, sleep, sleep disorders, and women's health. Therefore much has to be extrapolated from work that has been done about sleep disorders in women and sleep disorders in epilepsy.

There is a bidirectional influence of sleep and epilepsy on one another. Sleep itself, as well as sleep deprivation and fragmentation, has an effect on electrographic features, seizures, cognitive function, and quality of life in patients with epilepsy. Sleep disorders can exacerbate a person's seizures. Some seizure types seem to be potentiated in certain stages of sleep and wakefulness. Common perception is that the relationship between seizures and sleep is governed by sleep state itself; though time-of-day or circadian factors are also important. Both interictal discharges and seizures during sleep can disrupt sleep and decrease its restorative effect. Good seizure control, therefore, is of importance in promoting good sleep. One must also be cognizant of the effect of antiepileptic drugs (AEDs) on sleep architecture and daytime function. *In this chapter, ictal descriptive terminology and epilepsy classification are based on the classification scheme of the International League Against Epilepsy (ILAE) published in Epilepsia in 2010* [1, 2].

Women with Epilepsy, ed. Esther Bui and Autumn Klein. Published by Cambridge University Press.
© Cambridge University Press 2014.

Sleep stages

Sleep can be defined as a state of reversible alteration in the state of consciousness characterized by decreased responsiveness to the external environment, reduction in movement, typical posture, and eye closure. The sleep state is associated with predictable changes in physiology. Some of these include alterations in autonomic and endocrine functions, decreases in muscle tone, and characteristic electroencephalographic (EEG) changes. Sleep is actively regulated by neural processes, and in humans it occurs in a circadian pattern.

Sleep is not homogenous. It is characterized by two basic states: non-REM (NREM) sleep and rapid eye movement (REM) sleep. The EEG shows evidence of progressively more synchronized activity during NREM sleep, with increased slowing and increased amplitudes as sleep progresses [3]. NREM is further subdivided into stages N1, N2, and N3, according to the 2007 American Academy of Sleep Medicine manual which is in common usage now in sleep medicine [4]. This replaces the historical Rechtschaffen and Kales (R&K) sleep scoring rules [5]. Stage N1 represents light transitional sleep and is characterized by replacement of alpha in the posterior dominant rhythm by low-amplitude, mixed-frequency theta, as well as slow roving eye movements and vertex waves. Note that electroencephalographers traditionally consider slowing of the posterior dominant rhythm, diffuse theta activity, and slow roving eye movements as drowsiness, while the onset of sleep is defined by the appearance of vertex sharp waves [6]. Stage N2 represents consolidated sleep and is characterized by sleep spindles and K-complexes on the EEG. Stage N3 is fundamentally a homeostatic restorative component of sleep and is synonymous with slow-wave, delta, or deep sleep. Stage N3 incorporates both stage 3 and stage 4 sleep from the R&K rules, and is now defined as greater than 20% of the 30-second sample being comprised of generalized 0.5–2Hz, high-amplitude waves. REM sleep, also known as stage R, is characterized by a desynchronized EEG pattern with low-amplitude, mixed frequencies, as well as rapid eye movements and skeletal muscle atonia.

Physiologic mechanisms of sleep and epilepsy

Theoretical mechanisms that have been proposed to explain the interaction between sleep and epilepsy can be divided into the following categories: (1) shared neuronal circuits, (2) hypersynchronization, (3) hyperexcitability, (4) failure of normal inhibitory mechanisms, and (5) chemical mediators [3, 8].

The most well-known example of a shared neuronal substrate for sleep and epilepsy is the thalamic reticular neurons [8]. These gamma-aminobutyric acid or GABAergic neurons inhibit the thalamocortical neurons in the dorsal thalamus, which have glutamatergic projections to the cortex. Through the intrinsic oscillatory properties of the reticular neurons, sleep spindles are generated. However, if GABA-A-receptor-mediated inhibition is reduced, 3Hz spike-and-wave discharges characteristic of absence seizures can be produced.

As sleep progressively deepens, more sleep spindles and delta waves are seen on the EEG, reflecting synchronization activity as a feature of NREM sleep. Delta waves are mediated by a combination of the thalamocortical circuits described above and the cortex itself. Hypersynchronization is also a key feature of epilepsy. NREM synchronization can create an opportunity for an already hyperexcitable cortex to produce epileptic activity.

Cortical hyperexcitability is likely mediated by genetic factors and/or by acquired, often injury-related, mechanisms. Sleep arousals and microarousals may also increase cortical hyperexcitability, consistent with the observation that many seizures occur in this context. Malow and colleagues using depth electrodes demonstrated that seizures often precede (and therefore may cause) an arousal [3]. In addition, sleep deprivation enhances cortical hyperexcitability. For example, Scalise and colleagues used transmagnetic stimulation to demonstrate a reduction of intracortical inhibition after total sleep deprivation in seven normal subjects [12].

Failure of normal inhibitory mechanisms likely allows the propagation of seizure activity and may even result in status epilepticus. Inhibitory mechanisms are less effective during NREM sleep. In contrast, REM sleep is characterized by inhibition of thalamocortical synchronization and a reduction in interhemispheric impulses across the corpus callosum resulting in an anticonvulsant effect, with an overall reduction in interictal discharges and seizures [8].

Alterations in chemical mediators including neurotransmitters and neuropeptides in various sleep states are also important. Neurotransmitters and hormones change dramatically based on stage of normal sleep and circadian patterns. As such, this may influence cortical excitability.

Interactions between sleep and epilepsy
Sleep-wake timing of epileptic events

Clinical observations that there is a relationship between sleep and epilepsy date back to antiquity [7]. Over the last 100 years, investigators have looked at the sleep-wake timing of seizures in institutionalized patients and outpatients, and distinguished three general groups: those in whom seizures occurred mainly during sleep ("sleep epilepsies"), mainly during transition into wakefulness ("awakening" epilepsies), and both during wakefulness and sleep ("diffuse epilepsies") [8]. Both Gower and Janz noted an increased seizure frequency at sleep onset and at the end of sleep. Janz noted further differences in the seizure characteristics of these groups, namely, that the awakening epilepsies were usually primary generalized with onset in childhood, for example, absence seizures, juvenile myoclonic epilepsy, and generalized tonic-clonic seizure on awakening. Those with sleep epilepsies were more likely focal epilepsies with an idiopathic or symptomatic etiology and onset in adolescence or early adulthood, like nocturnal frontal lobe epilepsy and its autosomal dominant variant, benign epilepsy of childhood with centrotemporal spikes with or without occipital paroxysms, and continuous spike-and-wave discharges during slow-wave sleep. Lastly, those with diffuse epilepsies were most likely to be symptomatic cases and typically had poorer prognosis.

The following epilepsy syndromes are significantly associated with sleep: nocturnal frontal lobe epilepsy and autosomal dominant frontal lobe epilepsy (ADFLE), nocturnal temporal lobe epilepsy, benign childhood epilepsy with centrotemporal spikes (BECTS), Lennox–Gastaut syndrome (LGS) with nocturnal tonic seizures, and epileptic encephalopathy with continuous spike-and-wave discharges during sleep (CSWS) [9]. In terms of focal seizures, frontal lobe seizures are much more likely than temporal lobe seizures to occur during sleep. Temporal lobe seizures are more likely to secondarily generalize when they occur during sleep than during wakefulness.

Sudden unexpected death in epilepsy (SUDEP) is more likely to occur during sleep [10]. Other precipitating factors of SUDEP related to sleep should be considered, including worsening of autonomic dysfunction by comorbid obstructive sleep apnea (OSA), periodic limb movements of sleep (PLMS), sympathetic overstimulation during sleep after abrupt withdrawal of AEDs, and postictal central apnea and neurogenic pulmonary edema. Note that pregnant women may be uniquely tempted to discontinue their AEDs due to concerns about teratogenicity.

Sleep influences on interictal discharges

Further evidence for the interaction between sleep and epilepsy comes from the effect of sleep and sleep deprivation on the EEG. Most epileptic patients show increased interictal activity during sleep.

Generally, NREM sleep activates interictal epileptiform discharges [3], both in number and in spatial extent, while REM sleep inhibits interictal discharges. Discharges are more prominent during the first part of the night when NREM sleep is more abundant and consolidated. Discharges may be activated during NREM sleep in the late part of the night, possibly due to an increased number of sleep-stage shifts or due to reduced levels of anti-seizure medication.

For patients with primary generalized tonic-clonic seizures, the interictal discharges are most prominent during stages N1 and N2. For absence epilepsy, sleep activates the typical 3Hz spike-wave discharge. In partial onset seizures, interictal discharges are also activated during NREM sleep, but they also become more widespread. For temporal lobe epilepsy, interictal discharges when identified in REM sleep have a higher localizing value in temporal lobe epilepsy [28].

In a high percentage of patients with nocturnal epilepsies, the daytime EEG remains normal, emphasizing the importance of obtaining a sleep-deprived EEG with sleep if a routine EEG during wakefulness is normal and clinical suspicion of epilepsy persists. Sleep deprivation increases interictal discharges and seizures beyond the effect of sleep alone, but the exact mechanisms remain elusive. A sleep-deprived EEG increases the diagnostic yield when a diagnosis of epilepsy is considered [11].

Effect of seizures on sleep

It is well recognized that seizures produce postictal somnolence. However, they also cause sleep disruption by altering sleep-wake mechanisms. Seizures have been found to increase sleep fragmentation, sleep-stage shifts, and wakefulness after sleep onset. Other parameters may also be affected, including a decrease in sleep efficiency and in total sleep time. Otherwise, a reduction of REM sleep has been found in patients with primary or secondary generalized seizures and in those with nocturnal complex partial seizures. The severity of the seizure disorder usually correlates well with the severity of the sleep deficit. Nocturnal seizures have been associated with next day somnolence.

Conversely, improved seizure control with pharmacological or non-pharmacological treatment likely improves sleep parameters. Although detailed data are still lacking, it is thought that interictal discharges can cause repeated arousals and sleep fragmentation, resulting in excessive daytime sleepiness. Adequate treatment with AEDs can decrease the frequency of these discharges and potentially improve sleep quality. Surgical treatment of epilepsy that results in improved seizure control has been shown to improve sleep quality and excessive daytime sleepiness. The vagal nerve stimulator has been used for the treatment of refractory epilepsy, and is sometimes successful in treating the seizures and may help with daytime alertness. Unfortunately, in some patients it has caused sleep-disordered breathing, and patients should be monitored for this possible complication [20].

Effect of antiepileptic drugs on sleep

The exact effect of an individual AED on sleep can be difficult to determine. For a number of AEDs, the exact mechanisms of action are only partially understood [21]. In general, most AEDs are sedating. This is more notable with the barbiturates and benzodiazepines, but can also be seen with phenytoin, carbamazepine, gabapentin, and others. The newer AEDs can also cause sedation, though this is less frequently observed. Withdrawal of sedating AEDs may also lead to insomnia. Sedating AEDs, especially benzodiazepines and barbiturates, have to be used with care in patients with untreated obstructive sleep apnea, as it can worsen the problem. Some medications, such as topiramate, can assist sleep apnea by associated weight loss and are even theoretically beneficial in central sleep apnea given their carbonic anhydrase inhibition.

Hormonal influences on sleep

Women sleep differently than men. They spend more time in bed, sleep longer, have poorer subjective sleep quality, have less wakefulness after sleep onset, less light sleep and more slow-wave sleep, and are at higher risk of insomnia and restless legs syndrome after the onset of puberty [22]. Human studies of hormonal effects on women's sleep are scarce, partly due to significant barriers to study design [23].

Prenatal gonadal hormones alter brain development, with effects on receptor expression and neuronal networks that ultimately result in a phenotypically male or female brain. Recent animal data have suggested that sex-dependent differences in sleep are mediated by both hormone-dependent and hormone-independent mechanisms, and that the effects of sex steroids on sleep are gender-specific.

Estrogen

Reproductive hormones have neuroactive functions which are mediated through intracellular steroid receptors [24]. Many different cellular functions may be modulated, from neuronal excitability to neuroplasticity, and is discussed in greater detail in Chapter 4.

Estrogen seems to have a mainly neuroexcitatory role via inhibition of GABA and potentiation of glutamatergic conductance. Estrogen receptors are widely distributed throughout the brain, including several areas known to have a role in sleep-wake regulation, such as the prefrontal cortex, preoptic hypothalamus, locus ceruleus, paraventricular nucleus, lateral tegmentum of the pons, and the dorsal raphe nucleus. Estrogen also has effects on sleep architecture, mainly in decreasing REM sleep quantity.

Several lines of evidence are reviewed by Mong that suggest estradiol modulates adenosine and prostaglandin, known somnogens, at the level of the ventrolateral preoptic hypothalamus [22]. It may help to consolidate wakefulness, and thereby improve sleep, which is one of several possible mechanisms for the improvements in sleep quality in women taking hormone replacement therapy. Estradiol probably also plays a role in sleep-wake regulation via its effects on the suprachiasmatic nucleus (SCN). The SCN is the "master clock" that regulates all circadian aspects of physiology and behavior.

At a basic physiological level, estrogen also contributes to nasal congestion and airway edema, particularly during pregnancy, by increasing blood flow to the nose and upper airway and can precipitate frank obstructive apnea which can further affect sleep.

Progesterone

Progesterone exerts a mainly neuroinhibitory effect in the brain by promoting GABA and inhibiting glutamatergic conductance. It has anxiolytic and anticonvulsant properties, but in excess may cause sedation and depression. Many brain areas have progesterone receptors, and there is significant overlap with the estrogen receptors.

Progesterone increases non-REM sleep, possibly through an interaction between progesterone metabolites and GABA-A receptors which are found in the thalamocortical circuits. It is a potent respiratory stimulant and therefore can improve ventilation during sleep [25]. It also increases tone in the genioglossus muscle, a key upper airway dilator, which may reduce upper airway collapsibility during sleep. In menstruating women, the lowest rate of sleep-related respiratory events is seen during the luteal phase, when progesterone levels are highest. Theoretically, this means that obstructive sleep apnea can be falsely ruled out by a polysomnogram done at this point in the menstrual cycle. Postmenopausally, when progesterone levels are low, women are at increased risk of OSA. The withdrawal of progesterone, which may be as neuroactively potent as a sleeping medication, can lead to rebound insomnia perimenstrually.

Testosterone

Testosterone has been shown to affect sleep in men, and it may also play a role in sleep in women, specifically, in mediating menopausal sleep complaints and obstructive sleep apnea. However, studies of the effects of testosterone on women's sleep are rare, and this remains a complicated area because of conflicting results.

Support for the role of testosterone in mediating sleep in women comes from the effects on sleep-disordered breathing. Testosterone is known to down-regulate estrogen and progesterone receptors, which may weaken the progesterone respiratory stimulant effect. This becomes relevant in polycystic ovarian syndrome, which is associated with endogenous overproduction of testosterone and a higher apnea–hypopnea index (AHI), although insulin resistance may also play a role in the significantly increased prevalence of OSA in this population. Testosterone has been shown to alter respiratory functions in women during wakefulness, and may contribute to the increased risk of OSA in menopause [26].

The menstrual cycle and sleep

Subjective changes in sleep quality, as well as hypersomnia or insomnia at the time of menses or a few days before, are not uncommonly reported by women, but prospective studies have not been consistent. Women attribute sleep disruption during menses to physical discomforts such as cramps, bloating, breast tenderness, and headaches. However, consistent objective polysomnography (PSG) evidence of sleep disruption is lacking, despite documented differences in sleep architecture between the follicular and luteal phases.

Women with more severe dysmenorrhea are more likely to report sleep-related symptoms, including poor sleep quality. Baker et al. demonstrated PSG evidence of disrupted sleep with decreased sleep efficiency, increased wakefulness and stage N1 sleep in dysmenorrheic women during menses when compared to their own baseline [16].

Modest effects of oral contraceptive medications on sleep have been reported, including increased temperature, increased melatonin levels, less stage N3 sleep, as well as a reduced REM latency. These studies are limited by the heterogeneity of oral contraceptive preparations [16].

Certain sleep disorders have been noted to have a catamenial pattern. In the revised International Classification of Sleep Disorders (ICSD), menstrual-related hypersomnia and menopausal insomnia are considered [27]. Menstrual-related hypersomnia may be more common in the few months following menarche. Hormonal contraceptives may also have a role in managing these conditions.

Upper airway resistance is usually more severe during the follicular phase, and theoretically a diagnosis of sleep-disordered breathing can be missed if the PSG is performed during the luteal phase. The menstrual variability in the severity of sleep apnea may even necessitate varying the pressure of continuous positive airway pressure (CPAP) according to the patient's menstrual cycle.

Common sleep comorbidities in women with epilepsy

Epidemiology

Among both men and women, patients with neurological disorders, as well as patients with epilepsy, are more likely to self-report sleep disturbances than healthy people. Sleep architecture is frequently disrupted in patients with epilepsy. Epilepsy itself impairs quality of life, and comorbid sleep disturbances compound this effect [14]. Factors that are associated with sleep disturbances in this population include use of first generation AEDs and poor seizure control. Common complaints in patients with epilepsy are excessive daytime sleepiness (EDS), insomnia, and nocturnal behaviors. Women probably accumulate a sleep debt more quickly than men and take longer to recover from it [22]. However, they are also more likely to have sleep-state misperception, which manifests as believing they have less sleep or poorer quality sleep than what is objectively seen on PSG.

Excessive daytime sleepiness

In general, sleep deprivation is the most common cause of excessive daytime sleepiness [13]. Much of this sleep deprivation is voluntary and there is limited data on gender differences in EDS. Most adults require approximately 8 hours of sleep, but many adults, including patients with epilepsy, routinely sleep less than this. A heightened time of sleep deprivation is in the postpartum period, attributed to the care of a newborn. Education about adequate sleep time and good sleep hygiene is the first step in correcting this problem and avoiding a common trigger for seizures.

Other causes of excessive daytime sleepiness in patients with epilepsy include seizures, frequent epileptiform discharges on EEG, comorbid sleep disorders, and the effect of AEDs. A particularly common comorbid sleep disorder in patients with epilepsy is OSA. However, other primary sleep disorders like central sleep apnea, PLMS, and restless legs syndrome (RLS) are also often encountered. AEDs are notorious for causing sedation.

The effects of sleep deprivation go beyond sleepiness to affect quality of life, cognitive and neurobehavioral functions in normal individuals [14]. For example, a full night of sleep deprivation has been shown to result in cognitive impairment comparable to being legally intoxicated with alcohol [15]. Anxiety and depression are common in people with epilepsy [14] and this may reflect the high prevalence of sleep problems. Sleep loss is a significant contributor to the psychosocial comorbidity of epilepsy.

Insomnia

Insomnia has a prevalence of up to 50% on questionnaire-based studies among people with epilepsy, correlating with seizure frequency [14]. Malow found approximately 10% of those with refractory epilepsy have significant PLMS [7]. Diagnosis and treatment of the underlying disorders frequently improves sleep-related complaints, quality of life, and seizure frequency [7].

Insomnia is more common in women than in men across the lifespan independent of other factors. Insomnia can be divided into two basic types: sleep onset and sleep maintenance insomnia. Sleep onset and sleep maintenance insomnia often co-occur in the same individual, but it is a useful distinction for planning treatment strategies. It is particularly important to rule out restless legs syndrome in patients with sleep initiation difficulties and sleep-disordered breathing in those with sleep maintenance problems. After secondary causes of insomnia have been ruled out, including other primary sleep disorders that may require specific treatments and medication side effects, therapeutic options can be considered. Non-pharmacologic strategies are usually the mainstay of treatment, because of better long-term efficacy and none of the potential complications associated with medications. The role of pharmacotherapy is best reserved for the treatment of acute insomnia or as an adjunct to non-pharmacologic treatments. If a sedating antiepileptic medication is to be used, it should be used at night to help with sleep initiation.

All patients can be educated about good sleep hygiene. Patients are counseled on the importance of maintaining a regular sleep-wake schedule, minimizing caffeine and alcohol intake, avoiding caffeine, nicotine, bright light, and excessive fluid intake in the evenings, and ensuring the bedroom environment is conducive to sleep (quiet, cool, and dark). In certain scenarios, effective behavioral therapies include sleep restriction and stimulus control therapy. Sleep restriction and stimulus control are both based on the principles of classical conditioning. In general terms, sleep restriction eliminates naps and limits time in bed, and targets feeling sleepy as the signal to go to bed. Stimulus control is summarized by the statement "the bed is for sleep (and sex) only." Other behavioral interventions include relaxation techniques, meditation, hypnosis, and biofeedback.

In general, most, if not all, of the nonspecific prescription medications used in the treatment of insomnia are associated with some degree of tolerance over time. Psychological dependence is not uncommon with chronic daily use. Rebound insomnia can be managed by avoiding abrupt withdrawal of the medication and weaning one medication at a time at a very slow rate. This is especially important in the elderly in whom sedating medications are associated with an increased risk of falls. Off-label use of antidepressants for insomnia is common in clinical practice. This may be particularly helpful in patients with epilepsy where comorbid depression may be more frequent.

Sleep-disordered breathing (SDB)

Sleep-disordered breathing is a collective term which includes OSA, but also upper airway resistance syndrome, central apnea, and obesity-hypoventilation syndrome [16]. In the general population, this condition affects at least 4% of men and 2% of women. Malow found nearly one-third of patients with medically refractory epilepsy had sleep-disordered breathing on polysomnographic evaluation. This is associated with significant morbidity because it is an independent risk factor for hypertension and stroke amongst other complications [17].

OSA is caused by upper airway obstruction during sleep. This results in inadequate ventilation and relative hypercapnia and hypoxemia, which can rouse the patient from sleep in order to restore ventilation. Symptoms suggestive of the diagnosis include loud snoring, witnessed choking, gasping, frank apnea, morning headaches, unrefreshing sleep, and daytime sleepiness or fatigue. Risk factors for OSA include obesity, especially central adiposity, enlarged neck circumference (>16 inches in a woman, >17 inches in a man), and genetic and anatomical reasons for upper airway narrowing. PSG is used to diagnose OSA and to distinguish it from other sleep and sleep-breathing disorders.

Sleep, epilepsy, and breathing are interrelated, and the mechanisms by which OSA increases seizure frequency are outlined by Chokroverty and Montagna [8]. It is important to note that AEDs can worsen OSA. For example, valproate, vigabatrin, and gabapentin promote weight gain, which is a well-known risk factor for sleep apnea. Similarly, benzodiazepines and barbiturates can also be problematic because they cause decreased sensitivity to carbon dioxide and therefore oxygen desaturation, as well as relaxation of the upper airway musculature.

Treatment with continuous positive airway pressure helps to reduce cardiovascular risk, and it has also been suggested in numerous studies to decrease seizure frequency and improve seizure control [8]. In cases of mild OSA, weight loss or avoiding the supine position may be sufficient management. Other alternatives include surgical correction of airway anatomy and use of a dental appliance to advance the tongue or mandible and improve airway patency.

The prevalence of OSA in women in the US population has been documented to be half that of men, though the continuum of sleep-disordered breathing may be much more common than realized, and is certainly more common in women with epilepsy. The gender gap narrows in postmenopausal women because of the increased prevalence in this population. Women with SBD report more nonspecific symptoms and more commonly complain of fatigue than men do. They are also less likely to snore, and are more likely to complain of insomnia rather than sleepiness. Upper airway resistance syndrome is a less overt form of OSA where the airflow limitations do not result in oxygen desaturation, but causes arousals and therefore sleep fragmentation and daytime sleepiness. Common therapies include weight loss, positional therapy, and in more severe cases, a dental appliance or CPAP.

Restless legs syndrome (RLS) and periodic limb movement disorder (PLMD)

RLS is a clinical diagnosis characterized by unpleasant leg sensations that occur at rest and are associated with a strong urge to move. These symptoms are worse towards the end of the day and are relieved with movement. RLS is more common in women than men, and particularly more frequent in relation to pregnancy, as discussed below. Most patients with RLS have movements of the legs during sleep, called periodic limb movements of sleep (PLMS). Secondary causes such as iron deficiency, B12 deficiency, or diabetic neuropathy should be sought and corrected. Iron deficiency is particularly common in women given menstruation and pregnancy. In the setting of iron deficiency, iron supplementation is an effective treatment. The morbidity associated with RLS can be tremendous. Studies have found a reduction in quality of life related to RLS on par with suffering from a chronic medical condition like diabetes or heart disease [18]. Restless legs syndrome is associated with sleep initiation difficulties, and can reduce total sleep time. As sleep deprivation aggravates epilepsy, this may have significant consequences.

Treatment with dopaminergic agonists such as pramipexole is usually effective, in much smaller doses than that used in Parkinson's disease. The medication is taken an hour before bedtime. Minimal effective doses should be used to avoid sedating side effects or impulse control problems. Another common therapeutic option is gabapentin or pregabalin, which are particularly good options in the context of epilepsy. Anecdotal reports also suggest carbamazepine may be helpful [19].

In periodic limb movement disorder (PLMD), patients do not experience unpleasant leg sensations but rather develop involuntary leg kicks during sleep with associated insomnia or daytime sleepiness. It is important to ensure that upper airway resistance is not present on the polysomnogram, as it can cause excessive daytime sleepiness and can mimic isolated limb movements if signs of airflow limitation are missed. Treating the patient's sleep-disordered breathing (e.g., CPAP for a patient with OSA or upper airway resistance) is usually the first step, followed by re-evaluation for PLMS if needed.

Pregnancy and sleep

Pregnancy results in multisystemic changes which can have an effect on sleep. Sleep disruption can be caused by nocturia, gastroesophageal reflux disease (GERD), musculo-skeletal changes, discomfort, and psychosocial stressors.

Women in the first trimester report increased fatigue and daytime sleepiness, and often, total sleep time increases, although some report the onset of insomnia. PSG may show a reduction in slow-wave sleep. These symptoms are usually due to hormonal effects on sleep, but unmasking of a pre-existing sleep disorder should also be considered.

In the second trimester, total sleep time normalizes, but nocturnal awakenings increase, probably due to the emergence of nocturia and GERD as well as aggravation of sleep-disordered breathing. During the third trimester, nocturnal awakenings, fatigue, leg cramps, and shortness of breath all increase and are associated with a reduction in total sleep time. Women often try to compensate by napping or going to bed earlier. Sleep architecture changes with increased stage N1 sleep (a marker of sleep disruption), and decreased REM sleep and decreased stage N3 sleep are often seen.

The postpartum period has significant challenges to sleep as well, particularly with nighttime infant care. The amount of sleep disruption a woman experiences can depend on method of feeding, support from a spouse or others, the infant's sleep pattern, parity, and co-sleeping. PSG studies have shown increased nocturnal awakenings, increased wake time after sleep onset, lower sleep efficiency, and shortened REM latency [18]. However, hormo-nal and mood changes probably also play a role in sleep deprivation postpartum. For example, even in the absence of infant care postpartum, sleep does not return to pre-pregnancy baseline. Others have reported that a number of the nocturnal awakenings are not related to care of the infant. Many sleep medications are to be avoided in the context of pregnancy, and details are beyond the scope of this chapter.

Sleep-disordered breathing (SDB)

Pregnant women are at increased risk of developing SDB, especially in the third trimester. Increased levels of estrogen and progesterone cause airway edema and nasal congestion, which probably accounts for the progressively increasing risk of snoring over the course of pregnancy. Weight gain and reduced diaphragmatic excursion may also contribute.

Women who are hypertensive at the time of birth are more likely to be snorers. Snoring causes sleep fragmentation and may contribute to symptoms of daytime sleepiness. The mechanism for elevated blood pressure may be due to autonomic activation associated with the arousals from sleep-related respiratory events, preventing the normal circadian decrease in blood pressure overnight. Treatment of upper airway resistance syndrome and snoring with CPAP in women with pre-eclampsia can significantly reduce blood pressure.

Overt OSA is uncommon during pregnancy, but it is associated with intrauterine growth retardation and lower Apgar scores [18]. CPAP is the appropriate treatment for OSA and is considered safe in pregnancy.

Restless legs syndrome (RLS) and periodic limb movements in sleep (PLMS)

RLS occurs in 20–25% of otherwise healthy pregnant women. Iron deficiency can cause or aggravate RLS. Young women are often iron deficient and, in pregnancy, volume expansion and hematopoiesis increases iron requirements. Multivitamins that are routinely recommended in pregnancy often contain inadequate amounts of replacement iron, and additional supplementation is appropriate for symptomatic women or women who have had RLS in previous pregnancies. Ferritin levels and other iron indices are usually measured. Iron is the rate-limiting step in the synthesis of dopamine in the brain, and in non-pregnant populations, dopamine agonists can effectively treat RLS. Dopamine circuits in the brain have also been implicated in mood disorders, suggesting that there may be a relationship between iron loss, RLS, and peripartum mood disorders [18].

PLMS are often associated with restless legs syndrome, and these also increase in pregnancy. Both RLS and PLMS can cause sleep disruption, with RLS usually resulting in sleep onset insomnia. Nocturnal leg cramps should raise suspicion for PLMS, because these may represent the culmination of a series of occult periodic limb movements [18].

Conservative measures for the treatment of RLS and PLMS include reducing caffeine and sleep loss, and are often used preferentially in pregnancy. Reducing aggravating agents such as antidepressants may be considered. Iron management may be particularly important. Intravenous iron infusions may be an option for particularly symptomatic individuals. Dopamine agonists are the mainstay of treatment in non-pregnant populations. Opioids should be used with caution and are usually reserved for disabling refractory cases.

Menopause and sleep

Sleep complaints in the perimenopausal period are common and are present in up to half of women. Menopausal symptoms, particularly psychological changes and vasomotor symptoms like hot flashes and night sweats contribute to subjective sleep difficulties.

Sleep patterns are known to change with normal aging, and older people tend to awaken earlier and nap more frequently. Independent of this, it has been suggested that menopause may have an effect on melatonin, thereby advancing the circadian phase and leading to early morning awakenings. Many medical conditions and their treatments can have adverse effects on sleep and these become more common with age. Certain sleep disorders like OSA and restless legs syndrome increase with age.

Sleep-disordered breathing (SDB)

The risk of SDB increases about 4-fold at the time of menopause, independent of age and body mass index, for hormonal reasons related to progesterone and testosterone that have already been described [16]. It is important to note that OSA in older age can cause a syndrome of mild cognitive dysfunction, and in some cases people meet criteria for a dementia. Cognitive dysfunction due to OSA can sometimes be reversed with CPAP therapy. The OSA-associated risk of hypertension and stroke may further complicate comorbidities in older patients. The treatment for OSA in menopausal woman is the same as elsewhere, except there might be an expanded role for hormonal therapy in selected circumstances.

Insomnia

Although the relationship between menopause and insomnia continues to be debated, menopausal insomnia is considered in the revised ICSD [27]. It affects up to 60% of women. A possible mechanism for menopause-related insomnia is dysregulation of the GABA-A receptor due to fluctuations and decline in estrogen and progesterone levels [26].

OSA must be considered in the differential diagnosis of a perimenopausal woman complaining of insomnia, because of increased prevalence and atypical presentation with insomnia in this population. Restless legs syndrome is also more common with advancing age.

Non-HRT prescription medications such as fluoxetine, paroxetine, venlafaxine, and gabapentin have been reported to alleviate perimenopausal symptoms.

Hormone replacement therapy (HRT)

Estrogen hormone replacement therapy and combination hormone replacement therapy with estrogen and progesterone both have some efficacy in treating perimenopausal symptoms, and concomitant subjective sleep complaints usually also improve [16, 26]. HRT also seems to have a modest effect in the treatment of OSA: the Sleep Heart Health study showed that the prevalence of OSA and SBD in women receiving HRT was found to be half that of women not taking HRT. Again, the possible mechanism is progesterone-related respiratory stimulation and upper airway dilatation.

Importantly however, the Women's Health Initiative (WHI) trial showed harm with HRT. This randomized, placebo-controlled trial found an increased risk of vascular disease and cancer in woman taking conjugated equine estrogens with medroxyprogesterone [29, 30]. The study has been criticized for not including women with severe menopausal symptoms, who would have been expected to derive the most benefit.

Currently, most physicians look for alternatives to HRT for the treatment of menopausal insomnia. HRT may still have a role in the short-term treatment of women with severe menopausal symptoms, and in these circumstances benefit to short-term quality of life must be weighed against the risk of potential long-term harm. For some women the improvement in quality of life with HRT is dramatic. Estrogen is thought to mediate the harmful effects, and therefore the lowest effective dose of estrogen should be used, and HRT should be frequently reassessed to facilitate discontinuation when appropriate.

Approach to the woman with epilepsy and sleep complaints

Sleep complaints in women with epilepsy can be divided into three major categories: sleep during wake time (insomnia), wake during sleep time (hypersomnia), or unusual behaviors in sleep (parasomnia). The differential diagnoses for insomnias, hypersomnias, and even parasomnias share many overlapping etiologies. Table 3.1 outlines common primary sleep disorders with major examples, as well as hormonal and epilepsy factors that may influence diagnosis and management.

It is important to note that sleep disruption can lead to cognitive impairments, and drowsiness is of major concern in patients who need to maintain alertness for safety reasons such as driving. Treatment of the underlying sleep disorder may improve cognitive function

Table 3.1: A conceptual checklist for sleep-related comorbidities in women with epilepsy

International Classification of Sleep Disorders – 2	Category	Example
A – Major Sleep Disorders	Insomnia	Psychophysiological insomnia (conditioned insomnia)
	Sleep-related breathing disorders	Sleep apnea
	Hypersomnias	Behaviorally induced insufficient sleep syndrome
	Circadian rhythm disorders	Shift work sleep disorder
	Parasomnias	Sleep walking
	Sleep-related movement disorders	Restless legs syndrome
	Other sleep disorders	Environmental sleep disorder (e.g., noise)
B – Major Modifying Factors	Epilepsy syndrome	Juvenile myoclonic epilepsy and morning seizures
	Neurological or medical disorders	Associated brain lesions may affect sleep-wake machinery
	Medication and substance use	Benzodiazepines reduce slow-wave sleep
	Timing of medications	Sedating medications should be given before sleep
	Menstrual stage	Luteal phase hypersomnia
	Pregnancy stage	Increased restless legs associated with iron deficiency
	Menopause	Increase in sleep apnea
	Safety considerations	Driving

and quality of life. The treatment of sleep apnea, restless legs syndrome, and insomnia has been outlined above. Circadian rhythm disorder treatment modalities include behavioral management and phototherapy. Treatment of excessive daytime sleepiness depends largely on the underlying diagnosis. Non-pharmacological strategies that were outlined in a previous section for the treatment of insomnia can be applied here as well. Regularly scheduled naps can be helpful, and should be accommodated by employers and schools. Pharmacologic treatments include wakefulness-promoting medications, e.g., modafinil, and stimulants, e.g., methylphenidate, though the stimulants are concerning for an aggravating effect on epilepsy. Optimization of seizure control can improve sleep while optimization of sleep can improve seizure control.

Indications for sleep medicine consultation and polysomnography

Referral to a sleep specialist and polysomnography may be considered in the following circumstances:

- When a primary sleep disorder is suspected, especially sleep-disordered breathing, e.g., a history of snoring and sleepiness or witnessed apneas, etc.
- When the patient exhibits profound sleeplessness or sleepiness (Epworth Sleepiness Scale).
- Where the nocturnal diagnosis is in question: distinguishing seizures and parasomnias particularly with complex, or bizarre, nocturnal cases.
- When treatment options are limited due to comorbidities.
- When seizures or sleep symptoms are refractory to treatment.
- When safety concerns are present regarding nocturnal behaviors or alertness for driving.

If there is significant daytime sleepiness, daytime testing may be necessary in the form of multiple sleep latency test and the maintenance of wakefulness test. A multiple sleep latency test is used for the diagnosis of narcolepsy. A maintenance of wakefulness test quantifies the patient's ability to stay awake while sitting quietly in a dimly lit room typically for 40 minutes at a time for four or five attempts.

Conclusion

Though minimal research has focused on sleep disorders in women with epilepsy, clinicians can extrapolate from what is currently known about sleep disorders in patients with epilepsy and sleep disorders in women. Sleep disorders in epilepsy are common, and the incidence and presentation of sleep disorders in women differs from men. Sleep disorders and epilepsy can each exacerbate the other, therefore optimal treatment of both aspects can be expected to produce the best outcome. Pregnancy is a particularly high-risk time for women with epilepsy, and correction of sleep disorders with a few simple interventions can improve the health of mother and baby. Menopause also has significant implications for sleep. Simple interventions often make dramatic differences to patients and their families – it may be as simple as changing the timing of antiseizure medication dosing or sleeping in the lateral decubitus position. Sleep disorders in women can be associated with significant morbidity and deterioration in quality of life and therefore warrants attention.

References

1. Blume WT, Luders HO, Mizrahi E, et al. Glossary of descriptive terminology for ictal semiology: report of the ILAE task force on classification and terminology. *Epilepsia* 2001; 42:1212–8.

2. Berg AT, Berkovic SF, Brodie MJ, et al. Revised terminology and concepts for organization of seizures and epilepsies: report of the ILAE Commission on Classification and Terminology, 2005–2009. *Epilepsia* 2010; 51:676–85.

3. Sinha SR. Basic mechanisms of sleep and epilepsy. *J Clin Neurophysiol* 2011; 28:103–10.

4. Iber C. American Academy of Sleep Medicine. *The AASM manual for the scoring of sleep and associated events: rules, terminology, and technical specifications.* Westchester, IL: American Academy of Sleep Medicine, 2007.

5. Rechtschaffen A and Kales A. *A manual of standarized terminology, techniques and scoring system for sleep stages in human subjects.* US Government Printing Office, 1968.

6. Libenson MH. Visual analysis of the EEG: wakefulness, drowsiness, and sleep. In: *Practical approach to electroencephalography.* Philadelphia, IL: Saunders Elsevier, 2010; 5–30.

7. Vaughn BV and D'Cruz OF. Sleep and epilepsy. In: Carney PR, Berry RB, Geyer JD, eds. *Clinical sleep disorders.* Philadelphia, IL: Ovid Technologies Inc., Lippincott Williams & Wilkins, 2005; 403–19.

8. Chokroverty S and Montagna P. Sleep and epilepsy. In: Chokroverty S, ed. *Sleep disorders medicine: basic science, technical considerations, and clinical aspects,* 3rd edn. Philadelphia, IL: Saunders Elsevier, 2009; 499–529.

9. Kothare SV and Zarowski M. Sleep and epilepsy: common bedfellows. *J Clin Neurophysiol* 2011; 28:101–2.

10. Nobili L, Proserpio P, Rubboli G, et al. Sudden unexpected death in epilepsy (SUDEP) and sleep. *Sleep Med Rev* 2011; 15:237–46.

11. Glick TH. The sleep-deprived electroencephalogram: evidence and practice. *Arch Neurol* 2002; 59:1235–9.

12. Scalise A, Desiato MT, Gigli GL, et al. Increasing cortical excitability: a possible explanation for the proconvulsant role of sleep deprivation. *Sleep* 2006; 29:1595–8.

13. Boulos MI and Murray BJ. Current evaluation and management of excessive daytime sleepiness. *Can J Neurol Sci* 2010; 37:167–76.

14. van Golde EG, Gutter T and de Weerd AW. Sleep disturbances in people with epilepsy: prevalence, impact and treatment. *Sleep Med Rev* 2011; 15:357–68.

15. Arnedt JT, Owens J, Crouch M, et al. Neurobehavioral performance of residents after heavy night call vs after alcohol ingestion. *JAMA* 2005; 294:1025–33.

16. Driver HS and Sloan EP. Women's Sleep. In: Chokroverty S, ed. *Sleep disorders medicine: basic science, technical considerations, and clinical aspects,* 3rd edn. Philadelphia, IL: Saunders Elsevier, 2009; 644–53.

17. Redline S, Yenokyan G, Gottlieb DJ, et al. Obstructive sleep apnea-hypopnea and incident stroke: the sleep heart health study. *Am J Respir Crit Care Med* 2010; 182:269–77.

18. Kohn M and Murray BJ. Sleep and quality of life in pregnancy. In: Verster JC, Pandi-Perumal SR, Streiner D, eds. *Sleep and quality of life in medical illnesses.* Totowa, NJ: Humana Press; 2008, 497–504.

19. Trenkwalder C, Hening WA, Montagna P, et al. Treatment of restless legs syndrome: an evidence-based review and implications for clinical practice. *Mov Disord* 2008; 23:2267–302.

20. Hsieh T, Chen M, McAfee A and Kifle Y. Sleep-related breathing disorder in children with vagal nerve stimulators. *Pediatr Neurol* 2008; 38:99–103.

21. Roux FJ and Kryger MH. Medication effects on sleep. *Clin Chest Med* 2010; 31:397–405.

22. Mong JA, Baker FC, Mahoney MM, et al. Sleep, rhythms, and the endocrine brain: influence of sex and gonadal hormones. *J Neurosci* 2011; 31:16107–16.

23. Andersen ML, Alvarenga TF, Mazaro-Costa R, et al. The association of testosterone, sleep, and sexual function in men and women. *Brain Res* 2011; 1416:80–104.

24. Herzog AG. Neuroactive properties of reproductive steroids. *Headache* 2007; 47 (Suppl 2):S68–S78.

25. Saaresranta T and Polo O. Hormones and breathing. *Chest* 2002; 122:2165–82.

26. Soares CN and Murray BJ. Sleep disorders in women: clinical evidence and treatment strategies. *Psychiatr Clin North Am* 2006; 29:1095–113; abstract xi.

27. American Academy of Sleep Medicine. *The international classification of sleep disorders: diagnostic and coding manual,* 2nd edn. Westchester, IL: American Academy of Sleep Medicine, 2005.

28. Sammaritano M, Gigli GL and Gotman J. Interictal spiking during wakefulness and sleep and the localization of foci in temporal lobe epilepsy. *Neurology* 1991; 41 (2(Pt 1)):290–7.

29. Manson JE, Hsia J, Johnson KC, et al. Estrogen plus progestin and the risk of coronary heart disease. *N Engl J Med* 2003; 349:523–34.

30. Chlebowski RT, Kuller LH, Prentice RL, et al. Breast cancer after use of estrogen plus progestin in postmenopausal women. *N Engl J Med* 2009; 360(6):573–87.

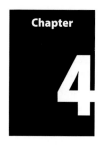

Chapter

4

Hormonal influences in women with epilepsy

Alberto Verrotti, Marianna Sebastiani, Alessandra Scaparrotta, and Carla Verrotti

Key points:

- Estrogen has primarily proconvulsant effects whereas progesterone has anticonvulsant effects
- Estrogen increases neuronal excitability via alterations in neurotransmitter function and structural changes in spine synapses, density, and shape
- Progesterone decreases neuronal excitability by modulating GABA-A receptors, reducing neuronal firing, suppressing kindling, and lessening epileptiform discharges
- Estrogen-to-progesterone ratio peaks during ovulation and menses resulting in potential seizure exacerbation, as can be seen in catamenial epilepsy
- Testosterone is thought to modulate seizure activity by its conversion to androstenediol (anticonvulsant) and estradiol (proconvulsant)

Introduction

Recognized since antiquity, the frequency and severity of epilepsy seems to be influenced by internal and environmental factors. At the end of the nineteenth century, various authors such as Sir Charles Locock and Gowers described the relationship between epileptic seizures and fluctuation in sex hormones, in particular during the menstrual cycle. Backstrom observed in seven patients that seizures appeared to be cyclical and were associated with changes in estrogen levels during ovulation [15]. Most studies found that seizure frequency increased close to the time of ovulation or menstrual flow. In the early 1950s, Laidlaw enrolled 50 patients with suspected menstrual-associated epilepsy and noted that 36 of them had an increase in monthly generalized tonic-clonic seizures, especially during the premenstrual, menstrual, and postmenstrual phases [35]. Both human and animal data suggest a strong influence of gonadal hormones on neuronal excitability. This influence of sexual hormones on the brain is noted to be strong to such an extent as to define a new type of epilepsy, called "catamenial epilepsy," deriving from the Greek word *katomenios* meaning "monthly." In fact, the main feature of this form of epilepsy is to cluster seizures around the time of menses or at other phases of the menstrual cycle [1]. For this reason, it is necessary to illustrate how steroid hormones and their metabolites can play a key role in the neuroendocrine control of neuronal excitability by biological effects.

Women with Epilepsy, ed. Esther Bui and Autumn Klein. Published by Cambridge University Press.
© Cambridge University Press 2014.

Influence of sexual hormones in the female brain

Sex hormones influence the brain from early development (organizational and nutritional effects) and modify its ongoing activity during adulthood (activational effects) [2]. The main female steroid hormones that affect brain function and its excitability are estrogen and progesterone. Moreover, due to their multifunctional actions, it should be considered that androgens, in particular androstenediols, share some properties of estrogen and progesterone metabolites. Deriving from cholesterol, sexual hormones are highly lipophilic; therefore, they easily cross the blood-brain barrier and diffuse through cell membrane, acting on nuclear receptors that are transcription factors. Moreover, the brain has the capacity to synthesize both gonadal hormones and their metabolites from cholesterol: these compounds are called neurosteroids and they can modulate different neurotransmitter pathways.

On the basis of the neuroactive properties of estradiol and progesterone and their relative levels during the menstrual cycle, Herzog et al. demonstrated that seizures do not occur randomly, but can cluster in specific parts of the menstrual cycle in one-third of women with epilepsy. The periodicity may differ between women with ovulatory and anovulatory cycles. As described in Chapter 8, three different patterns of catamenial epilepsy have been described: perimenstrual, periovulatory (in ovulatory cycles), and inadequate luteal phase (in anovulatory cycles) catamenial seizures [3].

Estrogen

Estradiol influences neuronal excitability, but not always in the same direction and as such, its role in seizure susceptibility is complex. Estrogen has proconvulsant and epileptogenic effects in the animal and human brain. Less well understood is its role in decreasing neuronal excitability with potential anticonvulsant effect [4].

Mechanisms of estrogen on neuronal excitability

The three main biologically active estrogens are estrone (E1), estradiol (E2), and estriol (E3). Postmenopausally, estrone is the principal estrogen and it is mainly formed by aromatization of the major androgen, androstenedione, in subcutaneous fat. In pregnancy, estriol is more abundant because it is synthesized in large quantities via placental aromatization of fetal androgen and by hydroxylation of estrone in the liver. However, the major estrogen in premenopausal women is estradiol. It represents the physiological ovarian hormone. Specifically, there are two isomers of estradiol, 17α-estradiol and 17ß-estradiol. The isoform considered bioactive in menstruating women is 17ß-estradiol, but the bioactivity of the 17α isomer should not be underestimated. Indeed, it is demonstrated that the 17α- and 17ß-estradiol both induce rapid morphological effects on the hippocampal area of animal models [4].

The effects of estrogens are mediated either via specific receptors (*classical genomic actions*) or as direct effects on the neurotransmitter receptors (*non-classical actions*). The classical genomic actions of estrogens are mediated by two distinct intracellular receptors, ERα and ERß: both estrogen receptor types have a similar structure, but different brain distribution and mediate different effects. ERα is distributed in the brain and reproductive organs of both females and males, whereas ERß is more widely distributed in the female brain. After diffusion into the cell, estrogens bind to intracellular receptors, forming a hormone receptor complex. The estrogen receptors are transcription factors that are transformed in active form and bind to DNA, leading to modulation of target genes and protein synthesis. This process requires 30 minutes to several hours (delayed effects), involving regulation of gene transcription [5].

However, an alternative pathway has been suggested because estrogens can also exert rapid and short-duration effects (seconds to a minute), that cannot easily be explained by genomic actions. Moreover, there are cellular responses to estradiol that are not blocked by pharmacological antagonists of nuclear estrogen receptors. Therefore, cellular effects of estrogen are thought to be mediated by a "membrane receptor." Although the nature of membrane receptors remains unclear, the possible mechanisms for these non-classical actions are: (a) changes in membrane fluidity; (b) action on membrane receptors; (c) regulation of GABA-A receptors on plasma membranes; (d) up-regulation of different factors by estrogens.

To better understand how estradiol may be able to act on neuronal excitability, many studies focus their attention on the limbic system (especially CA1 hippocampal pyramidal cells), cerebral cortex, and other regions important for seizure susceptibility. Estradiol appears to increase excitability involving synaptic structure and function. This mechanism may be due to estradiol capacity of decreasing gamma-aminobutyric acid or GABAergic inhibition and enhancing glutamate-mediated excitation through its N-methyl D-aspartate receptor (NMDA). Estradiol involves structural changes, such as the increase of the number of spine synapses, spine density, and spine shape. In particular, in ovariectomized animals, estrogen exposure increases the number and density of dendritic spines and excitatory synapses (within 12 to 24 hours) on hippocampal neurons through estradiol modulation of the NMDA receptor, leading to an increase of seizure susceptibility starting from the hippocampus. These results indicate the possibility that estrogen is involved in neuronal plasticity through the potentiation of postsynaptic function, leading to its relevant role of proconvulsant hormone [1].

However, estrogen is involved not only in postsynaptic effects. Chronic treatment with estradiol (1 or 10 nM) for 24 hours significantly increased high potassium (K)-induced glutamate release due to both phosphatidylinositol 3-kinase (PI 3-kinase) and mitogen-activated protein kinase (MAPK). Therefore, estradiol potentiates presynaptic function through the increase in release of neurotransmitter glutamate [6].

In the striatum, estradiol attenuates K-induced GABA release, inducing inhibitory effects. In the hippocampus, estradiol increases KA2, a kainic acid receptor subunit that induces a marked reduction in GABA release. This mechanism could mediate proconvulsant actions [4].

Moreover, estradiol could potentiate the increase in hippocampal acetylcholine (ACh) release, mediating effects on learning and memory. The relationship between estradiol and ACh release has also been shown in the frontal cortex of ovariectomized female rats [36]. Thus, it has been suggested that this hormone may have positive effects on cognitive function through stimulating cholinergic neurons.

Other studies found that estradiol could produce a concentration-dependent increase in norepinephrine release in the hypothalamus, involved in the regulation of female reproductive behavior. Zheng established the interaction between estradiol and striatal dopamine release, highlighting its possible effect on sensorimotor functions [7]. Table 4.1 shows some of the multiple actions of estrogens on the brain.

More recently, indirect mechanisms of estradiol on regulation of hippocampal seizure activity have been proposed, most notably, the relationship between estrogen

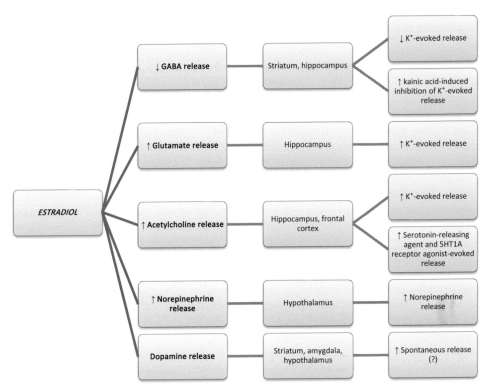

Figure 4.1: Effect of estradiol on neurotransmitter release and its particular effect on hippocampal system, playing a crucial role in neuronal plasticity and thus an important role in learning and memory. (↑) promote release; (↓) inhibit release (modified from reference 7).

and brain-derived neurotrophic factor (BDNF). Estrogen has a response element on the BDNF gene and it seems to up-regulate BDNF production. BDNF potentiates several of the glutamatergic pathways in hippocampus and other brain regions, acting like an agonist at neurotrophic tyrosine kinase receptors (trkB). In particular, trkB knockout mice are highly resistant to kindling epileptogenesis. Therefore, BDNF mediates estrogen actions on hippocampus excitability especially during the periovulatory period when estrogen rises, leading to a transient elevation in seizure frequency [4]. The effects summarized above support the idea that estradiol can increase excitability, working like a proconvulsant agent.

However, estradiol has also been shown to increase the levels of glutamic acid decarboxylase (GAD), the synthetic enzyme for GABA, increasing levels of GABA. Indeed, ERα receptors have been found in subsets of GABAergic neurons. Moreover, estradiol is able to increase the expression of neuropeptide Y (NPY) [4]. This anticonvulsant effect may not have been recognized in other studies due to the use of non-physiological endocrine state models and non-physiological doses of estradiol. Moreover, researchers have used different models of animals and with different endpoints. In light of this, current evidence suggests that estradiol influences on cortical excitability are more complex than simply proconvulsant.

The influence of estradiol on seizures

Preclinical studies

Animal models of epilepsy represent a key role in the identification of various mechanisms, pathophysiology, and discovery of antiepileptic drugs. Many studies are largely based on the utilization of acutely induced seizures in naive animals, but these conventional seizure models are not appropriate to test the different response to sex hormone fluctuation. More recent studies have designed specific animal models of catamenial epilepsy, in which it is possible to recreate a stimulation of the menstrual cycle and ovarian hormone-related changes in seizure susceptibility. Some of these types of models are made to mimic the luteal phase (including the pseudopregnancy, the chronic progesterone, and the progesterone withdrawal models), others administer exogenous hormones in ovariectomized rats, as if it were a normal ovarian cycle, still others first expose and then stop steroid hormone administration, as can be seen in catamenial seizure exacerbation [1].

Some early animal experiments demonstrated that estrogens decrease the electroshock seizure threshold or after-discharge threshold, using stimulus-evoked seizure threshold in rats [8]. Estrogens create new cortical seizure foci when applied topically, increasing cortical electrographic activity and promoting seizure. Estradiol administration to ovariectomized rats revealed proconvulsant effects, activating pre-existing cortical epileptogenic foci. Estradiol also potentiates seizures induced by chemoconvulsants, pentylenetetrazol (PTZ) and kainic acid.

As previously mentioned, the hippocampus is the region of the brain best studied for its relevant role in the generation and propagation of seizure activity. Hippocampal damage, known as hippocampal sclerosis, usually occurs following an initial precipitating event such as status epilepticus [37]. Loss of hilar and pyramidal neurons in the CA1 and CA3 regions lead to the irreversible damage of the hippocampus. New functional connections and reorganizations of hippocampal axon circuits occur and promote further seizures.

Estradiol increases the severity of chemically induced seizures. Indeed, acute administration of estradiol to experimental models of partial and limbic epilepsy enhances the frequency and severity of PTZ-induced seizures. It is important to remember that kainic acid can induce the damage of some structures of the brain, including the hippocampus, pyriform, entorhinal cortices, septum, amygdala, and thalamus. In experimental models of epilepsy, manipulations that affect the hippocampus can produce chronic seizures and alter electrical discharge of hippocampal neurons. An example of this effect is the intravenous administration of kainic acid to rats and the subsequent development of automatisms and limbic convulsion [9].

Other studies use kindling models in which the brains of experimental animals are repeatedly stimulated, usually with electricity or pilocarpine, to induce the seizures. In these models, estradiol has been demonstrated to facilitate not only kindling but also audiogenic seizures; chronic treatment of estradiol has a proconvulsant-like effect not only in female experimental models but also in male rodents [10]. Further, estradiol treatment facilitates hippocampus excitability in a subpopulation of neurons in ovariectomized female rats by prolonging the excitatory postsynaptic potential. Moreover, estradiol has been shown to alter electrolytes, vascular permeability, and blood-brain barrier because of its regulation of vascular endothelial growth factor expression [11].

Based on these studies, there is a general consensus that estradiol is "proconvulsant" and promotes seizure activity. However, although estradiol facilitates focally induced seizures, the effect of estradiol has been much more variable when seizures have been induced by systemic chemoconvulsants. There is evidence that supports lack of proconvulsant effect and even a "neuroprotective" effect. This protective effect of estrogens was first demonstrated independently by two experimental studies, guided by Veliskova et al. and Reibel et al. [12, 13]. Using chronic administration of estrogens in female rats (status epilepticus models), either anticonvulsant or no effect of estrogen on seizures was shown. Moreover, it has been highlighted that even low doses of estradiol can produce a protective effect. Subsequent studies confirmed the neuroprotective activity of estrogens, advancing the hypothesis that estradiol may protect neurons from seizure-induced damage [1]. Indeed, estradiol has been shown to increase the hippocampal levels of GAD, the synthetic enzyme for the inhibitory neurotransmitter GABA, and thus increase levels of GABA. Furthermore, estradiol seems to be involved in the modulation of NPY expression, increasing its expression in the dentate gyrus of the hippocampus. This interaction with inhibitory neurotransmitters could possibly be relevant to inhibition of seizures [14].

It is helpful to consider that some of these studies observed the *neuroprotective* effect of estradiol in non-physiological experimental models, such as ovariectomized female rats, or using aromatase inhibition in cultures of hippocampal neurons. Direct comparison is limited as studies differ in dosage paradigm, timing, sex of the models, and gonadal hormone status. What these results do highlight however is the complexity of the role of estrogen in seizures, that to date is not completely understood.

Clinical studies

As demonstrated in animal models, many studies have supported the key role estradiol plays in the exacerbation of seizures by decreasing seizure threshold or after-discharge threshold in women with epilepsy, while progesterone has an opposite effect. Backstrom observed a strong relationship between seizure susceptibility and an increase in estrogen-to-progesterone ratio, finding a peak of seizure frequency during the premenstrual and preovulatory phase and a decrease in the midluteal phase [15]. Another early study has shown that intravenous infusions of estrogen were associated with rapid interictal epileptiform activity in women with epilepsy, especially if given premenstrually. Furthermore, observations of hormonal fluctuations during the menstrual cycle have identified a periovulatory catamenial exacerbation, attributed to the increase of estradiol during the mid-cycle relative to a low progesterone level. Thus an increase in the ratio of estrogen-to-progesterone levels during the perimenstrual period may contribute to perimenstrual seizure exacerbation. Unfortunately, other clinical studies have demonstrated seemingly contradictory results. For example, Jacono et al. studied the possible relationship between levels of serum estrogen and levels of serum calcium (Ca^{++}) and frequency of seizures during the menstrual cycle. They noted that fewer seizures occurred during the mid-menstrual cycle, when estrogen levels are high and Ca^{++} level are low.

Other authors demonstrated the relationship between the effect of hormone replacement therapy in menopause and the catamenial seizure pattern. El-Khayat et al. dosed sex steroid concentrations in women with epilepsy and control subjects and found that serum concentration of estradiol in women with catamenial epilepsy is similar during the entire cycle compared to that of control subjects. Indeed, estradiol levels in women with catamenial epilepsy are lower in the perimenstrual phase than the midluteal and follicular phases. In the perimenstrual phase, progesterone levels are lower and the estrogen-to-progesterone ratio was higher in women with catamenial epilepsy [16]. Moreover, women

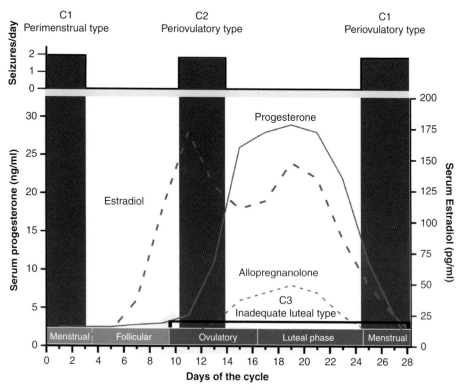

Figure 4.2: Serum hormone concentrations and seizure susceptibility during the menstrual cycle. Estradiol begins to increase during the second half of the follicular phase, reaching the peak at mid-cycle, while progesterone is only elevated during the luteal phase and declines before menstruation begins. Allopregnanolone, the progesterone-derived neurosteroid, is elevated in parallel to its hormone precursor. The upper middle figure illustrates the relationship between progesterone levels and seizure frequency. The area to the left and right represents the period of perimenstrual catamenial seizures. Day 1 is the onset of menstruation, and ovulation occurs 14 days before the onset of menstruation. The publisher for this copyrighted material is Elsevier, *Epilepsy Research*, Reddy, 2009.

with epilepsy often have anovulatory cycles and hypogonadism due to low sex hormone concentrations of both estrogens and progesterone (Figure 4.2).

Progesterone

Animal and human models of epilepsy have directly supported the relationship between ovarian steroids and seizure susceptibility. Specifically, progesterone appears to be anticonvulsant: it seems to reduce neuronal firing, suppresses kindling, lessens epileptiform discharges, raises the seizure threshold, and decreases interictal spikes caused by cortically-applied penicillin in most animal models. Progesterone is secreted by the corpus luteum in the ovary, by adrenal glands, and glial cells. It is quickly metabolized in the brain to 3α,5α-THP by 5α-reductase and 3α-hidroxysteroid dehydrogenase enzymes [2].

Mechanisms of progesterone on neuronal excitability

Progesterone receptors (PR), a member of the nuclear receptor superfamily of transcription factors, mediate physiological actions of progesterone and exist in two forms, PR-A and PR-B, which exhibit different physiological properties; they act as nuclear transcription factors, analogous to estrogens, transcribed from the same gene. In progesterone-responsive target cells, progesterone binds to cytoplasmic PRs and the hormone-nuclear receptor complexes translocate to the cell nucleus where they activate or silence the transcription of downstream gene networks, thus affecting the physiological response of the target cell [1].

Expressed in distinct brain regions, both PRs have similar affinities for progesterone. PR-A and PR-B may utilize distinct intracellular signaling pathways in response to progesterone-mediated activation versus ligand-independent activation, shown, for example, by dopamine activation of PRs via phosphorylation mechanisms, without progesterone. Several proteins, acting as co-activators or co-repressors, enhance or inhibit PR-dependent target transcription. The balance between progesterone-dependent and ligand-independent PR activation in different regions of the brain can be affected by reproductive state. Indeed, the effects of PR activation on neuronal excitability may vary with endocrine condition, maybe because the ratio of PR-A/PR-B expression is not constant from one region of the brain to another, regulated by circulating estradiol levels. Therefore, progesterone sensitivity is dependent on estrogen exposure.

The interaction between progesterone and estradiol has implications for the therapeutic use of progesterone in women with epilepsy. Progesterone administration may exert two effects: (1) actions on PRs, which depend on concurrent estradiol levels, and (2) actions at GABA-A receptors after conversion to allopregnanolone. Importantly, even the latter could depend on serum estradiol concentration, in part because estradiol alters GABA levels, GABA synthesis, and regulates the reversal potential of the GABA-A receptor by changing expression of KCC2, a potassium/chloride co-transporter [4].

Although the central nervous system is an important target for progesterone, with a wide distribution of PRs, progesterone's antiseizure effects are not related to interactions with classical PR. The hypothesis of more immediate antiseizure effects of progesterone is supported by the following evidence: (1) they occur rapidly (within minutes), which is inconsistent with delayed genomic actions of the hormone; (2) the seizure activity of progesterone is blocked by the PR antagonist RU486, a progesterone receptor antagonist; and (3) it is undiminished in PR knockout (PRKO) mice, generated by a null mutation of the PR gene that abrogates both the PR-A and PR-B subtypes [17]. Recently, several PRs' rapid signaling mechanisms have been identified in the brain. They consist of non-genomic "membrane-associated PRs" and short-latency effects of progesterone. However, the role of this membrane PR in seizure susceptibility has not been explored. To date, progesterone's rapid effect on the hippocampus slice excitability, blocked by the PR antagonist RU486, has been reported [18].

Utilizing the PRKO mouse model, progesterone was tested in three distinct models of epilepsy: the PTZ test, amygdala kindling, and maximal electroshock tests. In all three models, the anticonvulsant potency of progesterone was undiminished in PRKO mice, compared with control wild type mice. Indeed, progesterone had enhanced anticonvulsant potency in PRKO mice in the PTZ and amygdala kindling model of epilepsy. The antiseizure activity of progesterone in PRKO mice was reversed by pretreatment with finasteride, a 5α-reductase inhibitor that blocks the metabolism of progesterone to allopregnanolone. This and other studies support that theory 5α-reduced metabolites of progesterone, particularly allopregnanolone, are responsible for the seizure protection conferred by progesterone.

The influence of progesterone on seizure

Preclinical studies

From the first report of Hans Selye (1942), many successive animal studies confirmed the anticonvulsant properties and antiseizure activity of progesterone. Like neurosteroids, progesterone is inactive or requires high sedative doses to protect against seizures induced by glutamate receptor agonists, with elevation of seizure threshold following progesterone administration that is dose-dependent, lasting up to 2 hours post-progesterone. Therefore, during physiological conditions associated with high progesterone, seizure susceptibility is very low.

In animals, allopregnanolone seems to be the primary effector, because blockade of 5α-reductase (the enzyme that controls the first step in progesterone metabolism to allopregnanolone) delays the onset and decreases the incidence of PTZ-induced seizures. However, it is not always clear whether progesterone is responsible for these effects, or the effects are mediated through its metabolites. Interestingly, synthetic progestins do not necessarily have an anticonvulsant effect, but frequently contraceptives can increase seizure frequency. The different effects of contraceptives on seizures relative to "natural" progestins (like progesterone) are likely to be due in part to their inability to be converted to allopregnanolone [4].

Animal studies suggest that altered expression of GABA-A receptor subunits is at the basis of the increase in excitability following sudden loss of progesterone. GABA-A receptors are heteromeric complexes of various subunits, and subunit combination confers specificity for modulators such as allopregnanolone and benzodiazepines. Different GABA-A receptor combinations subserve distinct functions. GABA-A receptors with δ subunits subserve "tonic" inhibition, primarily mediated by ambient GABA release at extrasynaptic GABA-A receptors, creating an inhibitory "tone" that may reduce excitability in a widespread and continuous manner. Indeed, transgenic animals lacking δ subunits, or normal mice treated with antisense mRNA to the δ subunit, demonstrated decreased latency to seizures induced by kainic acid, and longer periods of seizures [38].

Changes in the expression of GABA-A receptor subunits associated with tonic inhibition during the normal ovarian cycle are observed in studies in laboratory mice, with subsequent alteration in the sensitivity of GABA-A receptors to modulators like allopregnanolone, as well as the degree of tonic inhibition. During the period of the cycle associated with elevated serum progesterone δ subunit expression is relatively high in the mouse, while low levels of the δ subunit were found when serum progesterone was low. In the same mice, tonic inhibition and seizure susceptibility was correlated with the levels of δ subunits. However, there may be a complex series of GABA-A receptor alterations that do not solely involve δ subunits, because γ2 subunit expression also differed between the two times of the cycle [19].

Indeed, the importance of other types of subunits is underscored by the fact that tonic inhibition is not only dependent on δ subunits; another subunit that appears to contribute to tonic inhibition is the α4 subunit, and this appears to be up-regulated in an animal model of progesterone withdrawal.

Clinical studies

Progesterone's ability to reduce seizures is also demonstrated by many clinical studies. Although the concentration of serum progesterone is clearly an important aspect, there is also evidence that the fluctuations in its concentration may be important. The natural cyclic variations in progesterone during the menstrual cycle in women with epilepsy can influence catamenial seizure exacerbation, with seizures decreasing in the midluteal phase when serum progesterone levels are high and a premenstrual increase in seizures when progesterone levels fall and the serum progesterone-to-estrogen ratio decreases.

Indeed, in women with catamenial epilepsy the midluteal phase serum progesterone concentrations were significantly lower, compared to control subjects, while estradiol levels were similar in both groups [16]. Therefore, the estradiol-to-progesterone ratio increased significantly in epileptic patients. In perimenstrual catamenial seizure ones, lower progesterone levels were observed compared to control levels. However, women with inadequate luteal type seizures showed significantly lower progesterone levels in the midluteal and menstrual phases, compared to patients with non catamenial seizures or to patients with the perimenstrual type. The "rapid decline" or the "withdrawal" of the antiseizure effects of progesterone can explain the premenstrual seizure exacerbations, as first suggested by Laidlaw in 1956 and successively confirmed in other human and animal studies.

Herzog reported the first clinical evidence that progesterone's therapeutic activity in catamenial epilepsy requires conversion to 5α-reduced metabolites such as allopregnanolone (3α,5α-THP) [20]. 3α,5α-THP may account for some antiseizure effects: better correlation between decreased seizure susceptibility in women with catamenial epilepsy and increased plasmatic 3α,5α-THP, rather than progesterone; increased seizures after inhibition of progesterone metabolism to 3α,5α-THP. How 3α,5α-THP produces its antiseizure effects is still a matter of debate, but probably this molecule acts via its agonist-like actions at GABA-A receptors. However, further studies are required to clarify whether progesterone or its metabolites are responsible for the observed anticonvulsant effects.

Neurosteroids: proconvulsant and anticonvulsant hormones

Neuroactive steroids, synthesized either de novo in neuronal and glial cells or in the peripheral endocrine glands, have been demonstrated to modulate many different effects on brain functions, mainly by specific membrane receptors. The most important neurosteroids directly synthesized into the brain are allopregnanolone, progesterone, pregnenolone, and their sulfate esters. Recent evidence indicates that neurosteroids are present mainly in principal neurons in many brain regions that are relevant to focal epilepsies, including the hippocampus and neocortex. Allopregnanolone is a positive modulator of GABA-A receptors. It has specific binding sites on the GABA-A receptor chloride ion channel, distinct from the binding sites for GABA, benzodiazepines, and barbiturates (Figure 4.2). Although the mechanism of how neurosteroids interact with the GABA-A receptor is unclear, two discrete binding sites have been identified. Neurosteroids have synaptic and extrasynaptic effects, playing an important role in setting the level of excitability by strengthening tonic inhibition during seizures due to high level of GABA. Thus, allopregnanolone and related neurosteroids can interact with both classical genomic steroid receptors and membrane receptors, having a modulatory influence on GABA-A receptor and seizure susceptibility. For example, animal studies have shown that prolonged exposure to allopregnanolone followed by withdrawal, such as that which occurs during menstruation, causes a marked increase in expression of a subunit of GABA-A receptor, enhancing neuronal excitability, seizure susceptibility, and benzodiazepine resistance [21]. Despite multiple animal models, few studies in humans are available to support a direct correlation

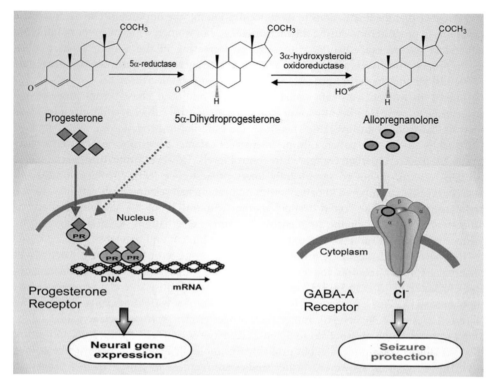

Figure 4.3: Molecular mechanism of progesterone action in seizure activity. There are two mechanisms by which progesterone affects seizure susceptibility: binding to progesterone receptors (PR), and metabolism to GABA$_A$ receptor-modulating neurosteroids. Neurosteroid allopregnanolone is synthesized from progesterone by two sequential A-ring reductions. The conversion of progesterone into allopregnanolone occurs both in peripheral tissues and in the brain. In addition, a small quantity of allopregnanolone is also produced locally within the brain from cholesterol, which is partly independent of its secretion from ovarian sources. Although allopregnanolone binds poorly to PRs, it could indirectly activate PRs by reconversion to 5α-dihydroprogesterone, which is a moderately potent PR agonist. Thus, PRs might play a role in the long-term actions of endogenous neurosteroids.

between allopregnanolone withdrawal and seizure exacerbation. However, as the main source of allopregnanolone is progesterone, decrease in progesterone levels around the perimenstrual phase would be expected to follow a drop in allopregnanolone, leading to potential seizure exacerbation. In contrast to allopregnanolone, pregnenolone sulfate is considered a proconvulsant steroid due to its property of inducing seizures and status epilepticus when administered systemically or directly into the brain. It has been demonstrated to inhibit the GABA-A receptor function and be able to moderate NMDA-glutamate receptors like agonists [22].

Androgenic neurosteroids and the influence on epileptogenesis

Regarding the role of androgens, it was demonstrated that testosterone and its main metabolic and active product dihydrotestosterone can influence ictal activity of the human brain. Androgen neurosteroids are not only metabolized by sequential reduction of testosterone and subsequently androstanediol *(androgen pathway)*, but testosterone is also readily aromatized to estradiol *(estrogen pathway)*. Indeed, testosterone is synthesized in the thecal interstitial cells of the ovary, and then converted to estradiol, which has a relevant excitatory effect, in the granulosa cells of the primordial follicle. Thus, the net effect of testosterone may become difficult to interpret.

Because of its similar structure to allopregnanolone, androstanediol seems to interact with GABA-A receptors and act as an anticonvulsant modulator. Some studies have demonstrated that the anticonvulsant effects of androstenediol occur too fast (within minutes) to be related to its interaction with classical androgen receptors. However, androstanediol is converted to dihydrotestosterone, which is a potent androgen receptor agonist. Moreover, dihydrotestosterone seems to have a neuroprotective effect on the brain [23].

Therefore, testosterone seems to have an influence on neural excitability and seizure susceptibility due to its "androgenic neurosteroids": androstanediol and estradiol. Regarding administration of androgens and modification of ictal activity, there is evidence to suggest that testosterone significantly lowers the seizure threshold, increases PTZ-induced seizures, and enhances the development of amygdala-kindled seizures [39]. Thus, testosterone may enhance catamenial seizure activity because testosterone secretion increases by approximately 4-fold at around the time of ovulation. Further evidence suggests that androgens may increase spine synapse density in the hippocampus in females and contribute to plastic changes over the course of the menstrual cycle [4].

On the other hand, the neurosteroid androstanediol was demonstrated to be a powerful antiseizure and neuroprotective agent by preclinical studies in animal models of epilepsy. This effect was shown against seizures induced by many GABA-A receptor antagonists, pilocarpine, and the maximal electroshock model. In intravenous PTZ tests, it produced a dose-dependent elevation of seizure threshold. Despite animal models supporting a neuroprotective role of androstanediol, there are no clinical studies that investigate its role in catamenial epilepsy to date.

In conclusion, testosterone is thought to modulate seizure activity by its conversion to androstanediol (anticonvulsant) and estradiol (proconvulsant). Therefore, an administration of aromatase inhibitors, which block the synthesis of estradiol from testosterone thus elevating relative androstanediol levels, may represent a possible treatment for epilepsy (Table 4.1)

Influence of antiepileptic drugs on sexual hormones

In women with epilepsy the treatment with certain antiepileptic drugs (AEDs) may increase the risk of reproductive endocrine disorders, although they may already have a higher prevalence of these diseases [24, 25]. AEDs may influence and alter the metabolism of some sex hormones and their binding proteins resulting in secondary complications [26], in particular, enzyme-inducing AEDs (EIAEDs)—such as phenobarbital (PB), phenytoin (PHT), and carbamazepine (CBZ) [27]. Among EIAEDs, increased serum levels of sex hormone-binding globulin (SHBG) and reduced serum concentrations of dehydroepiandrosterone (DHEAS), testosterone, free androgen index (FAI), and E2 have been reported [28, 29, 30]. In the late 1970s and 1980s a reduction of sex steroid levels, such as estradiol (E2) and DHEAS, was reported in female patients treated with some EIAEDs, suggesting that in women with epilepsy, abnormal serum sex hormone levels can be caused by the enzyme-inducing properties of certain AEDs. Indeed, EIAEDs can reduce biologically active sex hormone serum concentrations, such as E2 and testosterone, inducing hepatic cytochrome P450–dependent steroid hormone breakdown and production of SHBG [31].

Table 4.1: Sex hormones and their endogenous neurosteroids with anticonvulsant and proconvulsant properties

	Estradiol	Progesterone	Testosterone
Specific receptor sites	Especially hypothalamic and limbic	Especially hypothalamic and limbic	Especially hypothalamic and limbic
CNS-active metabolites	17ß-estradiol	Allopregnanolone	Estradiol, dihydrotestosterone, androstanediol
Membrane receptor modulation	GABA, NMDA, kainate, 5-HT3	GABA, NMDA, nicotinic acetylcholine, 5-HT3, kainate	GABA, NMDA, kainate, 5-HT3
Effects on neuronal excitability	↓ GABA synthesis; ↓ numbers of GABA-A receptor subunits; ↑ formation of new dendritic spines; ↓ electroconvulsive shock threshold; Creates new seizure focus when applied topically to the cortex; ↑ severity and duration of chemically induced seizures; Activates pre-existing epileptogenic foci	↑ GABA synthesis; ↑ numbers of GABA-A receptor subunits; Contrasts the effects of estradiol on dendritic spine density; ↑ electroconvulsive shock threshold; ↓ seizures induced by kindling, focal lesions, and alcohol withdrawal; ↑ threshold for seizures induced by chemical convulsants	Controversial, may exert pro- and anticonvulsant effects

↑: enhance; ↓: decrease

Low DHEAS levels have been reported in women taking CBZ, PHT, and PB in monotherapy or polytherapy [32, 33, 34]. Significant differences in E2 levels and in free estrogen index (FEI) were found between women on different AED regimens. Women with epilepsy who were taking EIAED polytherapy appeared to have lower levels E2 and FEI than patients treated with a single EIAED or non-enzyme-inducing AED (NEIAED) [33]. During CBZ treatment, a decrease of free testosterone serum levels due to an induction of SHBG was also documented, with a subsequent rise of free testosterone serum concentrations when patients were switched from CBZ to oxcarbazepine [27]. A more detailed discussion of AED influences on hormones can be found in Chapter 5.

References

1. Reddy DS. The role of neurosteroids in the pathophysiology and treatment of catamenial epilepsy. *Epilepsy Res* 2009; 85:1–30.

2. Verrotti A, Latini G, Manco R, et al. Influence of sex hormones in brain excitability and epilepsy. *J Endocr Invest* 2007; 30:797–803.

3. Herzog AG, Klein P and Ransil BJ. Three patterns of catamenial epilepsy. *Epilepsia* 1997; 38:1082–8.

4. Scharfman HE and MacLusky NJ. The influence of gonadal hormones on

neuronal excitability, seizures and epilepsy in the female. *Epilepsia* 2006; 47:1423–40.

5. Matthews J and Gustafsson JA. Estrogen signaling: a subtle balance between ERα and ERß. *Mol Interv* 2004; 3:281–92.

6. Yokomaku D, Numakawa T, Numakawa Y, et al. Estrogen enhances depolarization-induced glutamate release through activation of phosphatidylinositol 3-kinase and mitogen-activated protein kinase in cultured hippocampal neurons. *Mol Endocrinol* 2003; 17:831–44.

7. Zheng P. Neuroactive steroid regulation of neurotransmitter release in the CNS: action, mechanism and possible significance. *Prog Neurobiol* 2009; 89:134–52.

8. Stitt SL and Kinnard WJ. The effects of certain progestins and estrogen on the threshold of electrically induced seizure patterns. *Neurology* 1986; 18:213–16.

9. Lothman EW and Collins RC. Kainic acid induced limbic seizures: metabolic, behavioral, electroencephalographic and neuropathological correlates. *Brain Res* 1981; 218:299–318.

10. Edwards HE, Burnham WM, Mendonca A, et al. Steroid hormones affect limbic after-discharge thresholds and kindling rates in adult female rats. *Brain Res* 1999; 838:136–50.

11. Hyder SM, Huang JC, Nawaz Z, et al. Regulation of vascular endothelial growth factor expression by estrogens and progestins. *Environ Health Perspect* 2000; 108(Suppl 5):785–90.

12. Veliskova J, Velisek L and Galanopoulou AS. Neuroprotective effects of estrogens on hippocampal cells in adult female rats after status epilepticus. *Epilepsia* 2000; 41(Suppl 6):S30–S35.

13. Reibel S, André V, Chassagnon S, et al. Neuroprotective effects of chronic estradiol benzoate treatment on hippocampal cell loss induced by status epilepticus in the female rat. *Neurosci Lett* 2000; 281:79–82.

14. Nakamura NH, Rosell DR, Akama KT, et al. Estrogen and ovariectomy regulate mRNA and protein of glutamic acid decarboxylases and cation-chloride cotransporters in the adult rat hippocampus. *Neuroendocrinology* 2004; 80:308–23.

15. Bäckström T. Epileptic seizures in women related to plasma estrogen and progesterone during the menstrual cycle. *Acta Neurol Scand* 1976; 54:321–47.

16. El-Khayat HA, Soliman NA, Tomoum HY, et al. Reproductive hormonal changes and catamenial pattern in adolescent females with epilepsy. *Epilepsia* 2008; 49:1619–26.

17. Reddy DS, Castenada DA, O'Malley BW, et al. Antiseizure activity of progesterone and neurosteroids in progesterone receptor knockout mice. *J Pharmacol Exp Ther* 2004; 310:230–9.

18. Edwards HE, Epps T, Carlen PL, et al. Progestin receptors mediate progesterone suppression of epileptiform activity in tetanized hippocampal slices in vitro. *Neuroscience* 2000; 101:895–906.

19. Maguire JL, Stell BM, Rafizadeh M, et al. Ovarian cycle-linked changes in GABA-A receptors mediating tonic inhibition alter seizure susceptibility and anxiety. *Nat Neurosci* 2005; 8:797–804.

20. Herzog AG and Frye CA. Seizure exacerbation associated with inhibition of progesterone metabolism. *Ann Neurol* 2003; 53:390–1.

21. Gangisetty O and Reddy DS. Neurosteroid withdrawal regulates GABA-A receptor α4-subunit expression and seizure susceptibility by activation of progesterone receptor-independent early growth response factor-3 pathway. *Neuroscience* 2010; 170:865–80.

22. Williamson J, Mtchedlishvili Z and Kapur J. Characterization of the convulsant action of pregnenolone sulfate. *Neuropharmacology* 2004; 46:856–864.

23. Reddy DS. Testosterone modulation of seizure susceptibility is mediated by neurosteroids 3α-androstanediol and 17-estradiol. *Neuroscience* 2004; 129:195–207.

24. Verrotti A, la Torre R, Trotta D, et al. Valproate-induced insulin resistance and obesity in children. *Horm Res* 2009; 71:125–31.

25. Isojarvi J. Disorders of reproduction in patients with epilepsy: antiepileptic drug related mechanisms. *Seizure* 2008; 17:111–19.

26. Bauer J, Isojarvi JI, Herzog AG, et al. Reproductive dysfunction in women with epilepsy: recommendations for evaluation and management. *J Neurol Neurosurg Psychiatry* 2002; 73:121–5.

27. Verrotti A, D'Eqidio C, Mohn A, et al. Antiepileptic drugs, sex hormones, and PCOS. *Epilepsia* 2011; 52(2):199–211.

28. Jacobsen NW, Halling-Sorensen B and Birkved FK. Inhibition of human aromatase complex (CYP19) by antiepileptic drugs. *Toxicol In Vitro* 2008; 22:146–53.

29. Lossius MI, Taubøll E, Mowinckel P, et al. Reversible effects of antiepileptic drugs on reproductive endocrine function in men and women with epilepsy – a prospective randomized double-blind withdrawal study. *Epilepsia* 2007; 48:1875–82.

30. Hamed SA, Hamed EA, Shokry M, et al. The reproductive conditions and lipid profile in females with epilepsy. *Acta Neurol Scand* 2007; 115:12–22.

31. Isojärvi JI, Taubøll E and Herzog AG. Effect of antiepileptic drugs on reproductive endocrine function in individuals with epilepsy. *CNS Drugs* 2005; 19:207–23.

32. Galimberti CA, Magri F, Copello F, et al. Seizure frequency and cortisol and dehydroepiandrosterone sulphate (DHEAS) levels in women with epilepsy receiving antiepileptic drug treatment. *Epilepsia* 2005; 46:517–23.

33. Galimberti CA, Magri F, Copello F, et al. Changes in sex steroid levels in women with epilepsy on treatment: relationship with antiepileptic therapies and seizure frequency. *Epilepsia* 2009; 50:28–32.

34. Murialdo G, Galimberti CA, Gianelli MV, et al. Effects of valproate, phenobarbital, and carbamazepine on sex steroid setup in women with epilepsy. *Clin Neuropharmacol* 1998; 21:52–8.

35. Newmark ME and Penry JK. Catamenial epilepsy: a review. *Epilepsia* 1980; 21:281–300.

36. Chang Q and Gold PE. Switching memory systems during learning: changes in patterns of brain acetylcholine release in the hippocampus and striatum in rats. *J Neurosc* 2003; 23:3001–5.

37. Mathern GW, Babb TL and Armstrong DL. Hippocampal sclerosis. In: Engel J Jr, Pedley TA, eds. *Epilepsy: a comprehensive textbook*. Philadelphia, IL: Lippincott-Raven, 1997; 133–55.

38. Maguire JL, Stell BM, Rafizadeh M, et al. Ovarian cycle-linked changes in GABA(A) receptors mediating tonic inhibition alter seizure susceptibility and anxiety. *Nat Neurosc* 2005; 8:797–804.

39. Tan M and Tan U. Effects of testosterone and clomiphene on spectral EEG and visual evoked response in a young man with posttraumatic epilepsy. *Int J Neurosc* 2001; 106:87–94.

Antiepileptic drugs and hormones

Pavel Klein and Jaromir Janousek

Key points:
- Reproductive endocrine dysfunction is more common in women with epilepsy (WWE)
- Certain antiepileptic drugs (AEDs), especially enzyme-inducing AEDs, alter hormone levels and have been associated with infertility, amenorrhea, and oral contraceptive failure
- Alterations in glucose metabolism, weight fluctuations, and thyroid hormone levels have also been observed with specific AEDs
- Though controversial, valproic acid has been associated with polycystic ovarian syndrome
- AEDs, notably carbamazepine and oxcarbazepine, can alter serum sodium and osmolarity homeostasis in part, by influences to antidiuretic hormone (ADH) sensitivity

Introduction

There is a reciprocal relationship between hormones and some AEDs. Hormones, most notably gonadal steroids, affect metabolism and blood levels of certain AEDs, such as phenobarbital, carbamazepine, phenytoin, lamotrigine, and possibly levetiracetam. This impacts affected AED serum levels and seizure control during different phases of the menstrual cycle and during pregnancy. A number of AEDs, in turn, affect endocrine function, some in women only, others in both men and women. Effects of AEDs on hormones can be approached either by describing the effects of individual AEDs, or thematically, by hormonal systems affected. Because several AEDs may affect the same endocrine system, we have chosen the thematic approach in the present chapter. The impact of hormones on metabolism of AEDs in the context of catamenial epilepsy and pregnancy, and the effects of AEDs on hormonal contraceptives and on hormones related to bone metabolism, are discussed in separate chapters, as is the use of hormones as AEDs for treatment of epilepsy.

Effects of AEDs on reproductive endocrine system

In women with epilepsy, both epilepsy and anticonvulsant therapy may affect reproductive endocrine function and behavior. The impact of the disease is discussed in detail elsewhere

Women with Epilepsy, ed. Esther Bui and Autumn Klein. Published by Cambridge University Press.
© Cambridge University Press 2014.

in this book. Briefly, reproductive endocrine disorders are more common among WWE than in the general population [1, 2]. About 35% of menstrual cycles of women with epilepsy are anovulatory [3]. Women with temporal lobe epilepsy (TLE) have approximately 20% risk of developing polycystic ovarian syndrome (PCOS), and approximately 15% risk each of developing hypothalamic hypogonadism (HH), functional hyperprolactinemia, and premature menopause, compared to 5%, 1.5%, 1–2%, and 1% risk for the respective conditions in the general population [1, 2]. In addition, hyposexuality occurs in 30–60% of WWE. These conditions may contribute to reduced fertility and birth rate among women with epilepsy, which are about 70–90% of that expected in the developed countries [2, 4–6]. AEDs have been implicated in possible causation of some of these conditions, most notably PCOS and hyposexuality.

Infertility

Certain AEDs may reduce fertility. Specifically, in the monotherapy setting, phenobarbital use has been associated with reduced fertility [7]. In a recent study of 375 women with epilepsy followed prospectively in India, the infertility rate was 38.4% [7]. AED treatment included mainly phenobarbital, phenytoin, carbamazepine, and valproate, with only a small number of patients treated with newer AEDs. Infertility was least (7.1%) in the small cohort of women receiving no AED treatment. It increased to 31.8% with a single AED treatment, to 40.7% with 2 AEDs and to 60.3% with 3 AEDs.

Phenobarbital, phenytoin, and carbamazepine (PB, PHT, CBZ): These AEDs all induce hepatic cytochrome p450 enzymes, and are referred to as enzyme-inducing AEDs (EIAEDs). They increase hepatic gonadal steroid catabolism and hepatic synthesis of sex hormone-binding globulin (SHBG) [2]. SHBG binds gonadal steroids in serum, including 17-β-estradiol (estradiol) and testosterone. Because only the non-SHBG-bound gonadal steroids are active, SHBG regulates the bioactivity of gonadal steroids by determining their bound versus non-bound serum levels. WWE treated with PHT and CBZ have elevated serum SHBG concentrations and reduced levels of bioactive estradiol and testosterone [2], while WWE treated with PB have low serum estradiol levels without SHBG level change. With CBZ, the changes occur progressively over time (years) and are associated with the development of menstrual irregularities in 25% of women during the first 5 years of CBZ treatment [2, 8].

Polycystic ovarian syndrome (PCOS)
Valproic acid

PCOS is the commonest reproductive endocrine disease in the general population and the commonest cause of female infertility in the general population. In addition, PCOS increases the risk of developing metabolic syndrome. In 1993, Isojärvi and colleagues reported that in a study of 238 WWE, menstrual disturbances with polycystic ovaries and hyperandrogenism occurred more commonly in women with epilepsy treated with valproic acid (VPA, 45%) than in women treated with CBZ (19%) or other AEDs (8%) [9]. The effect was particularly marked in women who had started taking VPA before the age of 20, 80% of whom were affected [2]. The effect is reversible. Substitution of VPA with lamotrigine (LMT) or simple discontinuation of VPA leads to reversal of hyperandrogenism in both adult women and teenage girls [10, 11].

The finding has generated a lively controversy because a number of studies have failed to replicate the findings while other studies have corroborated them [2, 12, 13]. For instance, in a prospective cohort study aiming to repeat the comparison between WWE treated with VPA, CBZ, or no AEDs, Bauer et al. found the incidence of polycystic ovarian syndrome to be similar across the groups, 11.1% in VPA-treated, 10% in CBZ-treated, and 10.5% in untreated women, contradicting Isojärvi's findings [14].

Part of the controversy stems from different definitions used in different studies. The widely accepted NIH definition of PCOS consists only of: (i) ovulatory dysfunction (e.g., oligomenorrhea, amenorrhea, or polymenorrhea) and (ii) hyperandrogenism (symptomatic or biochemical), (iii) in the absence of other endocrinopathies [15]. It does not, paradoxically, include the morphological feature of polycystic ovaries (PCO) which was included in Isojärvi et al.'s original report and which was the main diagnostic criterion for PCOS in Europe until 2003 [15]. A woman may have PCO without either hyperandrogenism or menstrual irregularities, in which case the condition is called PCO and may not be associated with reproductive endocrine dysfunction. Thus a study that reports morphological polycystic ovaries with or without hyperandrogenism or oligomenorrhea differs from one that reports only the latter.

In addition, as already noted, epilepsy itself predisposes to PCOS. PCOS occurs in 20% of women with TLE *not* treated with VPA [1]. Among these women, PCOS occurs preferentially in women with *left-sided* TLE, suggesting a biological causation. Luteinizing hormone (LH) and follicle-stimulating hormone (FSH) are secreted from the anterior pituitary in a pulsatile manner in response to pulsatile release of gonadotropin-releasing hormone (GnRH) from the hypothalamus. The pulse frequency varies with phase of menstrual cycle and time of day, but is in general 6–8 pulses per hour. Frequency of the pulses affects ovarian gonadal synthesis: higher pulse frequency is associated with higher androgen secretion and lower pulse frequency with lower androgen secretion. Women with left-sided TLE have increased frequency of pulsatile secretion of GnRH and LH, presumably due to altered input from the amygdala and or hippocampus to the GnRH-releasing hypothalamic neurons [16, 17].

PCOS is more common in women treated with VPA for epilepsy than in women treated with VPA for bipolar affective disorder, although there is an effect in the latter group also [18]. This suggests that not only VPA but also the disease and the interaction of the disease with the medication may be important in causing PCOS in VPA-treated WWE.

Most of the studies evaluating a possible relationship between VPA and PCOS have been cross-sectional or prospective cohort studies. In the most recent and largest such study, Sahota et al. reported that among 427 consecutively evaluated WWE, PCOS (using the NIH criteria) was more common in WWE receiving VPA (11.8%) than those taking other AEDs (2.5%), independent of seizure type [19]. In the most definitive study of the possible role of VPA in PCOS to date, Morrell et al. compared 447 women without PCOS treated de novo with either VPA or with LMT in a prospective, randomized study. After 1 year of treatment, the VPA group had higher androgen levels or anovulation (36%) than the LMT group (23%). Nine percent of women on VPA developed new onset PCOS versus 2% on LTG [20].

On balance, then, the weight of the evidence suggests that VPA does induce hyperandrogenism and menstrual irregularities, possibly interacting with the physiological changes of epilepsy itself to produce the effect.

The mechanism by which VPA may cause hyperandrogenism and PCOS is not clear. In the general population, PCOS may arise as a result of at least two pathophysiological mechanisms: (a) central nervous system (CNS) effect, with altered LH/FSH secretion; and (b) peripheral effect, resulting from obesity and hyperinsulinemia.

(a) CNS effect: The biochemical hallmarks of PCOS are hyperandrogenism and increased blood levels of LH relative to FSH, with LH/FSH ratio of ≥ 3 during the early follicular phase. In PCOS, there is increased pulse frequency of LH by the anterior pituitary, suppression of FSH release, and an increased LH/FSH serum level ratio, all presumed to result from alteration in the pulsatile hypothalamic release of GnRH. The late luteal and early follicular phase increase in FSH release, which is essential for normal follicular development, is absent. This results in failure of follicular maturation and retention by the ovary of multiple immature follicles ("polycysts") [21]. The theca cells of the follicles produce androgens under the control of LH. In normal maturing follicles, androgens are converted to estrogens in the adjacent granulosa cells using FSH-controlled aromatase, the enzyme that converts androgens to estrogens. In PCOS, there is both basal and LH-stimulated increase in production of androgens by the theca cells, and reduced conversion of androgens to estrogens in the granulosa cells, resulting in increased androgen secretion by the follicle and hyperandrogenism [15].

(b) Peripheral effect: The majority of women with PCOS in the general population are obese [15, 21]. Obesity is associated with insulin resistance and elevated serum insulin level. Insulin stimulates follicular theca cells to produce androgens, again resulting in hyperandrogenism. High serum testosterone concentrations may in turn lead to arrest of follicular maturation and development of PCO.

In VPA-treated WWE with PCOS the proposed pathophysiological mechanisms have included: (a) effect on the hypothalamus/pituitary; (b) effect on insulin with or without weight gain; (c) direct effect on the ovary; and (d) inhibition of liver enzymes that catabolize androgens resulting in hyperandrogenism. More than one mechanism may be involved.

(a) CNS effect: While there have been several studies on the effect of VPA on neurotransmitters in the hypothalamus, no studies have evaluated possible VPA effect on GnRH or LH/FSH and LH/FSH ratio [13].

(b) Insulin/weight gain effect: Valproate causes weight gain. The majority (though not all) of VPA-treated women who have PCOS are obese. Weight gain is associated with and possibly caused by VPA-induced decrease in cellular sensitivity to insulin (insulin resistance), and increased blood levels of insulin, hyperinsulinemia. Interestingly, VPA induces hyperinsulinemia even in non-obese women [2]. Insulin has a direct effect on the ovary. It stimulates thecal androgen production, which is increased in hyperinsulinemia. In addition to insulin, insulin-like growth factor-1 (IGF-1) also stimulates thecal androgen production (reviewed in 2, 12). IGF-1 is bound in blood to its binding proteins, IGF-binding proteins (IGFBP). Insulin inhibits liver production of IGFBP-1, resulting in an increased serum level of free IGF-1 and stimulation of thecal androgen production. Androgens also circulate in blood either bound to proteins such as SHBG and albumin, or free. Insulin inhibits liver production of SHBG, resulting in an increased amount of circulating free androgens and hyperandrogenism [2, 12, 15]. However, it is unlikely that weight gain or hyperinsulinemia is the sole cause of VPA-related PCOS. PCO and hyperandrogenism occur also in VPA-treated non-obese women who have normal levels of insulin and IGFBP-1 [2]. In women with newly diagnosed epilepsy treated with VPA, an increase in serum testosterone and androstenedione levels occurs 1–3 months after VPA initiation in approximately 50% of cases, without associated weight gain [2]. In girls with epilepsy treated with VPA, hyperandrogenism develops without hyperinsulinemia [2]. Finally, pregabalin and gabapentin also cause weight gain but there have been no reports of associated increase in PCOS.

(c) Direct effect on the ovary: VPA induces polycystic ovarian morphology in rats. It increases basal and LH-stimulated production of testosterone in small follicles, stimulating ovarian theca cells to increase transcription of steroidogenic genes (CYP17 and CYP11A), and reduces conversion of testosterone to estradiol by suppressing aromatase activity in the granulosa cells [22, 23].

(d) VPA inhibits the hepatic P450 enzyme system, thereby reducing catabolism of androgens and increasing their blood levels, and inhibits hepatic production of aromatase, resulting in increased ovarian androgen secretion and levels [12].

Other AEDs

No other AEDs have been associated with PCOS in humans. It has been suggested that hepatic enzyme-inducing AEDs (EIAEDs) such as CBZ, PHT, and PB may protect against PCOS by causing *hypoandrogenism* [1, 17]. They may do this by inducing liver synthesis of: (a) SHBG, resulting in increased binding of testoterone by SHBG and reduced levels of free or bioavailable androgens; and (b) aromatase, with increased conversion of androgens to estrogens and reduction in androgen levels.

Among new AEDs, neither LMT nor levetiracetam (LEV) are associated with reproductive endocrine disorders [12]. In rats, chronic treatment with levetiracetam in high doses of 100–300 mg/kg/day increases serum testosterone and reduces serum estradiol levels, but this is not seen in LEV-treated women with epilepsy [24].

There are no data available for the other new AEDs (felbamate, gabapentin, tiagabine, topiramate, vigabatrin, and zonisamide).

Clinical implications: There are no evidence-based guidelines concerning VPA and PCOS and the use of VPA in women and girls of reproductive age. The following is the authors' personal perspective.

In women without obesity or clinical evidence of PCOS, VPA should be used on its anticonvulsant merits. PCOS should be discussed with the patient as a potential side effect together with other potential side effects. During VPA treatment, the patient should be monitored for body weight increase, appearance of hirsutism (face, extremities, abdomen, and breasts), and prolongation or irregularity of menstrual cycle (e.g., >35 days-long cycles). If any of these develop, substitution of VPA by another AED such as LMT, LEV, or OXC should be considered. In this setting, testing should include blood levels of total and free testosterone, androstenedione, bioactive testosterone, and sex hormone-binding globulin for evaluation of hyperandrogenism; menstrual cycle-day 3 LH and FSH blood levels, looking for elevated ratio of >3:1, the biochemical signature of PCOS; and menstrual cycle-day 20–22 serum progesterone level, looking for serum progesterone level of <5 ng/ml as evidence of anovulatory cycle. If abnormalities are found in these tests, a gynecological referral and ultrasound of the ovaries may be indicated.

We do not think that the potential side effect of PCOS is a reason not to use VPA when it is clinically indicated and there are no pre-existing conditions such as obesity or hirsutism to indicate an increased risk of PCOS.

Other reproductive endocrine dysfunction and AEDs

There have been reports of cases and a small case series of amenorrhea secondary to hypothalamic hypogonadism occurring in women treated with valproate [25]. VPA has also been reported to transiently arrest puberty in girls with epilepsy [2]. This has not been reported with other AEDs. Thus, if a woman treated with VPA develops menstrual irregularity, differential diagnosis includes not only PCOS but also hypothalamic hypogonadism. This presents as oligomenorrhea or amenorrhea as its sole manifestation, with associated low levels of estrogens (estradiol, estrone), androgens, and of LH and FSH.

No AEDs have been associated with the increased prevalence of premature menopause observed in women with epilepsy [26].

Sexuality

Hyposexuality is characterized by lack of libido and difficulty in achieving orgasm. Approximately 30–60% of WWE suffer from sexual dysfunction, including disorders of sexual desire and arousal, anorgasmia, dyspareunia, and vaginismus [27]. As with other reproductive endocrine dysfunction, this is likely due to a number of factors, including the disease, certain AEDs, and psychosocial factors.

Sexual dysfunction is more common in localization-related epilepsy (LRE)/focal seizures (64%) than in primary generalized epilepsy (PGE) (8%) [27, 28]. Women with LRE experience increased dyspareunia and vaginismus and sexual dissatisfaction, while women with PGE may experience more anorgasmia and sexual dissatisfaction [27]. Women with right-sided TLE are more likely to suffer from hyposexuality than women with left-sided TLE. This is associated with reduced serum testosterone levels, reduced frequency of LH pulsatile secretion, and increased risk of hypothalamic hypogonadism [17, 29].

Enzyme-inducing AEDs (EIAEDs)

Treatment with the EIAEDs CBZ, PHT, and PB is associated with hyposexuality [12, 28, 30]. The effect is likely mediated by their effect on serum levels of androgens and estrogens. Androgens and estrogens (mainly testosterone and estradiol) both stimulate libido and reproductive behavior. As already noted, EIAEDs increase hepatic SHBG synthesis and serum SHBG levels, and induce p450 enzymes involved in catabolism of gonadal steroids. This results in reduced circulating levels of bioactive estradiol and testosterone and the weak androgen dehydroepiandrosterone sulfate (DHEAS) [2]. Free testosterone, androstenedione, and DHEAS levels, and free estradiol and estrone levels, are reduced and serum SHBG levels are increased in women with epilepsy treated with EIAEDs compared with controls or women treated with non-EIAEDs [12, 30, 31]. The changes start to occur within 2 months after EIAED treatment initiation [2, 12], and increase with treatment duration. They are greater in women treated with more than one EIAED than in women treated with a single EIAED [31]. The effects are reversible [12]. Stopping CBZ decreases SHBG levels and increases serum concentrations of free and total testosterone [32]. Switching from CBZ to oxcarbazepine (OXC), which causes less hepatic induction, similarly reduces free testosterone levels [8, 12].

Other AEDs

Non-enzyme-inducing AEDs do not cause hypoandrogenism and have not been implicated in hyposexuality [12, 30, 31]. Women treated with VPA for bipolar affective disorder, however, have been reported to have severely decreased libido and anorgasmia (interestingly, even though their serum testosterone levels may be elevated). There are also case reports of gabapentin-associated anorgasmia [33]. Mechanisms of these effects have not been elucidated.

Clinical implications: Evaluations of hyposexuality in WWE should start with asking about the symptoms, which are not commonly discussed in the clinic. If symptoms of hyposexuality are present, further evaluations should include checking serum testosterone, free testosterone, estradiol, and SHBG levels. If free testosterone or testosterone levels are low and the patient's treatment includes an EIAED, consideration should be given to changing to a non-inducing AED. If this is not possible for reasons of seizure control, alternative therapeutic options include adjunctive treatment with testosterone, e.g. the daily transdermal patch (Androderm) or with long-acting (monthly) depot injection. An endocrinologist or a neuroendocrinologist should best administer these treatments.

Effects of AEDs on hormonal control of glucose and energy metabolism

Several AEDs affect body weight. Valproate, gabapentin, pregabalin, vigabatrin, and possibly carbamazepine may cause weight gain. Topiramate, zonisamide, and felbamate may cause weight loss, as can, infrequently, VPA [34]. The weight-changing effects of AEDs are not gender-specific, although VPA-related weight gain is more common in women.

Weight gain/glucose metabolism

Valproic acid

Treatment with valproic acid is associated with weight gain. This is more common in women, up to 50%, than in men, and is of greater magnitude in women [12, 35, 36]. Women treated with VPA crave carbohydrates more frequently than VPA-treated men (25.8% vs. 14.3%) [36]. In several prospective, randomized studies comparing VPA, CBZ, and TPM treatment in patients with new onset seizures treated for 24–56 weeks, VPA-treated patients had an average weight gain of 2–6 kg compared to CBZ and LMT weight gain (2.8% of baseline weight) [34, 35]. Body mass index (BMI) increase correlates with VPA levels [37]. The weight gain may start early, within the first 3 months of treatment, may increase during the first year of treatment, and then plateau off [35]. It is associated with an increase in plasma levels of insulin, leptin, and neuropeptide y (NPY, "hunger peptide") [35, 38] and with reduced levels of ghrelin ("satiety peptide"). There is an associated adverse impact on lipid profile, with increased triglyceride levels and reduced HDL levels [2]. Weight gain and increased insulin levels occur equally in women treated with VPA for epilepsy and for bipolar affective disorder, and are thus likely to be due to VPA rather than epilepsy [39].

Approximately 20–25% of VPA-treated women with epilepsy (45% of those with weight gain) may develop metabolic syndrome, a pre-diabetic condition characterized by central obesity, insulin resistance and elevated serum insulin levels, dyslipidemia, and hypertension [35, 40]. These women are at risk for developing both type 2 diabetes mellitus (DM) and cardiovascular disease.

While obesity is the biggest risk factor for type 2 diabetes mellitus, possible impact of VPA on DM risk, treatment, and disease course has not been systematically evaluated.

However, several case reports of VPA-related onset of DM have been published. In one case, addition of VPA treatment in a patient with bipolar affective disorder on antipsychotics lead to acute pancreatitis and acute onset of diabetic ketoacidosis which resolved with discontinuation of VPA [41]. In another report, three obese adolescents in whom VPA was added to antipsychotics developed type 2 DM [42].

The mechanism of VPA-induced weight gain appears to be related to insulin resistance [2]. VPA-treated WWE have increased plasma levels of insulin [2]. VPA-treated patients have higher plasma insulin level than control subjects with the same BMI [43]. The hyperinsulinemia may be due to VPA inhibition of liver metabolism of insulin rather than to increased insulin secretion: levels of insulin precursors, proinsulin, and peptide C, which indicate pancreatic insulin secretion, are the same in VPA-treated and control subjects [44]. Increased insulin level leads to increased glucose uptake into fat and liver cells, increased glycogen and fatty acid production, and weight gain. Increased cellular glucose uptake lowers blood glucose, which increases appetite and food intake. Fasting blood glucose levels in VPA-treated WWE are *low* (unlike in insulin resistance in type 2 diabetes, when they are high). Serum insulin and testosterone levels return to normal within 2 months of VPA discontinuation [10].

Gabapentin, pregabalin, vigabatrin

Gabapentin: While weight gain was not reported in the pivotal phase 3 studies of gabapentin (GBP), with 12-week long maintenance treatment and daily GBP doses of <1800 mg/day, in an open label study with higher doses of 1800–>3000 mg/day, long-term GBP treatment was associated with weight gain of >5% baseline body weight in 57% patients; 23% gained more than 10% (reviewed in [34]). There has been one report on GBP-induced *hypoglycemia* [45].

Pregabalin: 10–14% of patients treated with pregabalin in the pivotal randomized, double blind, placebo-controlled studies gained weight. Weight gain was dose-related, affecting 10% of patients treated with 150 mg/day versus 12–14% in patients treated with 600 mg/day [reviewed in [34]]. A recent review of 3,187 patients from 41 studies treated with pregabalin in doses of 150–600 mg/day for all indications, including seizures, painful neuropathy, and fibromyalgia, who were treated for 1 year, showed that 18.2% of patients experienced weight gain of ≥7%: 2.6% gained ≥7% of weight in the first 8 weeks of treatment, the remainder during the remainder of the 1 year of treatment [46]. In another review of six open label studies using pregabalin in adjunctive treatment of refractory epilepsy only, for up to 300 days, 20.8% patients gained weight. Weight gain typically became evident at the end of the first month of treatment. The rate of increase diminished after 4 months [47].

Vigabatrin: Weight gain is a common side effect of vigabatrin, occurring in approximately 10–15% of patients in both adjunctive monotherapy studies with weight gain of 4 kg noted over 1 year of treatment in one open label extension study [48].

Little is known of the pathophysiological mechanisms by which these AEDs may cause weight gain.

Weight loss

Topiramate

Topiramate (TPM) has been known to cause weight loss since the first pilot study which compared daily dosages of 1000 and 100 mg and showed a weight loss incidence of 43% and

13%, respectively [34, 45]. In the pivotal placebo-controlled studies of TPM adjunctive treatment in refractory LRE, 10% of patients had reduced appetite and weight loss [49, 50]. In an open label adjunctive TPM treatment study for 1 year and a median dose of 200 mg/day, weight loss was most common in patients with BMI >30, 7/8 of whom lost >5% of their body weight. There was associated food intake reduction by about 400 kcal/day, compared to 20-kcal/day intake reduction in the non-obese patients [49]. Weight loss with TPM is generally modest, in the order of 5% of BMI. It is more likely to occur in patients who are overweight, and is maximal after about 15–18 months of treatment. It can be higher when used in conjunction with other weight-losing medications such as phentermine. Recently, a combination of slow-release 46 or 92 mg topiramate/day with 7.5 or 15 mg phentermine has been approved by the FDA for weight loss treatment in the USA under the name Qsymia (7.5/46) or Qsymia (15/92). The higher dose of this combination led to a mean weight loss of 10.9% of baseline body weight over 56 weeks [51].

The mechanism of topiramate's weight-losing action is unknown. Topiramate reduces appetite. In animals, it reduces food intake and increases energy expenditure [52]. The anorexigenic effect may occur via enhancement of leptin and insulin-mediated signaling in the hypothalamus, and via reduction of NPY receptors in the hypothalamus [52].

In addition, topiramate increases insulin secretion by the pancreas and increases insulin-mediated glucose uptake, acting as both an insulin secretagogue and sensitizer in animal models of type 2 diabetes. Of interest, topiramate was initially developed as a hypoglycemic agent [53]. It increases, among others, insulin sensitization in adipocytes, resulting in a decrease in plasma glucose level. At 50 and 100 mg/kg/day it ameliorates streptozotocin-induced diabetes mellitus in rats, reducing blood glucose levels, increasing insulin levels, and increasing the number of pancreatic beta islets cells [54].

TPM has recently been evaluated in clinical studies for both weight loss and treatment of type 2 diabetes. TPM doses of 96–192 mg/day used in non-epileptic obese female and male patients with type 2 DM for 16–48 weeks as adjunctive treatment to diet and exercise in three separate studies, resulted in 6.6–9.1% baseline body weight reduction and 0.4 and 1.1% reduction in blood HbA1c levels [53, 55, 56].

Zonisamide, felbamate

Zonisamide: Weight loss effect is less with zonisamide (ZN) than with topiramate [34]. Twenty-two percent of patients with refractory LRE treated adjunctively with 400 mg zonisamide for 3 months in a placebo-controlled study lost weight [57]. A recent placebo-controlled study evaluated ZN and calorie-restricted diet for weight loss in obesity without epilepsy. After 1 year of treatment, mean weight loss was -4.4 kg for 200 mg/day dose and -7.3 kg for 400 mg/day, compared with -4 kg/day in the placebo arm; 22.4% and 32% of the 200 mg and 400 mg ZN-treated groups achieved 10% BMI reduction, compared to 8% in the placebo arm [58].

Felbamate: Felbamate has an anorexic effect. Seventy-five percent of patients with intractable seizures treated adjunctively with felbamate experienced weight loss, with mean weight loss of 3.2 kg (4% of body weight) after 23 weeks of treatment; 11% lost >8 kg. [45].

The mechanism of weight loss for zonisamide and felbamate are not known, nor are their possible effects on glucose and energy homeostasis.

Clinical implications: Weight gain, hyperinsulinemia, and metabolic syndrome should be considered as potential side effects when considering VPA treatment. VPA should not be used in obese patients with DM unless it is the only alternative. Obese patients without

DM should also be treated with VPA only after metabolic syndrome has been ruled out by establishing normal BP, and normal fasting serum insulin levels and lipid profile – and then also only if no alternative AED options exist. Patients started on VPA should have weight/ BMI checked before treatment initiation and regularly afterwards. We suggest checking weight monthly for the first 3 months and every 2 months for the rest of the first year of treatment. Should weight gain of >3kg occur, treatment of the weight gain as well as of seizures should be addressed. Weight-treating options include: (a) addition of topiramate or zonisamide to prevent further weight gain +/- assist with losing weight already gained while reinforcing antiseizure therapy; (b) aggressive dietary management; (c) discontinuing VPA or reducing VPA dose.

The weight-losing potential of topiramate and zonisamide can be beneficial in women with epilepsy with comorbidity of obesity/overweight and diabetes mellitus; or as adjunctive treatment in VPA-treated women with weight gain.

Effects of AEDs on thyroid hormones

Unlike the reproductive endocrine system, thyroid physiology is not impacted by epilepsy. It is, however, affected by several AEDs.

Enzyme-inducing AEDs (EIAEDs)

Thyroid function tests are frequently abnormal in patients of both genders treated with EIAEDs such as CBZ and PHT, and with oxcarbazepine – but not with VPA or other newer AEDs. In patients treated with CBZ, PHT, and OXC, thyroxine (T4) and free thyroxine (fT4) can be down to 70% of their normal values [45, 59]. Serum triiodothyronine (T3) and thyroid-stimulating hormone (TSH) are usually normal and the thyroid-releasing hormone (TRH) stimulating test is always normal [59]. Patients remain clinically euthyroid; the hormone alterations are not associated with clinical or subclinical hypothyroidism [45, 59]. The findings are common and occur in children also: 63% of CBZ-treated girls aged 8–18 and 67% of OXC-treated girls had T4 and fT4 levels below the lower limit of normal in one recent study [60]. Reduction of serum T4 and fT4 levels may start within 3 months of CBZ treatment initiation [61]. The changes remain for the duration of the treatment but values return to normal following discontinuation of CBZ or OXC, in the case of CBZ within 6 months of CBZ withdrawal [60, 61].

The changes may be due to several factors: increased conversion of T4 to T3, induction by EIAEDs of hepatic metabolism of thyroid hormones, competition by EIAEDs and thyroid hormones for thyroid-binding globulin (TBG), and reduction of TBG levels (which occurs more in women than in men).

Clinical manifestations of hypothyroidism with AEDs are rare [59]. In a survey in Germany, 3.9% of patients treated with classical AEDs were taking thyroid hormone supplementation, the same proportion as in the general population [45].

Other AEDs

VPA and newer AEDs without enzyme-inducing properties such as lamotrigine, topiramate, levetiracetam, gabapentin, and pregabalin (PGB) are not known to have a clinically relevant effect on thyroid function.

Clinical implications: Patients treated with EIAEDs or OXC who have low serum T4 +/- T3 are almost always clinically euthyroid. In asymptomatic patients, the changes are of little clinical importance and require no treatment. In thyroxine-substituted hypothyroid patients, the increased peripheral metabolism of thyroid hormones with CBZ may necessitate increasing the dose of thyroxine. Because clinically significant thyroid dysfunction is so uncommon with AED use, routine testing of thyroid function is not needed, except in patients with a pre-existing thyroid disorder or in patients with clinical evidence of hypo/hyperthyroidism. When thyroid function tests are obtained, findings of low total or free thyroid hormone levels do not require treatment adjustment if TSH is normal. If TSH levels are borderline, TRH stimulation tests may help in determining whether or not the patient is functionally hypothyroid. In this setting, evaluation by a neuroendocrinologist or endocrinologist may be warranted. In patients with clinically important thyroid dysfunctions, non-EIAEDs including VPA, LMT, LEV, GBP, and PGB can be used to substitute for EIAEDs or OXC.

Effects of AEDs on antidiuretic hormone/serum sodium/osmolarity homeostasis

As with energy balance, epilepsy does not appear to affect water and osmolarity homeostasis. Some AEDs do, however.

Oxcarbazepine and carbamazepine

OXC and CBZ treatment is associated with hyponatremia in both women and men. Hyponatremia is more common with OXC than with CBZ. The overall frequency of hyponatremia is approximately 3% for severe hyponatremia (Na ≤128 mEq/L) and 14% for mild hyponatremia (Na = 130–134 mEq/L) in CBZ-treated patients, and 8–12% and 25–30%, respectively, for OXC-treated patients [62, 63]. Hyponatremia is more likely to occur with advanced age (e.g., >65 years), in patients with concomitant use of diuretics or other sodium-depleting medications, angiotensin converting enzyme inhibitors and certain antidepressants, in women, and during menstruation. The importance of age is illustrated by frequency of severe hyponatremia (<125 mEq/L) in the patient database compiled from the pre-FDA approval studies: 0.4% in patients <17 years old, 3.8% in 18–64-year-old, and 7.3% in those ≥65 years. The degree of hyponatremia correlates loosely with OXC dose [63]. With CBZ, it is more likely to occur with CBZ serum levels above 6 mcg/ml. Changing from CBZ to OXC may result in reduction of serum sodium level [64].

An acute, dangerous form of OXC- or CBZ-induced hyponatremia may exist, when rate of serum Na fall exceeds 12 mEq/L/day, and levels of <125 mEq/L may be reached in ≤48 hours. This typically occurs postoperatively or with psychogenic polydipsia, especially in women during menstruation.

The pathophysiological mechanism of the hyponatremia has not been fully elucidated. It likely results from several actions of the AEDs: an increase in the sensitivity of renal tubular cells to ADH, a sensitizing effect on the osmolarity-sensing hypothalamic neurons, and possibly a direct effect on renal collecting tubular cells, with an increase in water reabsorption in the collecting tubule [63].

Phenytoin

By contrast, phenytoin (PHY) inhibits ADH release, and concomitant treatment of PHT in CBZ-treated patients with inappropriate ADH may reverse the latter [63].

Other AEDs

Valproate

There have been isolated reports of syndrome of inappropriate antidiuretic hormone secretion (SIADH) occurring with VPA. In one report, four women aged 57–88 years developed severe symptomatic hyponatremia or SIADH after starting VPA [65]. The mechanism by which VPA may cause hyponatremia or SIADH is unknown.

Levetiracetam

There have also been a couple of reports of SIADH and hyponatremia occurring in patients treated with levetiracetam, in one case subsiding with LEV discontinuation and recurring with LEV re-challenge [66]. In addition, LEV may increase the risk of developing hyponatremia in patients treated with OXC and, to a lesser degree, in patients treated with CBZ [63].

Clinical implications: Serum sodium levels should be checked in patients with pre-existing renal impairment or patients being treated with sodium-lowering agents prior to treatment initiation with oxcarbazepine or carbamazepine and then again after 2 weeks. It has been recommended monitoring should continue at monthly intervals for 3 months for OXC. Because of the rarity of hyponatremia with VPA and LEV, sodium levels do not need to be checked either before initiation of treatment or during treatment with these agents.

References

1. Herzog AG, Seibel MM, Schomer DL, et al. Reproductive endocrine disorders in women with partial seizures of temporal lobe origin. *Arch Neurol* 1986; 43:341–6.

2. Isojärvi JI. Reproductive dysfunction in women with epilepsy. *Neurology* 2003; 61(6 Suppl 2):S27–S34.

3. Cummings LN, Giudice L and Morrell MJ. Ovulatory function in epilepsy. *Epilepsia* 1995; 36:355–60.

4. Dansky LV, Andermann E and Andermann F. Marriage and fertility in epileptic patients. *Epilepsia* 1980; 21:261–71.

5. Wallace H, Shorvon S and Tallis R. Age-specific incidence and prevalence rates of treated epilepsy in an unselected population of 2,052,922 and age-specific fertility rates of women with epilepsy. *Lancet* 1998; 352:1970–73.

6. Artama M, Isojärvi JI, Raitanen J, et al. Birth rate among patients with epilepsy: a nationwide population-based cohort study in Finland. *Am J Epidemiol* 2004; 159:1057–63.

7. Sukumaran SC, Sarma PS and Thomas SV. Polytherapy increases the risk of infertility in women with epilepsy. *Neurology* 2010; 75(15):1351–5.

8. Isojärvi JI, Laatikainen TJ, Pakarinen AJ, et al. Menstrual disorders in women with epilepsy receiving carbamazepine. *Epilepsia* 1995; 36:676–81.

9. Isojarvi JIT, Laatikainen TJ, Pakarinen AJ, et al. Polycystic ovaries and hyperandrogenism in women taking valproate for epilepsy. *New Engl J Med* 1993; 329(19):1383–9.

10. Isojärvi JI, Rättyä J, Myllylä VV, et al. Valproate, lamotrigine, and insulin-mediated risks in women with epilepsy. *Ann Neurol* 1998; 43:446–51.

11. Mikkonen K, Vainionpää LK, Pakarinen AJ, et al. Long-term reproductive endocrine health in young women with epilepsy during puberty. *Neurology* 2004; 62:445–50.

12. Isojarvi J. Disorders of reproduction in patients with epilepsy: antiepileptic drug related mechanisms. *Seizure* 2008; 17:111–19.

13. Verrotti A, D'Egidio C, Mohn A, et al. Antiepileptic drugs, sex hormones, and PCOS. *Epilepsia* 2011; 52:199–211.

14. Bauer J, Jarre A, Klingmuller D, et al. Polycystic ovary syndrome in patients with focal epilepsy: a study in 93 women. *Epilepsy Res* 2000; 41:163–7.

15. Bentley-Lewis R, Ellen Seely E and Dunaif A. Ovarian hypertension: polycystic ovary syndrome. *Endocrinol Metab Clin North Am* 2011; 40:433–8.

16. Herzog AG, Coleman AE, Jacobs AR, at al. Interictal EEG discharges, reproductive hormones, and menstrual disorders in epilepsy. *Ann Neurol* 2003; 54:625–37.

17. Herzog AG. Disorders of reproduction in patients with epilepsy: primary neurological mechanisms. *Seizure* 2008; 17:101–10.

18. Rasgon NL, Altshuler LL, Fairbanks L, at al. Reproductive function and risk for PCOS in women treated for bipolar disorder. *Bipolar Disord* 2005; 7:246–59.

19. Sahota P, Prabhakar S, Kharbanda PS, at al. Seizure type, antiepileptic drugs, and reproductive endocrine dysfunction in Indian women with epilepsy: a cross-sectional study. *Epilepsia* 2008; 49:2069–77.

20. Morrell MJ, Hayes FJ, Sluss PM, at al. Hyperandrogenism, ovulatory dysfunction, polycystic ovary syndrome with valproate versus lamotrigine. *Ann Neurol* 2008; 64:200–11.

21. Speroff L, Glass RH and Kase NG. *Clinical gynecologic endocrinology and infertility.* 7th edn. Philadelphia, IL: Lippincott Williams & Wilkins, 2004.

22. Taubøll E, Gregoraszczuk EL, Kołodziej A, at al. Valproate inhibits the conversion of testosterone to estradiol and acts as an apoptotic agent in growing porcine ovarian follicular cells. *Epilepsia* 2003; 44:1014–21.

23. Nelson-DeGrave VL, Wickenheisser JK, Cockrell JE, at al. Valproate potentiates androgen biosynthesis in human ovarian theca cells. *Endocrinology* 2004; 145:799–808.

24. Svalheim S, Taubøll E, Luef G, at al. Differential effects of levetiracetam, carbamazepine, and lamotrigine on reproductive endocrine function in adults. *Epilepsy Behav* 2009; 16:281–7.

25. Margraf JW and Dreifuss FE. Amenorrhea following initiation of therapy with valproic acid. *Neurology* 1981; 31(Suppl): S159.

26. Klein P, Serje A and Pezzullo JC. Premature ovarian failure in women with epilepsy. *Epilepsia* 2001; 42:1584–9.

27. Morrell MJ and Guldner GT. Self-reported sexual function and sexual arousability in women with epilepsy. *Epilepsia* 1996; 37:1204–10.

28. Morrell MJ, Flynn KL, DoÇe S, et al. Sexual dysfunction, sex steroid hormone abnormalities, and depression in women with epilepsy treated with antiepileptic drugs. *Epilepsy Behav* 2005; 6:360–5.

29. Herzog AG, Coleman AE, Jacobs AR, at al. Relationship of sexual dysfunction to epilepsy laterality and reproductive hormone levels in women. *Epilepsy Behav* 2003; 4:407–13.

30. Morrell MJ, Flynn KL, Seale CG, at al. Reproductive dysfunction in women with epilepsy: antiepileptic drug effects on sex-steroid hormones. *CNS Spectr* 2001; 6:783–6.

31. Galimberti CA, Magri F, Copello F, at al. Changes in sex steroid levels in women with epilepsy on treatment: relationship with antiepileptic therapies and seizure frequency. *Epilepsia* 2009; 50: (Suppl 1):28–32.

32. Lossius MI, Taubøll E, Mowinckel P, et al. Reversible effects of antiepileptic drugs on reproductive endocrine function in men and women with epilepsy – a prospective randomized double-blind withdrawal study. *Epilepsia* 2007; 48:1875–82.

33. Harden CL. Sexuality in women with epilepsy. *Epilepsy Behav* 2005; 7(Suppl 2): S2–S6.

34. Ben-Menachem E. Weight issues for people with epilepsy – a review. *Epilepsia* 2007; 48(Suppl 9):42–5.

35. Verrotti A, D'Egidio C, Mohn A, at al. Weight gain following treatment with valproic acid: pathogenetic mechanisms and clinical implications. *Obes Rev* 2011; 12:e32–43.

36. El-Khatib F, Rauchenzauner M, Lechleitner M, et al. Valproate, weight gain and carbohydrate craving: a gender study. *Seizure* 2007; 16:226–32.

37. Abaci A, Saygi M and Yis U. Metabolic alterations during valproic acid treatment: a prospective study. *Pediatr Neurol* 2009; 41:435–9

38. Tokgoz H, Aydin K, Oran B, et al. Plasma leptin, neuropeptide Y, ghrelin, and adiponectin levels and carotid artery intima media thickness in epileptic children treated with valproate. *Childs Nerv Syst* 2012; 28:1049–53.

39. Chang HH, Yang YK, Gean PW, et al. The role of valproate in metabolic disturbances in bipolar disorder patients. *J Affect Disord* 2010; 124:319–23.

40. Verrotti A, Manco R, Agostinelli S, et al. The metabolic syndrome in overweight epileptic patients treated with valproic acid. *Epilepsia* 2010; 51:268–73.

41. Laghate VD and Gupta SB. Acute pancreatitis and diabetic ketoacidosis in non-diabetic person while on treatment with sodium valproate, chlorpromazine and haloperidol. *J Assoc Physicians India* 2004; 52:257–8.

42. Saito E and Kafantaris V. Can diabetes mellitus be induced by medication? *J Child Adolesc Psychopharmacol* 2002; 12:231–6.

43. Pylvänen V, Knip M, Pakarinen A, et al. Serum insulin and leptin levels in valproate-associated obesity. *Epilepsia* 2002; 43:514–7.

44. Pylvänen V, Pakarinen A, Knip M, et al. Characterization of insulin secretion in valproate-treated patients with epilepsy. *Epilepsia* 2006; 47:1460–4.

45. Steinhoff BJ. Optimizing therapy of seizures in patients with endocrine disorders. *Neurology* 2006; 67(Suppl 4): S23–S7.

46. Cabrera J, Emir B, Dills D, et al. Characterizing and understanding body weight patterns in patients treated with pregabalin. *Curr Med Res Opin* 2012; 28:1027–37.

47. Uthman BM, Bazil CW, Beydoun A, et al. Long-term add-on pregabalin treatment in patients with partial-onset epilepsy: pooled analysis of open-label clinical trials. *Epilepsia* 2010; 51:968–78.

48. Guberman A and Bruni J. Long-term open multicentre, add-on trial of vigabatrin in adult resistant partial epilepsy. The Canadian Vigabatrin Study Group. *Seizure* 2000; 9:112–8.

49. Ben-Menachem E, Axelsen M, Johanson EH, et al. Predictors of weight loss in adults with topiramate-treated epilepsy. *Obes Res* 2003; 11:556–62

50. Arroyo S, Dodson WE, Privitera MD, et al. Investigators randomized dose-controlled study of topiramate as first-line therapy in epilepsy. *Acta Neurol Scand* 2005; 112:214–22.

51. Allison DB, Gadde KM, Garvey WT, et al. Controlled-release phentermine/topiramate in severely obese adults: a randomized controlled trial (EQUIP). *Obesity (Silver Spring)* 2012; 20:330–42.

52. Caricilli AM, Penteado E, de Abreu LL, et al. Topiramate treatment improves hypothalamic insulin and leptin signaling and action and reduces obesity in mice. *Endocrinology* 2012; 153:4401–11.

53. Khanna V, Arumugam S, Roy S, et al. Topiramate and type 2 diabetes: an old wine in a new bottle. *Expert Opin Ther Targets* 2008; 12:81–90.

54. Shafik AN. Effects of topiramate on diabetes mellitus induced by streptozotocin in rats. *Eur J Pharmacol* 2012; 684:161–7.

55. Stenlöf K, Rössner S, Vercruysse F, et al. OBDM-OBDM-003 Study Group. Topiramate in the treatment of obese subjects with drug-naive type 2 diabetes. *Diabetes Obes Metab* 2007; 9:360–8.

56. Rosenstock J, Hollander P, Gadde KM, et al. OBD-202 Study Group. A randomized, double-blind, placebo-controlled, multicenter study to assess the efficacy and safety of topiramate controlled release in the treatment of obese type 2 diabetic patients. *Diabetes Care* 2007; 30:1480–6.

57. Faught E, Ayala R, Montouris GG, et al. Zonisamide 922 Trial Group. Randomized controlled trial of zonisamide for the

treatment of refractory partial-onset seizures. *Neurology* 2001; 57:1774–9.

58. Gadde KM, Kopping MF, Wagner HR, et al. Zonisamide for weight reduction in obese adults: a 1-year randomized controlled trial. *Arch Intern Med* 2012; 15:1–8.

59. Pennell PB. Hormonal aspects of epilepsy. *Neurol Clin* 2009; 27:941–65.

60. Vainionpää LK, Mikkonen K, Rättyä J, et al. Thyroid function in girls with epilepsy with carbamazepine, oxcarbazepine, or valproate monotherapy and after withdrawal of medication. *Epilepsia* 2004; 45:197–203.

61. Verrotti A, Laus M, Scardapane A, et al. Thyroid hormones in children with epilepsy during long-term administration of carbamazepine and valproate. *Eur J Endocrinol* 2009; 160:81–6.

62. Dong X, Leppik IE, White J, et al. Hyponatremia from oxcarbazepine and carbamazepine. *Neurology* 2005; 27:1976–8.

63. Lin CH, Lu CH, Wang FJ, et al. Risk factors of oxcarbazepine-induced hyponatremia in patients with epilepsy. *Clin Neuropharmacol* 2010; 33:293–6.

64. Isojärvi JI, Huuskonen UE, Pakarinen AJ, et al. The regulation of serum sodium after replacing carbamazepine with oxcarbazepine. *Epilepsia* 2001; 42:741–5.

65. Beers E, van Puijenbroek EP, Bartelink IH, et al. Syndrome of inappropriate antidiuretic hormone secretion (SIADH) or hyponatraemia associated with valproic acid: four case reports from the Netherlands and a case/non-case analysis of vigibase. *Drug Saf* 2010; 33:47–55.

66. Nasrallah K and Silver B. Hyponatremia associated with repeated use of levetiracetam. *Epilepsia* 2005; 46:972–3.

Genetic causes of epilepsies in women

Danielle Molinari Andrade

Key points:

- Important gender differences exist among different genetic epilepsy syndromes
- Epilepsy syndromes with mutations involving the X chromosome have distinct gender-dependent phenotypes (Rett syndrome, subcortical band heterotopia, epilepsy and mental retardation limited to females, and Aicardi syndrome)
- Idiopathic generalized epilepsy has a slightly higher incidence in females
- Juvenile myoclonic epilepsy (JME) has a female preference with some familial forms of JME having a predominantly maternal transmission

Introduction

The incidence of epilepsy and unprovoked seizures is slightly higher in males compared to females. This difference is mainly due to men's greater exposure to risk factors leading to lesional epilepsy and acute symptomatic seizures such as traumatic brain injury. Conversely, the most common form of epilepsy, idiopathic generalized epilepsy, which is genetically transmitted in most cases, has a slightly higher incidence in women and certain subtypes are commonly transmitted through the mother [1]. The epilepsy syndromes limited to females are frequently associated to mutated genes on the X chromosome. Here we describe the clinical and genetic factors associated to them.

Rett syndrome (RTT)

Clinical manifestations: Rett syndrome (RTT) is a neurodevelopmental disorder affecting mainly females [2]. The *MeCP2* gene is responsible for the majority of cases of RTT. Some patients with atypical, and rare patients with typical, RTT have mutations in *CDKL5* or less commonly *FOXG1* genes.

Classic (typical) RTT is characterized by early normal development (until 6–12 months) before the clinical symptoms appear. This is followed by a period of stagnation or regression in cognitive and social skills, loss of language, and loss of purposeful hand movements. Abnormal gait and growth failure also become evident in the following months and years [3, 4]. Microcephaly is an important, but not universal manifestation. Head circumference is

Women with Epilepsy, ed. Esther Bui and Autumn Klein. Published by Cambridge University Press.
© Cambridge University Press 2014.

normal until 3 months but falls to the 2nd percentile by 2 years. Length is also normal at birth but falls to the 5th percentile by 7 years [5].

Other manifestations include periods of inconsolable crying during early infancy. Later stereotypic (midline) hand movements, autism, constipation, gastroesophageal reflux, air swallowing, sleep cycle abnormalities, breathing problems (apnea and/or hyperventilation), and scoliosis can appear. Extrapyramidal disturbances are common and include: oculogyric crisis, dystonia, bruxism, proximal myoclonus, rigidity, bradykenisia, and hypomimia [6].

Epilepsy is frequently associated with RTT and negatively impacts the quality of life of patients and caregivers [7]. In typical RTT, seizures usually start between the ages of 3–20 years. Atypical RTT may manifest seizures from birth. Incidence of epilepsy varies between 48–86%, depending on the methodology and age of population studied [8, 9]. Given the complex nature of the condition, some paroxysmal events called seizures by parents are indeed non-epileptic events. Examples of such behaviors include: apnea, hyperventilation, behavioral arrest or "freezing" episodes, inappropriate screaming or laughter, dystonia, tremulousness, and limpness. Glaze and colleagues reported that only one-third of such parent-reported seizure behaviors were associated with ictal EEG findings [10]. Their subsequent study showed that a careful review of reported seizure behavior by clinicians determined that only 48% of the RTT participants were having seizures, in contrast to the parent report of 60% [9, 10].

Seizure characteristics: A large study of 528 patients with RTT looked at the seizure frequency in those with epilepsy. Frequency varied widely, with 1–2 seizures per year, monthly seizures, weekly seizures, and daily seizures in 36, 27, 20, and 11%, respectively. Those with more frequent seizures were overall more severely affected [9]. Seizures presenting in the first year of life are usually more difficult to control than seizures appearing later [11]. Seizure types include complex partial with multifocal onset, generalized tonic-clonic, atypical absences, myoclonic, and secondarily generalized seizures. Patients with atypical RTT due to *CDKL5* gene mutations may present with early onset infantile spasms and migrating focal seizures [8, 12]. Electrical status epilepticus during sleep (ESES) can be seen in up to 10% of patients [11].

There is no specific treatment for seizures in RTT. Carbamazepine and sulthiame have been proposed as good treatment options [13]. Others have favored lamotrigine and valproic acid (VPA) [14]. Given that VPA is a histone deacetylase (HDAC) inhibitor and RTT may be associated with HDAC dysfunction (see below), there are concerns that VPA may worsen the disease.

RTT prevalence is 0.5–0.75 per 10,000 girls worldwide [15–19]. So far there has been no evidence of any racial or ethnic predisposition.

Life expectancy: Analysis of a large database including RTT patients from the United States and Canada reveals that patients with RTT survive well into adulthood [20]. Therefore, adult neurologists should become familiar with the condition. Most patients with typical RTT live at least until 45 years of age. Patients with atypical forms may live longer. Cardiac abnormalities and frequent, pharmacoresistant seizures may increase the chances of sudden death.

Radiology/pathology: Most RTT brains are small and do not grow after 4 years of age. There is no evidence of brain degeneration. There is no evidence of macroscopic malformation of cortical development. However, there is a striking decrease in the dendritic trees of selected cortical areas, chiefly projection neurons of the motor, association, and limbic cortices. It is suggested that this may result from abnormalities of trophic factors [21].

Genetics

RTT is sporadic in more than 99% of cases, caused by de novo mutations. So far three genes have been shown to cause RTT: *MeCP2*, *CDKL5*, and *FOXG1*.

MeCP2

MeCP2 (methyl-CpG-binding protein 2) gene causes 50–95% of typical RTT cases, and up to 58% of atypical RTT cases. *MeCP2* maps to chromosome Xq28 [22]. *MeCP2* is a gene silencer by binding to methilated CpG islands in other gene's promoters and repressing their transcription [23, 24]. However, so far it is not clear which genes are affected by *MeCP2* [25, 26]. *MeCP2* associates to histone deacetylase (HDAC) in order to silence other genes. Since valproic acid is a HDAC inhibitor, some experts suggest that its use in patients with RTT may worsen phenotype.

Why RTT affects predominantly females

Given the random brain inactivation of one of the X chromosomes, it is likely that some *MeCP2* normal expression allows women to survive, while this is not enough to prevent the symptoms. Given that all *MeCP2* expressed in male embryos derive from the only X chromosome carrying the mutated gene, these embryos cannot survive. Possible exceptions are cases of Klinefelter syndrome, where a male has two X chromosomes, or mosaics.

MeCP2 duplication in men: a different syndrome. Although males with *MeCP2* deletion usually do not survive, duplication of this same gene causes a neurodevelopment disorder characterized by mild dysmorphic features (brachycephaly, midface hypoplasia, depressed nasal bridge), infantile hypotonia, developmental delay to profound mental retardation, absent or minimal speech. These patients also present with seizures (focal and/or generalized) and autism. Progressive spasticity of lower extremities as they age has been observed [27]. Frequent and severe respiratory infections are a common cause of death.

CDKL5

Mutations in the X-linked gene cyclin-dependent kinase-like 5 (*CDKL5*) cause an X-linked encephalopathy with early onset intractable epilepsy (atypical RTT) or a RTT-like phenotype [28, 29]. *CDKL5* mutations may also lead to a severe phenotype of early onset seizures and encephalopathy in boys [30].

CDKL5 and *MeCP2* genes' expression overlap during neural maturation and synaptogenesis. These two genes interact in vivo and in vitro. *CDKL5* possesses kinase activity and is able to autophosphorylate as well as to mediate *MeCP2* phosphorylation, suggesting that these two genes belong to the same molecular pathway [31]. Rare males with RTT-like symptoms have been shown to have *CDKL5* mutations [32].

FOXG1

Mutations in the *FOXG1* gene were identified in girls with congenital variant RTT (without a previous period of normal development). Head circumference is normal at birth but microcephaly is seen as early as 3 months [33–35]. However, some cases of typical RTT may also be caused by *FOXG1* mutations [35].

FOXG1 encodes a developmental transcription factor with repressor activities [36]. It maps to chromosome 14. Interestingly, there is also overlapping of expression of *FOXG1* and *MeCP2* genes in differentiating cortical compartments and neuronal subnuclear localization [33].

Subcortical band heterotopia (SBH)

SBH is also known as double cortex. This is a malformation of cortical development or neuronal migration disorder.

Clinical manifestations: Patients with SBH may have mild to moderate cognitive delay and frequently have seizures. Seizure types are varied, as is age of onset. Seizure and cognitive dysfunction severity are thought to be related to the thickness of the subcortical band. The overwhelming majority of affected patients are females, although some rare males have been described with SBH [37, 38].

Radiology/pathology: SBH is characterized by bilateral bands of heterotopic gray matter located in the white matter between the cortex and ventricles. The bands usually extend from the frontal to the occipital regions, usually with a frontal predominance (anterior-posterior gradient; see Figure 6.1). Rarely the bands are only frontal or only occipito-parietal. The heterotopic gray matter consists of a superficial zone of disorganized neurons, an intermediate zone of neurons with rudimentary columnization, and a deeper zone where

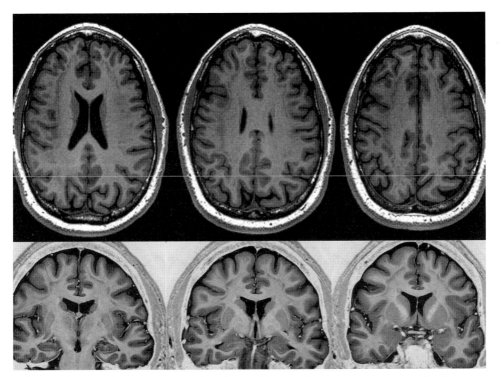

Figure 6.1: Subcortical band heterotopia. Bilateral areas of heterotopic gray matter are seen running the anterior-posterior axis, forming long bands. Courtesy of Dr. Timo Krings.

heterotopia may break into nodules. The overlying cortex is usually normal [39], although rarely SBH can merge frontally with the pachygyric cortex [40].

Genetics

The majority of patients with identified genetic mutations carry an abnormality on the X-linked *DCX* gene [41–45]. *DCX* mutations are seen in 100% of familial cases and in 53% [46] to 84% [47] of sporadic, diffuse, or anteriorly predominant band heterotopia cases. Multiplex ligation-dependent probe amplification has increased the detection of large genomic deletions in the *DCX* gene in patients with no identifiable mutations on gene sequencing [48, 49].

DCX codes for doublecortin, a protein expressed during embryogenesis in migrating neurons and in the cortical plate [44, 45, 50, 51]. Both *DCX* and *LIS1* (see below) appear to interact and to enhance tubulin polymerization in order to maintain proper microtubule function [52]. Microtubule proper functioning is necessary for neuronal migration and *DCX* appears to be regulated by phosphorylation through *CDK5* [53].

Why most SBH patients are female: The proposed mechanism is that in females the neurons with the mutant gene inactive (on the inactivated X chromosome) migrate normally to the cortex, and those neurons with the mutant gene active migrate abnormally to form the SBH. It is believed that surviving male embryos carrying mutations in the *DCX* gene develop lissencephaly instead of SBH. Rare cases of SBH in males were seen in patients with somatic mosaicism, suggesting that somatic mosaicism in males is the equivalent of X inactivation in females [37]. Some males may inherit a mutated *DCX* gene from their mothers. Interestingly, it was demonstrated that a few women with mild mental retardation, with or without epilepsy but with normal MRIs, had children affected with SBH. Some of these women had children with a mild phenotype, suggesting the mutation was mild also in the female carriers. However in another two families, the probands were severely affected, likely reflecting a severe mutation in the carrier mothers. Skewed X inactivation was observed in these carriers' lymphocytes. Although this same mechanism cannot be proven to occur in the brain, it might explain the heterogeneity in the female carriers [54].

Rare cases of posterior SBH are due to *LIS1* gene missense mutations [38] or mosaicism [55]. Rarely trisomy of 9p can lead to SBH [56].

Epilepsy and mental retardation limited to females (EFMR)

This condition is an X-linked disease that may be recognized by the analysis of large pedigrees with multiple affected females linked through unaffected male relatives [57]. The pattern of transmission is more difficult to recognize in small pedigrees with only one affected female.

Clinical manifestations: 67% of patients with EFMR have borderline intellect or intellectual disability varying from mild to profound. Obsessive features are seen in more than 30%, aggressive behavior in 25%, and autism spectrum disorders in 22% [58]. The early psychomotor development can vary from normal to severely abnormal. Some patients may have schizophreniform episodes in early adulthood. Interestingly, in one family five male obligate carriers had obsessive traits, and controlling, rigid, and inflexible personalities [59].

Seizures in EFMR usually start between 3–36 months of age. Initially, febrile seizures are seen in 63% of patients. However, subsequent seizures are mainly afebrile. Seizure types vary from hemimyclonic, complex partial, generalized tonic-clonic, atonic, myoclonic, and absence. In some families, patients stop having seizures after the age of 12 years. The clinical severity also varies. Some patients may have seizures controlled after a certain age, while others may have intractable seizures and several episodes of status epilepticus [58–60].

Genetics EFMR is caused by mutations in the protocadherin 19 (*PCDH19*) gene [60], which also localizes to the X chromosome. The protein encoded by this gene is a member of the delta-2 protocadherin subclass of the cadherin superfamily. The encoded protein is thought to be a calcium-dependent, cell-adhesion protein that is primarily expressed in the brain. Three transcript variants encoding different isoforms have been found for this gene [61].

Why EFMR affects only females?

This condition is different from those described above, where affected males would die in uterus. Here, the males with the mutation are usually normal and able to reproduce. Dibbens and colleagues proposed the following mechanism: "Since the *PCDH19* gene is subject to X inactivation, hemizygous transmitting males likely have a homogenous population of *PCDH19*-mutated cells, while affected females are likely to be mosaics comprising *PCDH19*-mutated cells and *PCDH19*-wildtype cells. This tissue mosaicism may scramble cell-cell communication which manifests clinically as EFMR. The absence of *PCDH19* function in males may be compensated by the related but non-paralogous procadherin gene *PCDH11Y*, a Y-chromosome gene expressed in human brain. *PCDH11Y* has a X chromosome paralogue, *PCDH11X*, that has strong sequence similarity" [61].

Aicardi syndrome

This is also a neurodevelopmental disorder affecting mainly girls.

Clinical manifestations: Aicardi syndrome (AS) is characterized by a triad of corpus callosum (partial or total) agenesis, infantile spasms and chorioretinal lacunae. Most patients have severe intellectual disability, malformation of cortical development, and vertebral and rib deformities.

Dysmorphic features are common and include: prominent premaxila, upturned nasal tip, decreased angle of the nasal bridge, and sparse lateral eyebrows. Externally apparent microphthalmia is present in up to 25% of cases [62].

Epilepsy in AS can range from mild (rarely) to very severe [63], with several forms of pharmacoresistant seizures. Seizures types include: infantile spasms, myoclonic, tonic, atonic, generalized tonic-clonic, atypical absence, complex partial, and reflex audiogenic seizures [64–67].

Radiology: The largest study of girls with AS showed that in addition to the known total or partial agenesis of corpus callosum, all patients had polymicrogyria that was predominantly frontal and perisylvian, and often associated with underopercularization. Periventricular nodular heterotopia was also present in all patients. Cerebellar abnormalities were seen in 95% of cases. Tectal enlargement was seen in 10 out of 23 cases studied. Single or multiple cysts were observed in 21 out of 23 cases [68].

Life expectancy: There is little information on the life expectancy of girls with AS. One report on 69 patients demonstrated a median age of survival of 18.5 (+/- 4 years).

Genetics AS is a sporadic disease. Given that almost all cases are seen in females, this condition is thought to be an X-linked disorder with lethality in the hemizygous male embryo. Some cases are associated with chromosomal translocations with breakpoints in the Xp22 region, however the specific causative gene has not been identified in that region [69]. The rare males with AS identified only recently were patients with Klinefelter syndrome (XXY), however, more recently one genotypic male (XY) was described with classic features of AS [70, 71]. In 2009, one case of classic AS was reported in a patient with monosomy 1p36 [72].

Juvenile myoclonic epilepsy (JME)

Clinical manifestations: Patients with JME present with myoclonic jerks, usually in the morning period, and generalized tonic-clonic seizures. Some atypical JME patients, especially those belonging to multiplex families, may have a history of absence or astatic (atonic) seizures in addition to myoclonus and generalized tonic-clonic seizures [78]. Seizure onset in typical JME patients is between 8 and 20 years and seizures usually continue for life [73].

Epidemiology: JME affects 10% of all patients with epilepsy, making it one of the most common epilepsy subtypes [73–75]. Although it affects both men and women, there is a female preference [76, 77]. In addition, some familial forms of JME have a maternal transmission [78].

Life expectancy: Normal. Unfortunately 74% of patients with JME for 20 years or more develop at least one unfavorable social outcome such as unemployment or unplanned pregnancy [79].

Radiology/pathology: No structural brain abnormalities are seen on routine MRI of patients with JME.

Genetics JME is one of the most heritable forms of epilepsy [80]; however, the precise mechanism of transmission is not clear [81–85]. Large efforts have been employed to identify the genetic basis of common epilepsies such as the idiopathic generalized epilepsies and specifically the JME subtype [73, 78, 80, 86–93]. JME is highly genetically determined, with concordance rates in monozygotic twins of up to 94% [73, 89, 94–98]. In extremely rare families (less than 1%) JME is inherited in Mendelian fashion, and in these families disease genes have been identified, including *EFHC1*, *CLCN2*, and *GABRA1* [81, 99, 100]. The vast majority of JME families are genetically complex. Not all multiplex families have "pure" JME [78, 82, 101, 102]. Multiplex families of JME probands are divided into: (i) families where all affected have classic JME (72%); (ii) families where some or most individuals present with childhood absence epilepsy which later evolves into JME as they grow older (18% of families); (iii) families where JME patients also develop adolescent onset absence seizures (7%); and (iv) families with JME individuals who also develop astatic (atonic) seizures (3%) [78]. In groups (i) and (ii) there is a higher maternal than paternal transmission. In groups (iii) and (iv) the maternal/paternal transmission rate is equal. No specific genes were associated with maternal/paternal transmission.

Conclusion

So far, genetic forms of epilepsy affecting mainly women are usually associated with several other clinical manifestations, especially cognitive delay. The majority of the known genes associated with these conditions localize to the X chromosome, and despite genetic heterogeneity, they have a simple Mendelian inheritance. Genetics of the more common and pure epilepsy syndrome of JME is much more complex, with unclear mechanisms affecting several genes.

To date, there is no specific treatment for these genetically determined seizures in women. Furthermore, most of these syndromes present in early childhood, and the long-term outcome is poorly known. Advances in molecular genetics research and diagnosis will lead to a better understanding of pathology, disease's natural history, and hopefully tailored treatment of seizures in these conditions.

References

1. Doose H and Neubauer BA. Preponderance of female sex in the transmission of seizure liability in idiopathic generalized epilepsy. *Epilepsy Res* 2001; 43:103–14.

2. Hagberg B and Hagberg G. Rett syndrome: epidemiology and geographical variability. *Eur Child Adolesc Psychiatry* 1997; 6(Suppl 1):5–7.

3. Hagberg B. *Rett syndrome: clinical and biologic aspects*. London: McKeith Press, 1992.

4. Hagberg B. The Rett syndrome: an introductory overview 1990. *Brain Dev* 1992; 14(Suppl):S5–S8.

5. Schultz RJ, Glaze DG, Motil KJ, et al. The pattern of growth failure in Rett syndrome. *Am J Dis Child* 1993; 147:633–7.

6. FitzGerald PM, Jankovic J and Percy AK. Rett syndrome and associated movement disorders. *Mov Disord* 1990; 5:195–202.

7. Bahi-Buisson N, Guellec I, Nabbout R, et al. Parental view of epilepsy in Rett Syndrome. *Brain Dev* 2008; 30:126–30.

8. Pintaudi M, Calevo MG, Vignoli A, et al. Epilepsy in Rett syndrome: clinical and genetic features. *Epilepsy Behav*; 19:296–300.

9. Glaze DG, Percy AK, Skinner S, et al. Epilepsy and the natural history of Rett syndrome. *Neurology* 2010; 74:909–12.

10. Glaze DG, Schultz RJ and Frost JD. Rett syndrome: characterization of seizures versus non-seizures. *Electroencephalogr Clin Neurophysiol* 1998; 106:79–83.

11. Nissenkorn A, Gak E, Vecsler M, et al. Epilepsy in Rett syndrome–the experience of a National Rett Center. *Epilepsia* 2010; 51:1252–8.

12. Archer HL, Evans J, Edwards S, et al. CDKL5 mutations cause infantile spasms, early onset seizures, and severe mental retardation in female patients. *J Med Genet* 2006; 43:729–34.

13. Huppke P, Kohler K, Brockmann K, et al. Treatment of epilepsy in Rett syndrome. *Eur J Paediatr Neurol* 2007; 11:10–16.

14. Jian L, Nagarajan L, de Klerk N, et al. Seizures in Rett syndrome: an overview from a one-year calendar study. *Eur J Paediatr Neurol* 2007; 11:310–7.

15. Kozinetz CA, Skender ML, MacNaughton N, et al. Epidemiology of Rett syndrome: a population-based registry. *Pediatrics* 1993; 91:445–50.

16. Bienvenu T, Philippe C, De Roux N, et al. The incidence of Rett syndrome in France. *Pediatr Neurol* 2006; 34:372–5.

17. Hagberg B. Rett's syndrome: prevalence and impact on progressive severe mental retardation in girls. *Acta Paediatr Scand* 1985; 74:405–8.

18. Kerr AM and Stephenson JB. Rett's syndrome in the west of Scotland. *Br Med J (Clin Res Ed)* 1985; 291:579–82.

19. Leonard H, Bower C and English D. The prevalence and incidence of Rett syndrome in Australia. *Eur Child Adolesc Psychiatry* 1997; 6(Suppl 1):8–10.

20. Kirby RS, Lane JB, Childers J, et al. Longevity in Rett syndrome: analysis of the North American Database. *J Pediatr* 2010; 156:135–8.

21. Armstrong DD, Dunn JK, Schultz RJ, et al. Organ growth in Rett syndrome: a postmortem examination analysis. *Pediatr Neurol* 1999; 20:125–9.

22. Amir RE, Van den Veyver IB, Wan M, et al. Rett syndrome is caused by mutations in X-linked MECP2, encoding methyl-CpG-binding protein 2. *Nat Genet* 1999; 23:185–8.

23. Nan X, Ng HH, Johnson CA, et al. Transcriptional repression by the methyl-CpG-binding protein MeCP2 involves a

histone deacetylase complex. *Nature* 1998; 393:386–9.

24. Jones PL, Veenstra GJ, Wade PA, et al. Methylated DNA and MeCP2 recruit histone deacetylase to repress transcription. *Nat Genet* 1998; 19:187–91.

25. Traynor J, Agarwal P, Lazzeroni L, et al. Gene expression patterns vary in clonal cell cultures from Rett syndrome females with eight different MECP2 mutations. *BMC Med Genet* 2002; 3:12.

26. Tudor M, Akbarian S, Chen RZ, et al. Transcriptional profiling of a mouse model for Rett syndrome reveals subtle transcriptional changes in the brain. *Proc Natl Acad Sci U S A* 2002; 99:15536–41.

27. Ramocki MB, Tavyev YJ and Peters SU. The MECP2 duplication syndrome. *Am J Med Genet A* 2010; 152A:1079–88.

28. Kalscheuer VM, Tao J, Donnelly A, et al. Disruption of the serine/threonine kinase 9 gene causes severe X-linked infantile spasms and mental retardation. *Am J Hum Genet* 2003; 72:1401–11.

29. Bahi-Buisson N, Nectoux J, Rosas-Vargas H, et al. Key clinical features to identify girls with CDKL5 mutations. *Brain* 2008; 131:2647–61.

30. Liang JS, Shimojima K, Takayama R, et al. CDKL5 alterations lead to early epileptic encephalopathy in both genders. *Epilepsia*; 52:1835–42.

31. Mari F, Azimonti S, Bertani I, et al. CDKL5 belongs to the same molecular pathway of MeCP2 and it is responsible for the early-onset seizure variant of Rett syndrome. *Hum Mol Genet* 2005; 14:1935–46.

32. Weaving LS, Christodoulou J, Williamson SL, et al. Mutations of CDKL5 cause a severe neurodevelopmental disorder with infantile spasms and mental retardation. *Am J Hum Genet* 2004; 75:1079–93.

33. Ariani F, Hayek G, Rondinella D, et al. FOXG1 is responsible for the congenital variant of Rett syndrome. *Am J Hum Genet* 2008; 83:89–93.

34. Mencarelli MA, Spanhol-Rosseto A, Artuso R, et al. Novel FOXG1 mutations associated with the congenital variant of Rett syndrome. *J Med Genet* 2010; 47:49–53.

35. Philippe C, Amsallem D, Francannet C, et al. Phenotypic variability in Rett syndrome associated with FOXG1 mutations in females. *J Med Genet* 2010; 47:59–65.

36. Murphy DB, Wiese S, Burfeind P, et al. Human brain factor 1, a new member of the fork head gene family. *Genomics* 1994; 21:551–7.

37. Poolos NP, Das S, Clark GD, et al. Males with epilepsy, complete subcortical band heterotopia, and somatic mosaicism for DCX. *Neurology* 2002; 58:1559–62.

38. Pilz DT, Kuc J, Matsumoto N, et al. Subcortical band heterotopia in rare affected males can be caused by missense mutations in DCX (XLIS) or LIS1. *Hum Mol Genet* 1999; 8:1757–60.

39. Harding AC. Malformations. In: Graham DI and Lantos PL, eds. *Greenfield's Neuropathology*, 7th edn. London: Arnold, 2002; 396–417.

40. Dobyns WB, Truwit CL, Ross ME, et al. Differences in the gyral pattern distinguish chromosome 17-linked and X-linked lissencephaly. *Neurology* 1999; 53:270–7.

41. des Portes V, Pinard JM, Smadja D, et al. Dominant X linked subcortical laminar heterotopia and lissencephaly syndrome (XSCLH/LIS): evidence for the occurrence of mutation in males and mapping of a potential locus in Xq22. *J Med Genet* 1997; 34:177–83.

42. Ross ME, Allen KM, Srivastava AK, et al. Linkage and physical mapping of X-linked lissencephaly/SBH (XLIS): a gene causing neuronal migration defects in human brain. *Hum Mol Genet* 1997; 6:555–62.

43. Sossey-Alaoui K, Hartung AJ, Guerrini R, et al. Human doublecortin (DCX) and the homologous gene in mouse encode a putative Ca2+-dependent signaling protein which is mutated in human X-linked neuronal migration defects. *Hum Mol Genet* 1998; 7:1327–32.

44. Gleeson JG, Minnerath SR, Fox JW, et al. Characterization of mutations in the gene

doublecortin in patients with double cortex syndrome. *Ann Neurol* 1999; 45:146–53.

45. des Portes V, Pinard JM, Billuart P, et al. A novel CNS gene required for neuronal migration and involved in X-linked subcortical laminar heterotopia and lissencephaly syndrome. *Cell* 1998; 92:51–61.

46. Gleeson JG, Luo RF, Grant PE, et al. Genetic and neuroradiological heterogeneity of double cortex syndrome. *Ann Neurol* 2000; 47:265–9.

47. Matsumoto N, Leventer RJ, Kuc JA, et al. Mutation analysis of the DCX gene and genotype/phenotype correlation in subcortical band heterotopia. *Eur J Hum Genet* 2001; 9:5–12.

48. Haverfield EV, Whited AJ, Petras KS, et al. Intragenic deletions and duplications of the LIS1 and DCX genes: a major disease-causing mechanism in lissencephaly and subcortical band heterotopia. *Eur J Hum Genet* 2009; 17(7):911–18.

49. Mei D, Parrini E, Pasqualetti M, et al. Multiplex ligation-dependent probe amplification detects DCX gene deletions in band heterotopia. *Neurology* 2007; 68:446–50.

50. Francis F, Koulakoff A, Boucher D, et al. Doublecortin is a developmentally regulated, microtubule-associated protein expressed in migrating and differentiating neurons. *Neuron* 1999; 23:247–56.

51. Gleeson JG, Allen KM, Fox JW, et al. Doublecortin, a brain-specific gene mutated in human X-linked lissencephaly and double cortex syndrome, encodes a putative signaling protein. *Cell* 1998; 92:63–72.

52. Caspi M, Atlas R, Kantor A, et al. Interaction between LIS1 and doublecortin, two lissencephaly gene products. *Hum Mol Genet* 2000; 9:2205–13.

53. Tanaka T, Serneo FF, Tseng HC, et al. Cdk5 phosphorylation of doublecortin ser297 regulates its effect on neuronal migration. *Neuron* 2004; 41:215–27.

54. Guerrini R, Moro F, Andermann E, et al. Nonsyndromic mental retardation and cryptogenic epilepsy in women with doublecortin gene mutations. *Ann Neurol* 2003; 54:30–37.

55. Sicca F, Kelemen A, Genton P, et al. Mosaic mutations of the LIS1 gene cause subcortical band heterotopia. *Neurology* 2003; 61:1042–6.

56. D'Agostino MD, Bernasconi A, Das S, et al. Subcortical band heterotopia (SBH) in males: clinical, imaging and genetic findings in comparison with females. *Brain* 2002; 125:2507–22.

57. Juberg RC and Hellman CD. A new familial form of convulsive disorder and mental retardation limited to females. *J of Pediatr* 1971; 79:726–32.

58. Hynes K, Tarpey P, Dibbens LM, et al. Epilepsy and mental retardation limited to females with PCDH19 mutations can present de novo or in single generation families. *J Med Genet* 2010; 47:211–16.

59. Scheffer IE, Turner SJ, Dibbens LM, et al. Epilepsy and mental retardation limited to females: an under-recognized disorder. *Brain* 2008; 131:918–27.

60. Depienne C, Bouteiller D, Keren B, et al. Sporadic infantile epileptic encephalopathy caused by mutations in PCDH19 resembles Dravet syndrome but mainly affects females. *PLoS Genet* 2009; 5:e1000381.

61. Dibbens LM, Tarpey PS, Hynes K, et al. X-linked protocadherin 19 mutations cause female-limited epilepsy and cognitive impairment. *Nat Genet* 2008; 40:776–81.

62. Sutton VR, Hopkins BJ, Eble TN, et al. Facial and physical features of Aicardi syndrome: infants to teenagers. *Am J Med Genet A* 2005; 138A:254–8.

63. King AM, Bowen DI, Goulding P, et al. Aicardi syndrome. *Br J Ophthalmol* 1998; 82:457.

64. Aicardi J. Aicardi syndrome. *Brain Dev* 2005; 27:164–71.

65. Rosser TL, Acosta MT and Packer RJ. Aicardi syndrome: spectrum of disease and long-term prognosis in 77 females. *Pediatr Neurol* 2002; 27:343–6.

66. Grosso S, Farnetani MA, Bernardoni E, et al. Intractable reflex audiogenic seizures

in Aicardi syndrome. *Brain Dev* 2007; 29:243–6.

67. Ohtsuka Y, Oka E, Terasaki T, et al. Aicardi syndrome: a longitudinal clinical and electroencephalographic study. *Epilepsia* 1993; 34:627–34.

68. Hopkins B, Sutton VR, Lewis RA, et al. Neuroimaging aspects of Aicardi syndrome. *Am J Med Genet A* 2008; 146A:2871–8.

69. Nielsen KB, Anvret M, Flodmark O, et al. Aicardi syndrome: early neuroradiological manifestations and results of DNA studies in one patient. *Am J Med Genet* 1991; 38:65–8.

70. Chen TH, Chao MC, Lin LC, et al. Aicardi syndrome in a 47, XXY male neonate with lissencephaly and holoprosencephaly. *J Neurol Sci* 2009; 278:138–40.

71. Zubairi MS, Carter RF and Ronen GM. A male phenotype with Aicardi syndrome. *J Child Neurol* 2009; 24:204–7.

72. Bursztejn AC, Bronner M, Peudenier S, et al. Molecular characterization of a monosomy 1p36 presenting as an Aicardi syndrome phenocopy. *Am J Med Genet A* 2009; 149A:2493–500.

73. Janz D. Epilepsy with impulsive petit mal (juvenile myoclonic epilepsy). *Acta Neurol Scand* 1985; 72:449–59.

74. Loiseau P and Duche B. Juvenile myoclonic epilepsy. *Rev Neurol* 1990; 146:719–25.

75. Panayiotopoulos CP, Obeid T and Tahan AR. Juvenile myoclonic epilepsy: a 5-year prospective study. *Epilepsia* 1994; 35:285–96.

76. Christensen J, Kjeldsen MJ, Andersen H, et al. Gender differences in epilepsy. *Epilepsia* 2005; 46:956–60.

77. Mullins GM, O'Sullivan S S, Neligan A, et al. A study of idiopathic generalised epilepsy in an Irish population. *Seizure* 2007; 16:204–10.

78. Martinez-Juarez IE, Alonso ME, Medina MT, et al. Juvenile myoclonic epilepsy subsyndromes: family studies and long-term follow-up. *Brain* 2006; 129:1269–80.

79. Camfield CS and Camfield PR. Juvenile myoclonic epilepsy 25 years after seizure onset: a population-based study. *Neurology* 2009; 73:1041–45.

80. Liu AW, Delgado-Escueta AV, Serratosa JM, et al. Juvenile myoclonic epilepsy locus in chromosome 6p21.2-p11: linkage to convulsions and electroencephalography trait. *Am J Hum Genet* 1995; 57:368–81.

81. Cossette P, Liu L, Brisebois K, et al. Mutation of GABRA1 in an autosomal dominant form of juvenile myoclonic epilepsy. *Nat Genet* 2002; 31:184–9.

82. Winawer MR, Rabinowitz D, Barker-Cummings C, et al. Evidence for distinct genetic influences on generalized and localization-related epilepsy. *Epilepsia* 2003; 44:1176–82.

83. Winawer MR, Rabinowitz D, Pedley TA, et al. Genetic influences on myoclonic and absence seizures. *Neurology* 2003; 61:1576–81.

84. Panayiotopoulos CP and Obeid T. Juvenile myoclonic epilepsy: an autosomal recessive disease. *Ann Neurol* 1989; 25:440–43.

85. Durner M, Sander T, Greenberg DA, et al. Localization of idiopathic generalized epilepsy on chromosome 6p in families of juvenile myoclonic epilepsy patients. *Neurology* 1991; 41:1651–5.

86. Andermann E. Multifactorial inheritance of generalized and focal epilepsy. In: Anderson VE, Hauser WA, Penry JK and Sing CF, eds. *Genetic basis of the epilepsies*. New York, NY: Raven Press, 1982; 355–74.

87. Matthes A and Weber H. Clinical and electroencephalographic family studies on pyknolepsy. *Dtsch Med Wochenschr* 1968; 93:429–35.

88. Metrakos JD and Metrakos K. Childhood epilepsy of subcortical ("centrencephalic") origin. Some questions and answers for the pediatrician. *Clin Pediatr (Phila)* 1966; 5:537–42.

89. Metrakos K and Metrakos JD. Genetics of convulsive disorders. II. Genetic and electroencephalographic studies in centrencephalic epilepsy. *Neurology* 1961; 11:474–83.

90. Metrakos K and Metrakos JD. Is the centrencephalic EEG inherited as a dominant? *Electroencephalogr Clin Neurophysiol* 1961; 13:289.

91. Blandfort M, Tsuboi T and Vogel F. Genetic counseling in the epilepsies. I. Genetic risks. *Hum Genet* 1987; 76:303–31.

92. Jayalakshmi SS, Mohandas S, Sailaja S, et al. Clinical and electroencephalographic study of first-degree relatives and probands with juvenile myoclonic epilepsy. *Seizure* 2006; 15:177–83.

93. Tsuboi T and Christian W. On the genetics of the primary generalized epilepsy with sporadic myoclonias of impulsive petit mal type. A clinical and electroencephalographic study of 399 probands. *Humangenetik* 1973; 19:155–82.

94. Berkovic SF, Howell RA, Hay DA, et al. Epilepsies in twins: genetics of the major epilepsy syndromes. *Ann Neurol* 1998; 43:435–45.

95. Corey LA, Pellock JM, Kjeldsen MJ, et al. Importance of genetic factors in the occurrence of epilepsy syndrome type: a twin study. *Epilepsy Res* 2011; 97:103–11.

96. Lennox WG and Lennox MA. *Epilepsy and related disorders*. Boston, MA: Little, Brown, 1960.

97. Lennox WG. Sixty-six twins affected by seizures. *Assoc Rev Nerv Ment Dis Proc* 1947; 26:11–34.

98. Pal DK, Strug LJ and Greenberg DA. Evaluating candidate genes in common epilepsies and the nature of evidence. *Epilepsia* 2008; 49:386–92.

99. Suzuki T, Delgado-Escueta AV, Aguan K, et al. Mutations in EFHC1 cause juvenile myoclonic epilepsy. *Nat Genet* 2004; 36:842–9.

100. Haug K, Warnstedt M, Alekov AK, et al. Mutations in CLCN2 encoding a voltage-gated chloride channel are associated with idiopathic generalized epilepsies. *Nat Genet* 2003; 33:527–32.

101. Winawer MR, Marini C, Grinton BE, et al. Familial clustering of seizure types within the idiopathic generalized epilepsies. *Neurology* 2005; 65:523–8.

102. Wirrell EC, Camfield CS, Camfield PR, et al. Long-term prognosis of typical childhood absence epilepsy: remission or progression to juvenile myoclonic epilepsy. *Neurology* 1996; 47:912–18.

Epilepsy in girls during childhood and adolescence

Cristina Y. Go and O. Carter Snead, III

Key points:

- Epilepsy is the most common neurological disease in childhood and adolescence
- Developmental changes influence choice of antiepileptic drugs (AEDs)
- AED with side effects involving hormonal dysregulation, aesthetic changes, neurocognitive dysfunction, and bone metabolism should be carefully considered in this age group
- Unique psychosocial factors in childhood and adolescence add a greater complexity in the treatment of epilepsy
- Transition from pediatric to adult epilepsy care is an important but under-developed aspect of epilepsy care

Introduction

Epilepsy, defined as recurrent spontaneous seizures [1], is the most common neurologic disease in childhood and adolescence. Adolescence can be defined either as an actual age range, or as the period from onset of puberty until the achievement of economic independence [9]. The age range varies, according to the literature, from 10–18 years. The annual incidence of newly diagnosed epilepsy in children and adolescents aged 1 month to <15 years in developed countries ranges from 53–97/100,000, with the highest incidence in the first year of life and decreasing after the tenth year of life [2–5]. About 55% of these cases are focal epilepsies, 12–39% are generalized epilepsies, and another 12–29% are of undetermined classification. For the most part there is no apparent statistical difference in incidence rates of epilepsy between boys and girls [3]. However, some epilepsy syndromes such as childhood absence epilepsy (CAE), juvenile myoclonic epilepsy (JME), and certain genetic disorders associated with epilepsy (Rett syndrome, Aicardi syndrome) are more common in girls [6, 7].

Medical issues
Hormones and epilepsy

Reproductive endocrine disorders are more common in females and males with epilepsy than the general population of similar age. This may be due to the epilepsy itself as well as the effect of AEDs. Polycystic ovarian syndrome (PCOS) occurs in 10–25% of females

Women with Epilepsy, ed. Esther Bui and Autumn Klein. Published by Cambridge University Press.
© Cambridge University Press 2014.

with epilepsy not treated with AEDs compared to 5–6% of females in the general population. Some studies have suggested that ictal and interictal epileptiform discharges, especially those arising from the temporolimbic areas, can lead to impairment or disruption of the GnRH pulsatile release and its effect on the hypothalamic-pituitary axis [21]. For a more detailed discussion see Chapter 5. The result of this neuroendocrine cascade is an increase in the luteinizing hormone/follicle-stimulating hormone (LH/FSH) ratio and development of immature follicles that are deficient in aromatase, which normally converts androgens to estrogens, thereby causing hyperandrogenism and PCOS [20]. The effects of the anticonvulsant drug valproic acid (VPA) on the female's reproductive endocrine health have been studied extensively. Long-term use in adolescent girls with epilepsy after menarche was associated with increased testosterone levels [21], an effect not seen in girls before menarche, which implies that VPA may induce laboratory and/or clinical symptoms of hyperandrogenism in postmenarcheal girls, similar to adult women. This may be associated with PCOS and menstrual irregularities. Although other AEDs have also been associated with PCOS features, Sahota et al. reported that it is significantly higher in women taking VPA than those taking other AEDs (11.8% vs. 2.5%), independent of seizure types [22].

Adverse effects associated with antiepileptic drugs

The presence of adverse effects from AEDs contributes greatly to medication compliance. Many of these side effects are due to age-related pharmacokinetics.

The most common idiosyncratic reaction from lamotrigine (LTG) is a rash, which is seen in 10–20% of patients. Young age, concurrent use of VPA, high dose, and rapid escalation are risk factors. Children have increased cytochrome P450 (CYP)-catalyzed metabolism compared to adults. This increased CYP of metabolism of LTG in children could increase reactive metabolites and result in a higher incidence of rash [23].

VPA is a widely used and very effective AED in many epilepsy syndromes, which can cause transient sedation, tremors, reversible thrombocytopenia, and GGT elevation. In addition to PCOS, there can be serious side effects, including pancreatitis, coagulopathy, bone marrow suppression, encephalopathy, and hepatotoxicity that can, rarely, be fatal [24]. VPA-induced hepatotoxicity may be due to pre-existing or undiagnosed inborn errors of metabolism, mitochondrial disorders, VPA-induced inhibition of beta-oxidation, or direct toxicity from VPA metabolites [23]. VPA-induced carnitine deficiency may be responsible for the hepatotoxicity and hyperammonemia [25]. Supplementation with carnitine may result in subjective and objective improvements in patients on VPA [26]. VPA-induced encephalopathy has been described in children and adults [27, 28], possibly due to a direct toxic effect of VPA at high levels. However, patients with underlying inborn errors of metabolism are at risk, even when taking VPA at therapeutic levels. There are also cases of pseudoatrophy of the brain and mental deterioration with VPA monotherapy [29, 30]. Fortunately, this condition is reversible when VPA is discontinued.

Cosmetic adverse effects from AEDs can greatly contribute to the low self-esteem of adolescent females. Weight gain (discussed below) can be seen with VPA and carbamazepine (CBZ), in addition to alopecia that occurs in 5–10% of patients taking VPA, and can be distressing. Phenytoin (PHT) is often associated with gingival hyperplasia, facial acne, and coarsening, excessive hair growth on the face and arms, all of which can alter the body image of adolescents.

Cognitive adverse effects are common complaints of more developmentally intact children and adolescents using AEDs although these can also be seen in those with underlying cognitive impairment. Topiramate (TPM) has been associated with a negative impact on cognition consistent with subjective complaints of patients and objective assessments by neuropsychological scores in multiple domains, especially in verbal IQ, verbal fluency, and verbal learning [31]. Improvements in these domains were noted when TPM was withdrawn or the dose reduced. For patients who are showing signs of cognitive problems associated with AED use, it is important to consider reducing dose or switching to a different AED in an effort to balance seizure control and AED-related cognitive side effects.

AEDs are also associated with behavioral and mood adverse effects. Levetiracetam is a well-tolerated and effective medication that is increasingly being used in various epilepsy syndromes. However, there are numerous reports of behavioral side effects ranging from insomnia, agitation, anxiety, emotional lability, and hyperactivity to hallucinations and frank psychosis. It is seen in up to 13% of patients, especially those with pre-existing developmental and behavioral challenges. The US FDA issued an alert in 2008 regarding the risk of suicidal thoughts and behavior with AED use. Preliminary analysis of data from 199 placebo-controlled clinical trials of 11 AEDs suggested an increased risk of suicide and suicidal symptoms compared to patients treated with placebo. The risk of suicidal thoughts and behavior was 0.43% on drug therapy and 0.22% on placebo, which corresponds to an estimated 2.1/1000 more patients in the treatment group. This was seen as early as the first week of therapy and did not decrease for the duration of the clinical trials. This effect was not specific to a specific AED or class of AED. An enhanced awareness of this risk will enable the physician to increase communication about emotional health with patients and their families and also advocate early treatment of the symptoms when these emerge.

AEDs and the endocrine system

Late childhood and especially adolescence is a period marked by rapid physical growth and skeletal and genital maturation. The epilepsy itself can affect these maturational changes as well as concurrent AED use. Physicians managing children with epilepsy need to be aware of the potential effects of AEDs on the endocrine system.

AEDs can cause disturbances in thyroid homeostasis by altering the biosynthesis, secretion, metabolism, and excretion of thyroid hormones. Both CBZ and phenobarbital (PB), but not VPA, have been reported to be associated with a reduction in triiodothyronine (T3) and thyroxine (T4). Given that even minor changes in thyroid metabolism can lead to somatic symptoms and cognitive problems [33], some patients may benefit from L-thyroxine treatment [34], and consultation with a neuroendocrinologist or endocrinologist would be recommended.

Weight gain is an important issue, not just because of its long-term impact on health but also as a source of self-image problems, especially in the female adolescent. Several AEDs have been associated with weight gain, including gabapentin (GBP), CBZ, pregabalin, vigabatrin (VGB), and most especially, VPA. Weight gain is the most common reported adverse effect of VPA. It occurs within the first 3 months of therapy and peaks at the sixth month [35]. Although genetic and nutritional factors play a role in weight gain, VPA appears to cause weight gain due to its effect on insulin and leptin. On the other hand, TPM can cause weight loss, which is associated with reduced leptin/adiponectin (L/A) ratio [36].

Bone mineral density increases throughout childhood and adolescence, peaking at 20 years of age. In children with epilepsy, factors that can influence bone health include limitation of physical activity associated with many symptomatic epilepsies. There is also an association between AEDs and bone disease. Reduction in 25-OHD levels and increased bone turnover [38] can be seen in patients taking both enzyme-inducing and enzyme-inhibiting AEDs [37]. These effects may be observed even following a relatively short period of therapy, i.e., 2 years. Although it is important to ensure adequate vitamin D and calcium intake, more standardized studies are needed to determine the effectiveness of vitamin D and calcium supplementation and clarify the utility of bisphosphonate therapy. Bone health is further discussed in Chapter 22.

Another important endocrine aspect of AED therapy involves the use of oral contraceptives. AEDs, especially the enzyme-inducers like CBZ, PB, and PHT may decrease the efficacy of oral and injectable contraceptives by increasing sex hormone-binding globulin, causing a decrease in free, biologically active fraction of the hormone. Therefore, when counseling adolescent females on contraception use, it is critically important to inform them of this potential interaction, and recommend either contraceptives with 50 ug or more of the estrogen component or use of alternative means of contraception such as the intrauterine device (IUD). Contraceptive options are discussed in Chapter 10.

Seizure control

Approximately 10–40% of children with epilepsy will continue to have seizures despite optimal medical management [39–41]. Factors that contribute to AED failure include, but are not limited to, the choice of appropriate AED for the type of epilepsy used, side effects, and medication compliance. When a patient fails two AEDs appropriate for the seizure type and at adequate doses, the probability of achieving seizure control with a third drug is only 5–10% [42]. For these patients, a timely referral to a tertiary epilepsy center for diagnostic evaluation may lead to other treatment options, which may include diet therapy, neurostimulation devices, and epilepsy surgery. Carefully selected children and adolescents with medically refractory epilepsy may benefit from early surgical intervention to avoid the negative effects of on going seizures, side effects from AED, and can potentially improve the quality of life for the child and their families [43].

Psychosocial issues

Adolescence in females is heralded by a number of dramatic physical changes such as the development of breasts and onset of menarche. Equally dramatic emotional and behavioral changes occur during adolescence in females that can all be impacted by epilepsy. These include risk-taking behaviors, striving for independence and self-empowerment, sexuality, relationships, growth to adulthood, and the development of self-esteem.

The spontaneous, recurrent seizures that characterize epilepsy pose a significant burden for adolescents because of their unpredictable nature. The adverse effects of chronic AED therapy can also be devastating to the adolescent. For example, an adolescent who experiences seizures in public has a greater sense of embarrassment and loss of self-esteem. Seizures may also prevent adolescents from developing the same degree of independence as their peers because of safety concerns, further impairing self-esteem.

Risk-taking behaviors are a common feature of adolescence in both males and females [10], and in combination with epilepsy and AED therapy, have the potential to create challenges in epilepsy care. For example, the increased prevalence of sexual activity may contribute to unintended pregnancy with a potential for teratogenic effects of anti-epileptic drugs and sexually transmitted diseases. As well, young females with epilepsy and underlying developmental delay may be vulnerable to physical and sexual abuse. In terms of other risk-taking behavior, the use of alcohol and illicit drugs, both prevalent amongst female adolescents, have the potential to be exacerbated in the presence of epilepsy, but may also make seizures worse and have significant drug–drug interactions with whatever AED the patient is taking. Bullying is often a major problem for the child and adolescent with epilepsy, especially when their peers have misinformation about their medical condition.

Cognitive, behavioral, and mood effects associated with epilepsy

Academic underachievement is a common problem seen in the pediatric patient with epilepsy. The type of seizure and epilepsy syndrome, underlying cause of epilepsy, age at onset, severity of seizures, gender, home environment, and psychosocial factors all can contribute to neuropsychological deficits that put the child at risk for adverse academic outcomes [11–13]. Children and adolescents with epilepsy have a significant risk for comorbid attention deficit hyperactivity disorder (ADHD), which often is associated with derangements in working memory.

There is some evidence for gender differences in the psychosocial comorbidities of epilepsy in children and adolescents, with males with epilepsy being more at risk for academic underachievement [11], although male adolescents with neurologic conditions appear to have higher achievement scores compared to their female counterparts [14].

A high seizure burden, as indicated by frequency and severity of ictal events, is well known to be a risk factor for neurocognitive impairment in children and adolescents with epilepsy. In addition, interictal epileptiform discharges also may be contributory. For example, continuous spike-waves during slow-wave sleep (CSWS) are almost always associated with cognitive and behavioral regression even when clinical seizures are apparently under control. Similarly, absence epilepsy, which is more common in females and typically considered to be a "benign" childhood epilepsy syndrome, is associated with lower scores of measures of general cognitive functioning and visuospatial skills, even in those with well-controlled clinical seizures compared to controls.

Behavioral problems are 3–5 times higher in children with epilepsy compared to the general population [15, 16]. Depression in children and adolescents with epilepsy is often unrecognized and contributes to poor long-term psychosocial outcomes [17]. The risk of suicide is greater in depressed youth with epilepsy than the general population and the prevalence is higher among young females than males (8.1% vs. 4.6%) [10].

Quality of life

Quality of life of patients and their families is almost invariably adversely impacted by epilepsy, to a degree not seen by other chronic medical conditions such as asthma [18].

Factors that contribute are the stigma of the diagnosis, seizure control, and cognitive, behavioral, and psychosocial issues arising from the underlying cause of the epilepsy and/or its treatment. Seizure severity and the female gender are particularly associated with increased risk for Quality of Life (QOL) problems [18].

Transition to adult care

The transition of care from a pediatric neurologist to an adult provider can pose many challenges for the physician, the patient, and their families. It is not simply a physical transfer of the patient and their health care records but also one that needs to be carefully planned with the objective of improving the young adult's skills in navigating the adult health care system, providing autonomy and planning for long-term needs [45]. This is especially challenging for patients with special needs. A questionnaire-based study of pediatric and adult neurologists in Quebec, Canada showed that most pediatric neurologists do not have a patient transition program or policy in place, with most of the responders agreeing that the transition process was poorly coordinated [44]. The most commonly identified barriers to transition included, but are not limited to: (1) young patients not always ready to assume medical decision-making responsibilities; (2) parents and care givers who remain excessively protective and do not understand privacy issues of the young adult patient; and (3) the patients not knowing how to navigate the adult health care system. This gap in care is seen universally and presents a major source of frustration, not only for the transitioning adolescents but also for the adult neurologists taking over their care.

Summary

The management of girls and female adolescent patients with epilepsy presents many challenges that include the age of the patient, the underlying cause of epilepsy, the presence of psychosocial comorbidities, any attendant cognitive disability, and both gender-specific and generic side effects of the medications used to control the seizures. Each of these factors has the potential to impact adversely upon QOL measures of the patients and their families. Awareness of these challenges will allow better communication between the physician and the patients they are caring for and will facilitate the process of establishing goals of treatment, as well as better planning for transition from pediatric to adult care and, in the end, improve the overall health and QOL of this unique population.

References

1. Guidelines for epidemiologic studies on epilepsy. *Epilepsia* 1993; 34(4): 592–6.

2. Freitag C, May T, Pfafflin M, et al. Incidence of epilepsies and epileptic syndromes in children and adolescents: A population-based prospective study in Germany. *Epilepsia* 2001; 42(8):979–85.

3. Granieri E, Rosati G, Tola R, et al. A descriptive study of epilepsy in the district of Copparo, Italy, 1964–1978. *Epilepsia* 1983; 24(4):502–14.

4. Hauser WA and Kurland LT. The epidemiology of epilepsy in Rochester,

Minnesota, 1935 through 1967. *Epilepsia* 1975; 16(1):1–66.

5. Hauser W, Annegers J and Kurland L. Incidence of epilepsy and unprovoked seizures in Rochester, Minnesota: 1935–1984. *Epilepsia* 1993; 34(3): 453–68.

6. Morrell M. Seizures and epilepsy in women. In: PW K, ed. *Neurologic disease in women*. New York, NY: Demos, 1998.

7. Thomas P, Genton P, Gelisse P, et al. Juvenile myoclonic epilepsy. In: Roger J, Bureau M, Dravet C, et al., eds. *Epileptic syndromes in infancy, childhood and adolescence*, 4th edn. Montrouge, France: John Libbey Eurotext, 2005; 367–88.

8. Genton P, Salas PJ, Tunon A, et al. Juvenile myoclonic epilepsy and related syndromes: clinical and neurophysiological aspects. In: Malafosse A, Genton P, Hirsch E, et al., eds. *Idiopathic generalized epilepsies: clinical, experimental and genetic aspects*. London: John Libbey, 1999; 253–265.

9. Gentry JH and Campbell M. *Developing adolescents: a reference for professionals*. Association AP, 2002.

10. Eaton DK, Kann L, Kinchen S, et al. Youth risk behavior surveillance – United States, 2009. *Morb Mortal Wkly Rep Surveill Summ* 2010; 59(5): 1–142.

11. Austin J, Huberty T, Huster G, at al. Academic achievement in children with epilepsy or asthma. *Dev Med Child Neurol* 1998; 40(4):248–55.

12. Wirrell E, Camfield C, Camfield P, et al. Long-term psychosocial outcome in typical absence epilepsy: sometimes a wolf in sheeps' clothing. *Arch Pediatr Adolesc Med* 1997; 151(2): 152–8.

13. Fastenau P, Shen J, Dunn D, et al. Neuropsychological predictors of academic underachievement in pediatric epilepsy:

moderating roles of demographic, seizure, and psychosocial variables. *Epilepsia* 2004; 45(10):1261–72.

14. Howe G, Feinstein C, Reiss D, et al. Adolescent adjustment to chronic physical disorders – I. Comparing neurological and non-neurological conditions. *J Child Psychol Psychiatry Allied Discip* 1993; 34(7): 1153–71.

15. Caplan R, Siddarth P, Gurbani S, et al. Psychopathology and pediatric complex partial seizures: seizure-related, cognitive, and linguistic variables. *Epilepsia* 2004; 45(10):1273–81.

16. Rodenburg R, Stams GJ, Meijer AM, et al. Psychopathology in children with epilepsy: a meta-analysis. *J Pediatr Psychol* 2005; 30(6):453–68.

17. Ettinger AB, Weisbrot DM, Nolan EE, et al. Symptoms of depression and anxiety in pediatric epilepsy patients. *Epilepsia* 1998; 39(6):595–9.

18. Austin J, Huster G, Dunn D, et al. Adolescents with active or inactive epilepsy or asthma: a comparison of quality of life. *Epilepsia* 1996; 37(12): 1228–38.

19. Herzog AG, Coleman AE, Jacobs AR, et al. Interictal EEG discharges, reproductive hormones, and menstrual disorders in epilepsy. *Ann Neurol* 2003; 54:625–37.

20. Bilo L, Meo R, Valentino R, et al. Characterization of reproductive endocrine disorders in women with epilepsy. *J Clin Endocrinol Metab* 2001; 186:2950–6.

21. De Vries L, Karasik A, Landau Z, et al. Endocrine effects of valproate in adolescent girls with epilepsy. *Epilepsia* 2007; 48(3): 470–7.

22. Sahota P, Prabhakar S, Kharbanda PS, et al. Seizure type, antiepileptic drugs, and reproductive endocrine dysfunction in Indian women with epilepsy: a cross-sectional study. *Epilepsia* 2008; 49: 2069–77.

23. Anderson G. Children versus adults: pharmacokinetic and adverse-effect differences. *Epilepsia* 2002; 43(Suppl 3): 53–9.

24. Koenig SA, Buesing D, Longin E, et al. Valproic acid-induced hepatopathy: nine new fatalities in Germany from 1994 to 2003. *Epilepsia* 2006; 47(12): 2027–31.

25. Raskind J and El-Chaar G. The role of carnitine supplementation during valproic acid therapy. *Ann Pharmacother* 2000; 34(5):630–8.

26. De Vivo D, Bohan T, Coulter D, et al. L-Carnitine supplementation in childhood epilepsy: current perspectives. *Epilepsia* 1998; 39(11):1216–25.

27. Gerstner T, Buesing D, Longin E, et al. Valproic acid induced encephalopathy – 19 new cases in Germany from 1994 to 2003 – a side effect associated to VPA-therapy not only in young children. *Seizure* 2006; 15(6):443–8.

28. Zaret BS and Cohen RA. Reversible valproic acid-induced dementia: a case report. *Epilepsia* 1986; 27(3):234–40.

29. Guerrini R, Belmonte A, Canapicchi R, et al. Reversible pseudoatrophy of the brain and mental deterioration associated with valproate treatment. *Epilepsia* 1998; 39(1):27–32.

30. McLachlan RS. Pseudoatrophy of the brain with valproic acid monotherapy. *Can J Neurol Sci* 1987; 14(3):294–6.

31. Thompson PJ, Baxendale SA, Duncan JS, et al. Effects of topiramate on cognitive function. *J Neurol Neurosurg Psychiatry* 2000; 69(5):636–41.

32. Tanaka K, Kodama S, Yokoyama S, et al. Thyroid function in children with long-term anticonvulsant treatment. *Pediatr Neurosci* 1987; 13(2):90–4.

33. Jensovsky J, Ruzicka E, Spackova N, et al. Changes of event-related potential and cognitive processes in patients with subclinical hypothyroidism after thyroxine treatment. *Endocr Regul* 2002; 36(3): 115–22.

34. Monzani F, Del Guerra P, Caraccio N, et al. Subclinical hypothyroidism: neurobehavioral features and beneficial effect of L-thyroxine treatment. *Clin Investig* 1993; 71(5):367–71.

35. Demir E and Aysun S. Weight gain associated with valproate in childhood. *Pediatr Neurol* 2000; 22(5):361–4.

36. Li HF, Zou Y, Xia ZZ, et al. Effects of topiramate on weight and metabolism in children with epilepsy. *Acta Paediatr* 2009; 98(9):1521–5.

37. Toledano R and Gil-Nagel A. Adverse effects of antiepileptic drugs. *Semin Neurol* 2008; 28(3):317–27.

38. Verrotti A, Greco R, Latini G, et al. Increased bone turnover in prepubertal, pubertal, and postpubertal patients receiving carbamazepine. *Epilepsia* 2002; 43(12):1488–92.

39. Berg A, Shinnar S, Levy S, et al. Early development of intractable epilepsy in children: a prospective study. *Neurology* 2001; 56(11): 1445–52.

40. Camfield C, Camfield P, Gordon K, et al. Outcome of childhood epilepsy: A population-based study with a simple predictive scoring system for those treated with medication. *J Pediatr* 1993; 122(6): 861–8.

41. Dlugos D, Sammel M, Strom B, et al. Response to first drug trial predicts outcome in childhood temporal lobe epilepsy. *Neurology* 2001; 57(12): 2259–64.

42. Kwan P and Brodie M. Early identification of refractory epilepsy. *New Engl J Med* 2000; 342(5):314–9.

43. Go C and Snead, III OC. Pharmacologically intractable epilepsy in children: diagnosis and preoperative evaluation. *Neurosurg Focus* 2008; 25(3):e2.

44. Oskoui M and Wolfson C. Current practice and views of neurologists on the transition

from pediatric to adult care. *J Child Neurol* 2012; 27(12):1553–8.

45. American Academy of Pediatrics AAoFP, American College of Physicians-American Society of Internal Medicine. A consensus statement on health care transitions for young adults with special health care needs. *Pediatrics* 2002; 110 (Suppl):1304–6.

Catamenial epilepsy

Sima Indubhai Patel and Nancy Foldvary-Schaefer

Key points:

- Catamenial epilepsy is the exacerbation of seizures in relation to the menstrual cycle
- Factors contributing to catamenial seizures may include hormonal fluctuations and metabolic changes influencing antiepileptic drug (AED) levels
- Estrogen is mainly proconvulsant, progesterone is mainly anticonvulsant
- In women who ovulate, catamenial seizures can occur perimenstrually (C1 pattern) or periovulatory (C2 pattern); in women who have anovulatory cycles, catamenial seizures can occur during the luteal phase (C3 pattern)
- Therapies for catamenial seizures include optimization of AEDs, non-hormonal therapies, hormonal therapies, and neurosteroids

Introduction

The term "catamenial" is derived from the Greek word "katamenios" meaning monthly. *Catamenial epilepsy* consists of patterns of seizure occurrence due to the variation in sex hormone secretion across the menstrual cycle. In ancient times the cyclical occurrence of epileptic seizures, like menstruation cycles, was attributed to the phases of the moon. In 1857, at a meeting of the Royal Medical and Chirurgical Society, Sir Charles Locock first described the relationship between epileptic seizures and the menstrual cycle. He described "a form of epilepsy to which special notice had not been drawn and which he had been in the habit of regarding as hysterical epilepsy ... confined to women ... connected to menstruation ... with paroxysms that only occurred at the menstrual period or except in the case of great mental excitement" [1]. In 1881, Gowers described the first series of menstruation-related seizures, in which he noted in 46 of 82 women, "the attacks were worse at the monthly periods" [1]. In recent years the pathophysiology, classification, and treatment of catamenial epilepsy have broadened – the subject of several comprehensive reviews [1].

The menstrual cycle

The normal menstrual cycle is depicted in Figure 8.1 [1]. Cycle duration ranges from 24 to 35 days, with the average interval between menstrual periods being 28 days. The menstrual cycle is divided into the follicular phase, ovulation, and the luteal phase.

Women with Epilepsy, ed. Esther Bui and Autumn Klein. Published by Cambridge University Press.
© Cambridge University Press 2014.

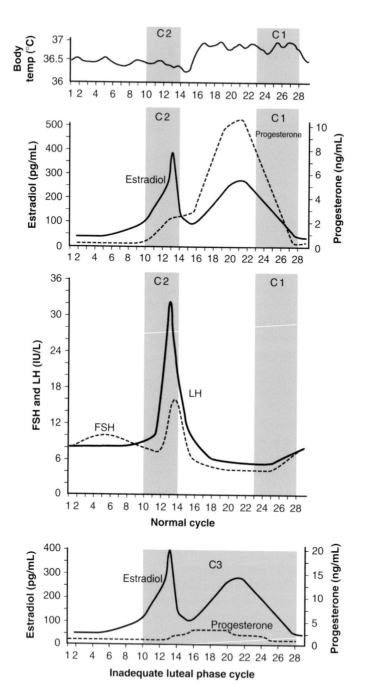

Figure 8.1: Schematic of the menstrual cycle and patterns of catamenial epilepsy. The top three panels depict the normal menstrual cycle. The inadequate luteal phase cycle (lower panel) is defined by progesterone levels less than 5 ng/ml. Patterns of seizure expression include the perimenstrual (C1), periovulatory (C2), and inadequate luteal phase (C3) types.

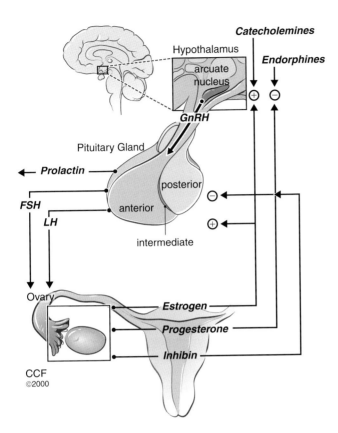

Figure 8.2: The hypothalamic-pituitary-ovarian axis regulates the interactions between neurohormones, gonadotropin-releasing hormone, pituitary gonadotropins, and the gonadal steroids through a feedback loop mechanism.

By convention, day 1 is the first day of menses and ovulation occurs approximately on day 14. The follicular phase begins at the onset of menses and ends near the luteinizing hormone (LH) surge. The luteal phase begins on the day of the LH surge and ends on day 1 of the next cycle.

The menstrual cycle is the expression of a complex neuroendocrinological system known as the hypothalamic-pituitary-ovarian axis. The hypothalamic-pituitary-ovarian axis regulates the interactions between neurohormones, gonadotropin-releasing hormone (GnRH), pituitary gonadotropins, and the gonadal steroids through a feedback loop mechanism (Figure 8.2). Synthesized in the medial basal hypothalamus, GnRH is secreted in a pulsatile manner from nerve terminals at the median eminence into the portal system and delivered to the anterior pituitary. Normal menstrual function is dependent on the pulsatile secretion of GnRH within a critical range of amplitude and frequency. The pulsatile release of GnRH stimulates secretion of follicle-stimulating hormone (FSH) and LH from the anterior pituitary. FSH promotes follicular growth; LH stimulates ovulation and maintenance of the corpus luteum. FSH and LH regulate the production of estrogen and progesterone, which in turn influences the release of the gonadotropins from pituitary cells. Abnormal FSH secretion during the follicular phase results in diminished follicular development and inadequate corpus luteum formation and function. This condition is known as the inadequate luteal phase (ILP) or anovulatory cycle. In the ILP, the estrogen-producing function remains unimpaired but the corpus luteum is defective in progesterone production causing variability in menstrual cycle duration due to sustained elevation of estrogen relative to progesterone (Figure 8.1). ILP cycles occur in over 25% of women.

Pathophysiology of catamenial epilepsy
Hormonal influences

Although multiple mechanisms of catamenial epilepsy have been postulated, a cumulating body of evidence supports that seizures are influenced by the physiological variation in sex hormone secretion during the menstrual cycle. Both estrogen and progesterone exert significant effects on seizure threshold. The anticonvulsant effects of progesterone and proconvulsant properties of estrogen have been demonstrated in animal studies and in humans, and extensively reviewed in Chapter 4 and elsewhere [2, 3].

Estrogen

There are three biologically active estrogens: 17β-estradiol (E2), estriol, and estrone. Estrogens are highly lipophilic, capable of crossing the blood-brain barrier. The principal estrogen in premenopausal women is E2; estrone predominates in the postmenopausal period and estriol during pregnancy. Estradiol facilitates pentyletetrazol-(PTZ) and kainic acid-induced seizures and accelerates kindling following limbic network stimulation in animal models of epilepsy [4, 5]. Administration of intravenous conjugated estrogen to 16 women produced an increase in the frequency of epileptic discharges in 11 cases and clinical seizures in 4 [1]. A significant positive correlation between secondary generalized seizures and elevated estrogen-to-progesterone (E/P) ratio was found, peaking in the premenstrual and preovulatory periods in ovulatory cycles and declining in the midluteal phases of six women with epilepsy [6]. In three anovulatory cycles, seizure frequency correlated positively with E2 levels only.

The mechanism by which estrogen exerts proconvulsant effects is incompletely elucidated. While E2 enhances glutamate receptor-mediated excitatory neurotransmission and decreases GABAergic inhibition [7], recent work suggests that estrogen has anticonvulsant properties through transcriptional regulation of neuropeptides [3]. Therefore, the effect of estrogen on seizure threshold may depend on factors not yet fully understood, such as epilepsy type and localization and pathologic substrate.

Progesterone

The anticonvulsant effects of progesterone are primarily attributed to its metabolite allopregnanolone [8, 9]. Progesterone is first metabolized to 5α-dihydroprogestrone by the enzyme 5α-reductase, and then to allopregnanolone by 3α-hydroxysteroid oxidoreductase. The rate-limiting step in the conversion of progesterone to allopregnanolone is dependent on the enzyme 5α-reductase. The use of a 5α-reductase inhibitor in an animal model of catamenial epilepsy demonstrated that the anticonvulsant effect of progesterone depends upon the conversion of progesterone to allopregnanolone. Both progesterone and allopregnanolone potentiate GABA-A-mediated inhibition of neurons by increasing the frequency and duration of chloride channel opening at GABA-A receptors. At physiologic and pharmacologic levels, allopregnanolone is a more potent modulator of GABA-A receptors than progesterone [2, 8, 9]. Elevated concentrations of allopregnanolone and progesterone increase seizure threshold in kainic acid, PTZ, and pilocarpine animal models [2]. In addition to modulating GABA-A inhibition, allopregnanolone acts as an antagonist at the glutamate receptor. Many investigators attribute the perimenstrual seizure susceptibility in women with catamenial epilepsy to the precipitous drop in progesterone and rise in E/P ratio at the end of the luteal phase [2, 9].

Water balance

In the early twentieth century, observations of the association between cerebral edema and convulsions led to a series of experiments investigating the effect of water ingestion on seizures. In patients with epilepsy the antidiuretic hormone vasopressin and excessive water ingestion provoked seizures, while negative water balance produced by fluid restriction had the opposite effect. It was proposed that water retention during menstruation might be an underlying mechanism of the perimenstrual seizure exacerbation in some women with epilepsy [10]. However, no significant difference in sodium metabolism, total body water, or body weight was found between women with perimenstrual seizures and healthy controls, or between epileptic women with and without catamenial epilepsy [11].

Antiepileptic drug metabolism

Another proposed mechanism underlying seizure susceptibility in relation to the menstrual cycle is the impact of gonadal steroids on AED metabolism. Like gonadal steroids, many of the AEDs are metabolized by hepatic cytochrome P450 enzymes. Endogenous steroids and enzyme-inducing AEDs have bidirectional interactions, thereby affecting each other's serum concentrations. Similarly, like hormones, lamotrigine (LTG), and to a lesser extent oxcarbazepine, are eliminated via glucurondation by the hepatic uridine 5'-diphosphate (UDP)-glucuronosyltransferases (UGTs), rendering their metabolism vulnerable to the influence of sex steroids [11]. This interaction can theoretically produce clinically relevant fluctuations in AED concentrations across the menstrual cycle leading to seizures or signs of toxicity. The extent to which this occurs in clinical practice is uncertain.

In a study investigating these relationships in women taking phenytoin (PHT) mono-therapy or in combination with phenobarbital, despite higher daily dosage, women with perimenstrual seizures had lower PHT serum concentrations and greater fluctuations in concentrations across the cycle than women without catamenial seizures [1, 12]. Women with perimenstrual seizures were more likely (55% vs. 14%) to have a 30% or greater reduction in PHT concentration on day 28 of the cycle. Phenobarbital concentrations did not vary significantly. The reduced PHT concentration corresponded to an increase in seizure frequency in the perimenstrual period. In another group of women with peri-menstrual seizures, fluctuations in salivary PHT and carbamazepine concentrations were found with lower concentrations during the period of seizure susceptibility [13].

Variations in LTG and valproic acid (VPA) serum concentration levels secondary to endogenous steroid fluctuations across the menstrual cycle have also been investigated [14]. Declines of 8.3% in VPA and 31.3% in LTG serum concentration during the midluteal phase compared to the mid-follicular phase were found without associated clinical correlations. Further work is needed to fully elucidate the pharmacokinetic relationships between endogenous steroids and newer AEDs [13].

Definitions and prevalence

Catamenial epilepsy has been historically defined as the occurrence of seizures around menses or an increase in seizures in relation to the menstrual cycle. Using this definition, the prevalence of catamenial epilepsy varies from 10–78%, with significant methodological differences between studies [1, 15]. Many early studies relied on self-reports or seizure diaries over a single cycle, or were limited to institutionalized or medically refractory patients. Individual perceptions of how seizures relate to menses can be inaccurate. One study found only 12.5% of women met the criteria for catamenial epilepsy by having ≥75% of seizures over a 10-day period beginning 4 days before menses, yet 78% claimed to have seizures triggered by menses [1, 15].

Although an increase in seizures immediately before and during menses is the most prevalent pattern, some women have cyclical seizures during other phases of the menstrual cycle. Three distinct patterns of catamenial epilepsy are illustrated in Figure 8.1, assuming a 28-day cycle [1, 15]. The perimenstrual (C1) pattern is characterized by a greater seizure frequency prior to (days 24–28) and during menstruation (days 1–3) compared with the mid-follicular (days 4 to 9) and midluteal (days 15–23) phases in ovulatory cycles. An increase in seizures during the perimenstrual phase is attributed to the abrupt withdrawal of progesterone prior to menstruation. In a multicenter progesterone trial, the perimenstrual pattern of seizure occurrence (C1) was significantly more prevalent among women with temporal lobe epilepsy (TLE) than extra-temporal or multifocal epilepsies [16]. The peri-ovulatory (C2) pattern is defined as a greater seizure frequency during the ovulatory phase (days 10 to 14) compared with the mid-follicular and midluteal phases in ovulatory cycles. Seizures having this pattern are attributed to the mid cycle estrogen surge. In the luteal

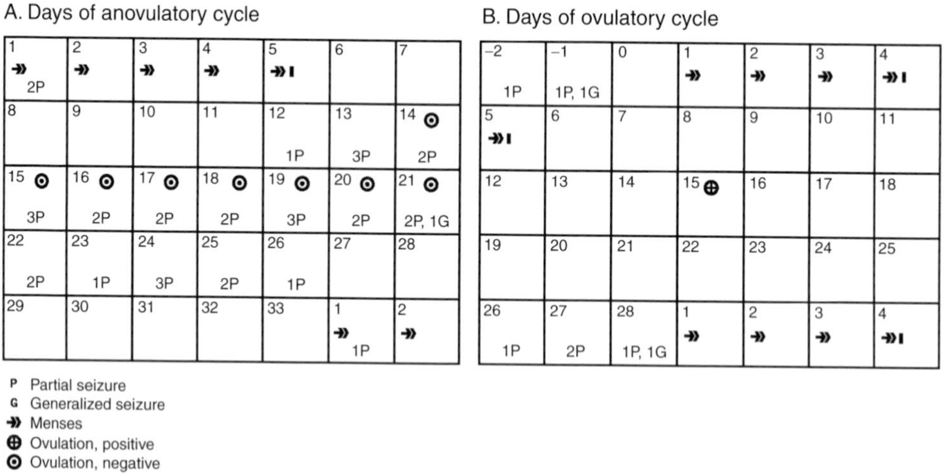

A. Days of anovulatory cycle

1 ➤➤ 2P	2 ➤➤	3 ➤➤	4 ➤➤	5 ➤➤ I	6	7
8	9	10	11	12 1P	13 3P	14 ◎ 2P
15 ◎ 3P	16 ◎ 2P	17 ◎ 2P	18 ◎ 2P	19 ◎ 3P	20 ◎ 2P	21 ◎ 2P, 1G
22 2P	23 1P	24 3P	25 2P	26 1P	27	28
29	30	31	32	33	1 ➤➤ 1P	2 ➤➤

B. Days of ovulatory cycle

-2 1P	-1 1P, 1G	0	1 ➤➤	2 ➤➤	3 ➤➤	4 ➤➤ I
5 ➤➤ I	6	7	8	9	10	11
12	13	14	15 ⊕	16	17	18
19	20	21	22	23	24	25
26 1P	27 2P	28 1P, 1G	1 ➤➤	2 ➤➤	3 ➤➤	4 ➤➤ I

P Partial seizure
G Generalized seizure
➤➤ Menses
⊕ Ovulation, positive
◎ Ovulation, negative

Figure 8.3: Impact of ovulatory status on seizure control in a young female with medically refractory left perirolandic epilepsy. Seizures started at the age of 10 around menarche and were characterized by a cramping or gripping sensation in the right leg followed by right-leg clonic movements, occasionally evolving to a generalized motor seizure. MRI revealed a left parietal malformation of cortical development. Seizures were exacerbated prior to and during menstruation and menstrual cycles were irregular until she reached the age of 20 years. A representative calendar month at 16 years of age (A) shows an anovulatory cycle with frequent seizures, predominantly in the second half of the cycle. Ovulatory cycles became increasing prevalent and by 20 years of age, seizures improved dramatically without change in AED therapy (B).

pattern (C3), seizure frequency is greater during the ovulatory, midluteal, and menstrual phases than during the mid-follicular phase in women with ILP cycles.

When catamenial epilepsy was defined as a 2-fold increase in seizure frequency during a particular phase of the cycle, approximately one-third of women with TLE met the criteria [16]. Using less stringent criteria, 71% of women with ovulatory cycles had perimenstrual or periovulatory patterns (most having both) and 78% of women with ILP cycles showed the luteal pattern. Some women with epilepsy have both ovulatory and anovulatory cycles, including approximately one-third of women with TLE [17]. Anovulatory cycles are common in females under 20 years of age. Seizure frequency is greater during anovulatory cycles, with a significant proportional correlation between the frequency of secondary generalized motor seizures and the E/P ratio [17]. Figure 8.3 illustrates the variation in seizure frequency between ovulatory and ILP cycles in an adolescent with medically refractory epilepsy.

Diagnosis

The diagnosis of catamenial epilepsy is established through documentation of menses, ovulatory status, and patterns of seizure occurrence. There are several ways to confirm ovulation [18]. For the purposes of characterizing seizure patterns, ovulation is usually documented using measurements of basal body temperature (BBT) or commercially available urinary LH kits. Basal body temperature is measured with a basal body thermometer immediately after the morning awakening. Ovulation is documented by a rise of at least 0.7° F on BBT charts. LH urinary kits detect a surge of LH 32–36 hours prior to ovulation. Testing days vary based on individual menstrual cycle length; for a normal 28-day cycle testing should start on day 12. Women are encouraged to test for the LH surge in the morning prior to any activity, at the same time for 10 consecutive days, or until a LH surge is detected. More sophisticated measurements of ovulation include documentation of a midluteal progesterone serum concentration greater than 3 ng/mL, a ≥90% decrease in volume of the dominant follicle on transvaginal ultrasound, or a secretory phase endometrium on endometrial biopsy. ILP cycles are suspected by a BBT rise of <11 days, midluteal progesterone level <5ng/mL, or an out-of-phase endometrial biopsy of >2 days. Ovulation is more difficult to document in very short (<23 days) and long (>35 days) cycles.

Management strategies

Various approaches have been proposed for the treatment of catamenial seizures, virtually all of which are based on small, unblinded series or anecdotal reports. The best initial approach is to optimize therapy with conventional AEDs that are appropriate for the epilepsy syndrome. When conventional therapy proves to be ineffective, alternative approaches may be considered.

Non-hormonal therapies

Cyclical antiepileptic drugs

Antiepileptic drugs, particularly benzodiazepines (BZDs) are often prescribed for intermittent use in women with catamenial epilepsy. Clobazam is the only BZD studied in this population. Recently approved in the USA for use in patients with Lennox–Gastaut syndrome, clobazam is a 1,5-BDZ purported to be less sedating than older BDZs having a 1,4 configuration. The effects of clobazam were studied in a double blind, placebo-controlled, crossover study in 24 women with refractory perimenstrual seizures [19]. Clobazam 20–30 mg/day was administered for 10 days beginning 2–4 days before menstruation for one cycle. Efficacy was defined as seizure freedom in patients with fewer than four seizures per month or >50% reduction in women with more frequent seizures. Clobazam was effective in 14 of 18 evaluable cases (78%), of which 8 women responded to only clobazam and 6 responded to both placebo and clobazam. Three women initially did not respond to either treatment, but had seizure remission with a second trial of clobazam at a higher dosage (30 mg/day). Efficacy for 6 months to 3.5 years was achieved in 13 cases and tolerance was not observed in 9 women treated for ≥ 1 year [20]. Sedation and depression were the most common adverse effects.

Adjusting the dosage of maintenance AEDs during seizure exacerbations in women with catamenial epilepsy has not been adequately investigated. Monthly seizure frequency declined from eight to one in a woman taking valproic acid when dosage was increased intermittently to treat perimenstrual seizures [21]. Changes in maintenance therapy should be carefully considered as the risk of patient and provider errors may increase.

Acetazolamide

Acetazolamide (AZ) is an unsubstituted sulfonamide and potent inhibitor of carbonic anhydrase that produces an accumulation of carbon dioxide in the brain. In a maximum electro shock rat model, AZ raised seizure threshold and decreased seizure susceptibility [22]. AZ has been used to treat catamenial epilepsy for nearly 50 years on the basis of anecdotal reports, even though efficacy has not been clearly demonstrated. The diuretic effects of AZ was proposed as a mechanism of action; however, body weight, sodium metabolism, and total body water during menses were not different in women with and without catamenial seizures, and total body water was unchanged once seizures were controlled with the drug [10].

In a retrospective analysis of 20 women with perimenstrual seizures, AZ (mean daily dose 347 mg) produced a significant reduction in seizure frequency in 40% of cases [23]. An initial dose of 4 mg/kg (not to exceed 1g/day) administered in 1–4 divided doses for 5 to 7 days immediately before and during menstruation is recommended. Adverse effects include paresthesias, drowsiness, ataxia, nausea, vomiting, malaise, anorexia, fatigue, diuresis, intermittent dyspnea, depression, hyperchloremic metabolic acidosis, dysgeusia, renal calculi, and aplastic anemia. The efficacy of AZ is limited by the development of tolerance due to the induction of increased amounts and activity of carbonic anhydrase in glial cells and the production of additional glial cells. Tolerance may be reduced with cyclical dosing regimens surrounding the time of seizure exacerbation [23].

Hormonal therapy
Oral contraceptives

While commonly prescribed for the treatment of perimenstrual seizures, evidence of efficacy of oral contraceptive agents in catamenial epilepsy is lacking. In the only double blind, placebo-controlled study, the oral synthetic progestin norethisterone was ineffective in nine women with perimenstrual seizures treated over 4 months [24]. Given the variable pharmacokinetic interactions between AEDs and hormones, judicious patient education is required when prescribing these agents to sexually active female patients. Patients interested in using hormonal contraception agents should be encouraged to review potential pharmacokinetic interactions with their epilepsy provider and gynecologist. A detailed discussion of contraception in women with epilepsy can be in found Chapter 10.

Medroxyprogesterone acetate

Medroxyprogesterone acetate (MPA) is a progesterone derivative that reduces seizures in some women with epilepsy. Depot-MPA (Depo-Provera) is typically administered as a 150 mg intramuscular injection every 3 months. MPA increases progestin levels, thereby effectively blocking the LH surge and ovulation. It is an appropriate contraceptive choice for women who are noncompliant or cognitively impaired and for those at risk of estrogenic side effects. Adverse effects include irregular menstrual bleeding, nausea, breast tenderness, weight gain, and depression. Long-term treatment often results in amenorrhea and osteoporosis.

The effectiveness of MPA in the treatment of catamenial epilepsy was studied in 14 women, all but one having focal epilepsy [25]. Subjects were treated with oral MPA 10 mg, 2–4 times daily. Six women who did not become amenorrheic were treated with depot-MPA 120–150 mg at 6- to 12-week intervals. At a mean follow-up of 12 months, a 39% reduction in monthly seizures was achieved. No significant adverse effects were reported; however women who received depot-MPA had a delay in the resumption of normal menstruation of 3–12 months [25].

Natural progesterone

Natural progesterone is the most extensively investigated hormonal agent for treatment of catamenial epilepsy. Distinct from cyclic oral progestin (synthetic progestogen) that lacks proven efficacy in seizure reduction [24, 25], natural progesterone has had some evidence in its anticonvulsant properties. Initial studies involving women with TLE treated with progesterone lozenges or vaginal suppositories for 3 months produced a reduction in average monthly seizure frequency of 54–68% and a sustained reduction of 62–74% after 3 years of therapy [26–28]. Adverse effects, including transient fatigue and depression, resolved within 48 hours of dose reduction. Complex partial and generalized motor seizures were reduced to a similar degree. Reduction in seizures was greater in women with ILP cycles (59%) compared with perimenstrual seizures (49%). In a single case of absence epilepsy, seizure control deteriorated during progesterone treatment [26–28]. Whether the effectiveness of hormonal therapy differs in women with generalized and focal epilepsies remains undetermined.

The efficacy and safety of adjunctive, cyclic natural progesterone therapy versus placebo in the treatment of intractable focal seizures was recently studied in 294 women stratified by catamenial (n =130) and noncatamenial (n =164) status [29]. Treatment consisted of progesterone 200 mg, 3 times daily, on days 14–28 of cycles. There was no difference in proportions of ≥50% responders between progesterone and placebo for catamenial and noncatamenial groups. However, the level of perimenstrual (C1) seizure exacerbation was a significant predictor of progesterone response, with the reduction in seizure frequency increasing the degree of C1 tendency from 26–71% for progesterone versus 25–26% for placebo.

Progesterone dosing should be individualized to achieve serum concentrations of 5–25 ng/ml [8]. These levels may be achieved with a total daily dose of 300–600 mg divided 2–3 times per day, as illustrated in Figure 8.4. Therapy is initiated at a dose of 100 mg, 2–3 times daily, on days 14–25, titrated to 200 mg, 3 times daily, if tolerated and seizures persist.

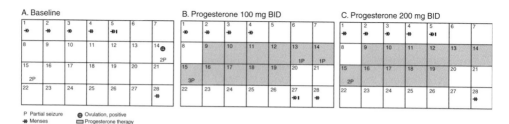

Figure 8.4: Effect of natural progesterone in the treatment of catamenial epilepsy. Shown are seizure calendars of a 37-year-old woman with periovulatory seizure exacerbation (C2). Seizure onset occurred after her third pregnancy, with episodes of hot flashes associated with staring at midcycle, and occasionally prior and during menstruation, that were initially misdiagnosed as manifestations of postpartum depression and anxiety. EEG showed left temporal epileptic discharges and MRI revealed a slight dysmorphism of the left hippocampal formation without signal change. Menstrual cycle duration was 28–30 days and ovulation occurred consistently on day 14. Over 80% of seizures occurred during the ovulatory phase (A). Natural progesterone 100 mg bid taken on days 9–19 reduced seizures (B). Seizures were completely controlled for several years with a dose of 200 mg bid (C).

The dose is reduced to 50% on days 26–27 and 25% on day 28. Enzyme-inducing AEDs may increase progesterone metabolism or vice versa, thereby affecting AED serum concentrations. Therefore, therapeutic drug monitoring is recommended. Adverse effects of progesterone include sedation, nausea, emotional depression, asthenia, breast tenderness, weight gain, constipation, and irregular vaginal bleeding. These effects are reversible with reduction in progesterone dosage. Oral natural progesterone is available in 100 and 200 mg capsules and 200 lozenges (Freedom Drug 1–781–595–0991 or 1–800–660–4283). Lozenges should be allowed to dissolve under the tongue or between the gum and cheek. In the case of early menses, oral progesterone should not be abruptly discontinued, but tapered over 3 days.

Neurosteroids

Ganaxolone, 3α-hydroxy, 3β-methyl-5α-pregnan-20-one, is a neurosteroid and a synthetic analogue of allopregnanolone that modulates the GABA-A receptor complex and possesses anticonvulsant properties [2]. The beta methylation of ganaxolone inhibits reconversion back to progestin. An important distinction between allopregnanolone and ganaxolone is that while they share the same binding profile, ganaxolone does not appear to generate metabolites that have significant classical nuclear steroid hormone activity. Ganaxolone trials have been completed in adults with complex partial seizures and pediatric patients with infantile spasms. Moderate reduction in seizures was achieved in two women with perimenstrual seizures treated with ganaxolone 300 mg twice daily on days 21–23 of treatment cycles [30].

Other hormonal agents

Isolated reports of the antiestrogen clomiphene citrate, synthetic androgen danazol, and synthetic gonadotropin analogues triptorelin and goserelin suggest some potential in treating catamenial epilepsy, although confirmatory investigations are needed. Clomiphene citrate 25–100 mg administered on days 5–9 of treatment cycles reduced seizures by at least 50% in 10 of 12 women with TLE and by >90% in 5 cases [31]. Transient adverse effects including vasomotor flushes, abdominal distension or pain, breast discomfort, nausea, vomiting, and visual disturbances occurred in six cases, all resolving with drug withdrawal. The synthetic androgen danazol eliminates the gonadotropin surge of FSH and LH, producing a high androgen and low estrogen state. It successfully controlled seizures in a woman with cerebral endometriosis and catamenial epilepsy [32]. The synthetic GnRH agonist triptorelin was administered at 3.75 mg intramuscularly at 4-week intervals for 12 months, producing a significant improvement in 7 of 10 women with refractory perimenstrual seizures and amenorrhea, including seizure remission in three cases [33]. Adverse effects including hot flashes, headache, and weight gain were observed in eight cases. Treatment with the LH-releasing hormone agonist goserelin markedly reduced the frequency of status epilepticus in a woman with primary generalized epilepsy [1, 34].

Conclusions

Catamenial epilepsy is a common disorder, affecting one-third of women with epilepsy. Three distinct patterns of seizure susceptibility have been described. The pathophysiology of this disorder has not been entirely elucidated; however studies suggest that the abrupt withdrawal of progesterone is operative in women with perimenstrual seizures (C1), and a state of hyperestrogenism plays a role in periovulatory (C2) and luteal phase (C3) patterns. While various treatment approaches have been proposed, evidence of effectiveness is based largely on small, uncontrolled series or anecdotal observations. A recent multicenter randomized controlled trial found progesterone to be most efficacious than placebo in women with perimenstrual seizures, with efficacy increasing with the degree of C1 exacerbation.

References

1. Foldvary-Schaefer N, Harden C, Herzog A, et al. Hormones and seizures. *Cleve Clin J Med* 2004; 71(Suppl 2):S11–S8.

2. Reddy DS. Role of neurosteroids in catamenial epilepsy. *Epilepsy Res* 2004; 62 (2–3):99–118.

3. Veliskova J, De Jesus G, Kaur R, et al. Females, their estrogens, and seizures. *Epilepsia* 2010; 51(Suppl 3):141–4.

4. Woolley CS. Estradiol facilitates kainic acid-induced, but not flurothyl-induced, behavioral seizure activity in adult female rats. *Epilepsia* 2000; 41(5):510–5.

5. Hom, AC and Butterbough, GG. Estrogen alters the acquisition of seizures kindled by repeated amygdala stimulation or pentylenetetrazol administration in ovariectomized female rats. *Epilepsia* 1986; 27:103–8.

6. Backstrom T. Epileptic seizures in women related to plasma estrogen and progesterone during the menstrual cycle. *Acta Neurol Scand* 1976; 54(4):321–47.

7. Woolley CS and McEwen BS. Estradiol regulates hippocampal dendritic spine density via an N-methyl-D-aspartate receptor-dependent mechanism. *Neurosci* 1994; 14(12):7680–7.

8. Herzog AG. Hormonal therapies: progesterone. *Neurotherapeutic* 2009; 6(2):383–91.

9. Frye CA. Effects and mechanisms of progestogens and androgens in ictal activity. *Epilepsia* 2010; 51 (Suppl 3):135–40.

10. Ansell B and Clarke E. Epilepsy and menstruation: the role of water retention. *Lancet* 1956; 271(6955):1232–5.

11. De Wildt SN KG, Leeder JS and Van Den Anker JN. Glucuronidation in humans. Pharmacogenetic and developmental aspects. *Clin Pharmacokinet* 1999; 36(6):439–52.

12. Rosciszewska D, Buntner B, Guz I, et al. Ovarian hormones, anticonvulsant drugs, and seizures during the menstrual cycle in women with epilepsy. *J Neurol Neurosurg Psychiatry* 1986; 49(1):47–51.

13. Herkes G and Eadie, MJ. Possible roles for frequent salivary AED monitoring in the management of epilepsy. *Epilepsy Res Suppl* 1990; 6:146–54.

14. Herzog AG, Blum AS, Farina EL, et al. Valproate and lamotrigine level variation with menstrual cycle phase and oral contraceptive use. *Neurology* 2009; 72(10):911–4.

15. Herzog AG, Klein P and Ransil BJ. Three patterns of catamenial epilepsy. *Epilepsia* 1997; 38(10):1082–8.

16. Quigg M, Smithson SD, Fowler KM, et al. Laterality and location influence catamenial seizure expression in women with partial epilepsy. *Neurology* 2009; 73(3):223–7.

17. Herzog AG, Fowler KM, Sperling MR, et al. Variation of seizure frequency with ovulatory status of menstrual cycles. *Epilepsia* 2011; 52(10):1843–8.

18. Speroff L, Glass RH and Kase NG. *Clinical gynecologic endocrinology and infertility.* Philadelphia, PA: Lippincott Williams & Wilkins, 1999.

19. Feely M, Calvert R and Gibson J. Clobazam in catamenial epilepsy. A model for evaluating anticonvulsants. *Lancet* 1982; 2(8289):71–3.

20. Feely M and Gibson J. Intermittent clobazam for catamenial epilepsy: tolerance avoided. *J Neurol Neurosurg Psychiatry* 1984; 47(12):1279–82.

21. Krishnamurthy BS and Schomer DL. Weekly fluctuation and adjustment of antiepileptic drugs to treat catamenial seizures. *Epilepsia* 1998; 39 (Suppl 6):179.

22. Anderson RE, Howard RA and Woodbury DM. Correlation between effects of acute acetazolamide administration to mice on electroshock seizure threshold and maximal electroshock seizure pattern, and on carbonic anhydrase activity in subcellular fractions of brain. *Epilepsia* 1986; 27(5):504–9.

23. Lim LL, Foldvary N, Mascha E, et al. Acetazolamide in women with catamenial epilepsy. *Epilepsia* 2001; 42(6):746–9.

24. Dana-Haeri J and Richens A. Effect of norethisterone on seizures associated with menstruation. *Epilepsia* 1983; 24(3):377–81.

25. Mattson RH, Cramer JA, Caldwell BV, et al. Treatment of seizures with medroxyprogesterone acetate: preliminary report. *Neurology* 1984; 34(9):1255–8.

26. Herzog AG. Progesterone therapy in women with epilepsy: a 3-year follow-up. *Neurology* 1999; 52(9):1917–8.

27. Herzog AG. Progesterone therapy in women with complex partial and secondary generalized seizures. *Neurology* 1995; 45(9):1660–2.

28. Herzog A. Intermittent progesterone therapy of partial complex seizures in women with menstrual disorders. *Neurology* 1986; 36:1607–10.

29. Herzog A, Fowler KM, Smithson SD, et al. For the Progesterone Trial Study Group. Progesterone vs placebo therapy for women with epilepsy: a randomized clinical trial. *Neurology* 2012; 78(24):1959–66.

30. McAuley J, Moore JL, Reeves AL, et al. A pilot study of the neurosteroid ganaxolone in catamenial epilepsy: clinical experience in two patients. *Epilepsia* 2001; 42:85.

31. Herzog A. Clomiphene therapy in epileptic women with menstrual disorders. *Neurology* 1988; 38:432–4.

32. Bauer J, Wildt L, Flugel D, et al. The effect of a synthetic GnRH analogue on catamenial epilepsy: a study in ten patients. *J Neurol Neurosurg Psychiatry* 1992; 239:284–6.

33. Ichida M, Gomi A, Hiranouchi N, et al. A case of cerebral endometriosis causing catamenial epilepsy. *Neurology* 1993; 43(12):2708–9.

34. Vilos GA, Hollett-Caines J, Abu-Rafea B, et al. Resolution of catamenial epilepsy after goserelin therapy and oophorectomy: case report of presumed cerebral endometriosis. *J Minim Invasive Gynecol* 2011; 18(1):128–30.

Fertility in women with epilepsy

Mark Quigg

Key points:

- Women with epilepsy (WWE) have lower fertility compared to the general population
- Signs of infertility may include menstrual irregularity, obesity, hirsutism, and galactorrhea
- Infertility in WWE is likely multifactorial attributed to psychosocial factors, decreased libido, and neuroendocrine alterations secondary to seizures and antiepileptic drugs (AEDs)
- The hypothalamic-pituitary-gonadal axis (HPG-axis) and feedback inhibitory mechanisms play a key part in infertility among WWE
- Reversible/treatable causes of infertility should be identified and addressed if WWE wish to conceive

Introduction

Infertility is usually not just a disorder of individuals but a disorder of couples. Infertility is the failure to conceive after regular intercourse in women who are not using contraception for a duration of 1 year for women <35 years and 6 months for those >35 years [1]. Epidemiological data suggest that about 10–15% of all couples will experience difficulties to conceive (primary infertility) or to conceive the full number of children they want (secondary infertility) [1–3].

Fertility is also an important concern of WWE and their families. Historically, constraints on reproductive rights – bans on marriage and having children – were important factors in the ability of WWE to bear children. For example, state laws in the USA allowed forcible sterilization of WWE until 1956, while in the UK people with epilepsy were not allowed to marry until 1970 [4]. Until 1999, epilepsy was grounds for annulment of marriage in India [5].

Although these laws are obsolete, social considerations may continue to influence decisions on childbearing. With these confounders in place, determining the biological effects of epilepsy, seizures, and AEDs on fertility of WWE is not straightforward. The purpose of this review is to summarize the epidemiological data on infertility in WWE, describe some of the social and biological constraints on fertility experienced in the epileptic population, and to review the evaluation and treatment of infertility in WWE.

Women with Epilepsy, ed. Esther Bui and Autumn Klein. Published by Cambridge University Press.
© Cambridge University Press 2014.

Epidemiology of infertility in WWE

Table 9.1 summarizes selected epidemiological studies of fertility in WWE. Studies vary in the measurements of fertility, with some reporting the number of children (live births per patient or by patient-years) and others the proportion of women successfully concluding a pregnancy (proportion of women with at least one birth). To standardize the comparison of different studies, Table 9.1 and the discussion below uses a normalized "fertility rate," the proportion of observed fertility to expected in the units as defined by each study.

Most studies that assess fertility in WWE use public health databases. These studies [6–9], with one exception [10], demonstrate decreased fertility among WWE with a range of 61–86% lower than controls. The earliest compared WWE and women without epilepsy within the Mayo clinic catchment area between 1935–1974 [6]. WWE had 71.0 live births (per 1,000 person-years) compared to 82.9 live births in non-epileptic controls for a fertility rate of 86%. The largest study consisted of >2 million people sample in the UK National Health database between 1990–1995 [7]. Fertility was lower among WWE (47.1 (95% confidence interval (CI), 42.3–52.2) live births per 1,000 women aged 15–45 per year) compared to controls (62.1 live births). Therefore, fertility in WWE in this sample was ~75% that of the non-epileptic population. Another nationwide cohort study conducted in Finland compared live birth rates of WWE and those without between 1985–2001 [8]. This study showed a fertility rate of 61%. A Finnish study confined to a single hospital confirmed the wider study with 59% of WWE between ages 16–39 bearing at least 1 child compared to 77% of controls for a fertility rate of 76% [9]. One national health system-based study from Iceland conflicts with the above studies. Olafsson et al. reported that, between 1960 and 1964, 209 WWE had 2.0 live births per patient, no different from age-matched controls [10].

Several prospective studies followed WWE through a period of time to directly observe birth rates. Overall, these studies [11–13] show similar ranges of fertility in WWE (55–73%) as the retrospective health care-database studies. Jalava et al. followed WWE and compared them to two control groups [13]. The first control group was constructed from a sample of 100 age-matched women selected at random from a Finnish health care database. Another control group (n = 100) came from the health care rolls of a large corporation. The WWE were subdivided into those with and without "epilepsy-only": i.e., idiopathic or cryptogenic epilepsy without cognitive impairment or symptomatic cause. The 99 women with "epilepsy only" had live birth rates of 0.97, whereas randomized controls had birth rates of 1.77 and the "employee controls" had birth rates of 1.61, for fertility rates of 55–60%, respectively. Another prospective study performed in India tracked a group of WWE who were anticipating pregnancy and compared characteristics of those who became pregnant and those who did not [12]. Thirty-eight percent of women remained infertile, a rate nearly double that of a non-epileptic comparison obtained from the same region's census board. A US study used a novel design of surveying a group of WWE about their overall pregnancy history compared to a control group of their asymptomatic oldest female siblings [11]. Women were included only if they had been married at least once. WWE had a fertility rate of 70% compared to their non-epileptic sisters.

In summary, most studies, whether based in the examination of large health care databases or in the prospective following of cohorts, demonstrate that fertility in WWE occurs at a rate of about 75% of that expected.

Table 9.1: Studies of fertility rates in women with epilepsy (WWE)

First author	Year	Country	Design	N	Duration of sample or study (years)	WWE sample	Control sample	Fertility rate WWE	Fertility rate controls	Fertility ratio
Webber [6]	1986	USA	Retro	220	44	All WWE between 1935–74 Rochester, MN	All women without epilepsy	71.0 LB per 1,000 person-years	82.9 LB per 1,000 person-years	0.86
Jalava [13]	1997	Finland	Pro	100	35	Clinic sample	Age-matched national health survey N = 99,	0.97 LB per woman	1.77 LB per woman,	0.55
						Clinic sample	Age-matched employee survey N = 100		1.61 LB per woman	0.60
Olafsson [10]	1998	Iceland	Retro	209	5	All WWE Iceland National Health	Age-matched non-epileptic sample N = 418	2.0 LB per woman	2.0 LB per woman	1.00
Wallace [7]	1998	UK	Retro	7626	5	All WWE age 15–45 National Health	All women without epilepsy age 15–45	47.1 LB per 1,000 women	62.1 LB per 1,000 women	0.75
Artama [8]	2004	Finland	Retro			All WWE 1985–2001 age 15–45 National Health	All women without epilepsy age 15–45	0.54 LB per woman	0.88 LB per woman	0.61
Schupf [11]	2006	USA	Retro	581	lifetime	Clinic sample: WWE who had been married at least one	Female siblings who had been married N = 170	1.4 LB per woman	2.0 LB per woman	0.70
Viinikainen [9]	2008	Finland	Retro	286	1	All WWE age 16–39 National Health	Public health database	59% with at least 1 LB	77% with at least 1 LB	0.76
Sukumaran [12]	2010	India	Pro	375	1–10	Clinic sample	Public health database	61.8% with at least 1 LB	84.9% with at least 1 LB	0.73

Fertility ratio = fertility rate of WWE/controls; design = retro(spective) or pro(spective); LB = live births

Etiology of infertility in WWE
Social factors and stigma

In the Mayo study of long-term trends in fertility from 1935 to 1974, the authors noted that infertility in WWE changed through the decades. Infertility in WWE was most marked in the decades after World War II (1945–1964, the postwar "baby boom"), when fertility of the population as a whole jumped and fertility of WWE lagged [6]. Similar findings were seen in the cohort study by Schupf et al. [11].

The social stigma of epilepsy may be one reason WWE demonstrate relatively low rates of fertility. Two studies based in India examined perceptions of epilepsy and marriage. From interviews of 400 WWE in rural India, onset of epilepsy before 20 years of age reduces the chances of patients finding a spouse among those who disclose their diagnosis to family or community members [14]. This relationship between age of onset and delay in marriage (and hence, possibly reduced fertility) was confirmed in the Indian population in a second study that showed WWE are less likely to get married, to be older when married, and have higher rates of "withheld marriage" (spinsterhood). On the other hand, the large majority of women (95%) do not disclose their diagnosis before marriage. Perhaps lack of disclosure is one factor that accounts for higher rates of divorce compared to national means as observed in this study. Decreased marriage rates have been observed in other cultures. In a survey of 100 WWE in Canada [15], the marriage rate was 83% that expected. Early onset of seizures was the main demographic factor noted to worsen chance of marriage. The stigma against marriage was the main finding in a Hong Kong survey; in a non-epileptic sample, 94% of respondents thought it appropriate for people with epilepsy to marry, one-third thought it inappropriate to marry a person with epilepsy if the proposed spouse was their own child [16]. The rates of marriage were also evaluated in the previously discussed Finnish study [13]. Compared to controls with an 83% marriage or significant cohabitation rate, only 60% of WWE achieved marriage or cohabitation over the duration of the study; WWE were 3.6-fold more likely to remain single. In contrast, the Icelandic study—one in which fertility of WWE was not impaired compared to controls—found no disadvantage in rates of marriage of WWE [10].

Patients with cognitive impairment may not have the means to independently marry and raise children. The studies in India [12], Finland [9], and Iceland [10] all found worse birth rates among WWE who had comorbid mental retardation or cerebral palsy.

Once married, choices in childbearing in WWE appeared to play a small but real role in the Indian cohorts. For example, 2% of married WWE chose not to have children for fear of transmitting the disease [8]. Abortion as a method of regulating fertility has not been widely investigated in WWE. The only study in Table 9.1 that measured voluntary abortion rates found that less than 5% of WWE had abortions compared to the Indian national average of 6% [8].

Sexual desire and mood

Problems with mood and libido may affect fertility in WWE. For example, even in WWE who have the appropriate social possibility of conceiving children, they may do so less frequently because of decreased sexual desire or depressed mood. Morrell et al. studied sexual function and hormones in women with epilepsy aged 18–40 with partial or generalized epilepsies compared to non-epileptic controls [17]. Questionnaires examined sexual experience, arousability, anxiety, and depression; the questionnaires were then compared to endocrine assessments. Compared to controls, women with partial epilepsy had significantly impaired sexual function, lower degrees of self-reported arousal, and worse depression scores. Women with generalized epilepsy were less impaired overall, but still reported decreased arousal. Women taking enzyme-inducing AEDs were most affected. Hormonal measurements that correlated with sexual dysfunction were estradiol (negatively correlated with sexual anxiety), and dehydroepiandrostone (negatively correlated with sexual dysfunction and lack of arousal). Furthermore, the associations among low libido, low testosterone, and use of enzyme-inducing AEDs are also observed in men with epilepsy [18].

Direct biological effects

The interactions between epilepsy, neuroendocrine regulation of the hypothalamic-pituitary-gonadal axis (HPG-axis, see Figure 9.1), and AEDs are complex and lay outside the broad answers that epidemiology can provide. A direct role for epilepsy in the pathogenesis of infertility is suggested by the differences in fertility according to epilepsy syndrome, the high rate of reproductive disorders in those with epilepsy, the acute disruption of normal hypothalamic-pituitary activity by seizures and interictal discharges [19–21], the physiologic and clinical effects of laterality of epileptic foci [19–21], and the chronic effects of the epileptic lesion on menstrual function that correct after successful epilepsy surgery [22].

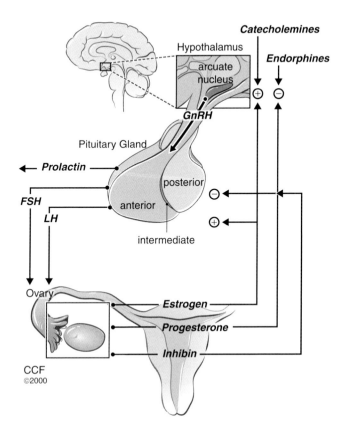

Figure 9.1: The hypothalamic-pituitary-ovarian axis regulates the interactions between neurohormones, gonadotropin-releasing hormone, pituitary gonadotropins, and the gonadal steroids through a feedback loop mechanism.

Epilepsy syndrome

Several of the surveys in Table 9.1 evaluated the effects on fertility by epilepsy syndrome. Epidemiology studies are not consistent in demonstrating that epilepsy syndrome has on effect on fertility. Some show, however, that fertility is most affected in the case of remote symptomatic epilepsy compared to idiopathic/cryptogenic epilepsy. For example, Schupf et al., in their study of WWE compared to their healthy sisters [11], found that the effects of infertility were highest in partial rather than generalized epilepsies, a difference that was most marked before diagnosis of epilepsy. Similar findings were seen in the large population study by Webber et al. [6].

In comparison, the Icelandic survey, in addition to finding no disadvantage in fertility in WWE, also found no differences between those with partial versus generalized epilepsies [10]. When WWE with idiopathic/cryptogenic epilepsy were compared with controls, there was no difference in the number of children or number of partners overall, nor were there differences when stratified by seizure type or age at diagnosis. Patients with remote symptomatic epilepsy, when mental retardation (MR) or cerebral palsy (CP) were excluded, also had an equal rate of live births to controls. Differences from controls only emerged in patients with MR/CP, from which only 8% of women bore children [10]. A large effect of MR/CP on infertility was also seen in the Finnish population (type of epilepsy was not measured) [9].

A prospective study of an Indian cohort similarly found that the type of epilepsy had no significance in fertility rates [12]. Demographic factors that were associated with infertile WWE included older age and lower educational status (perhaps reflective of severity of epilepsy rather than a direct effect of education).

In comparison to epidemiological studies, studies investigating HPG-axis function focus on those with temporal lobe epilepsy, partly because of availability of patients in tertiary clinics and partly because of evidence of the importance of temporolimbic connections in hypothalamic dysfunction [19]. For example, prolactin, a hormone that usually rises more than 2-fold after partial seizures of temporal lobe origin, is less likely to rise after simple partial seizures that spare the limbic system [21].

Reproductive disorders in WWE

WWE have higher than expected rates of disorders that directly affect fertility, and these disorders have been either directly linked or have enough evidence to infer that they are present largely because of disruption of normal function due to the epileptic condition (including AED use) or epileptic seizures. These disorders include polycystic ovary syndrome (PCOS), hypothalamic hypogonadism, functional hyperprolactinemia, and premature menopause [23].

Polycystic ovary syndrome (PCOS)

PCOS is defined as a hyperandrogenic state with obesity, hirsutism, and chronic amenorrhea or oligomenorrhea affecting about 5% of women in the general population. In a series of 50 consecutive women with temporolimbic epilepsy, Herzog et al. found that 20% were affected with PCOS [24]. Another study of women with generalized epilepsy found an incidence of 15% [24]. Although AED use may be an important factor in the development of PCOS, some women in these studies were not taking AEDs, suggesting that the epileptic condition is sufficient for neuroendocrine dysfunction.

Hypothalamic hypogonadism

Hypothalamic hypogonadism, or inadequate stimulation of ovarian function due to insufficient or disordered secretion of gonadotropins, results in infertility and amenorrhea or oligomenorrhea, and has been reported to occur in 12% of a sample of women with temporal lobe epilepsy, compared to a rate of 1.5% in the general population [24].

Hyperprolactinemia

Hyperprolactinemia theoretically may be a factor in infertility in active epilepsy. Hyperprolactinemia may cause polymenorrhea, oligomenorrhea, or amenorrhea, as well as poor fertility, galactorrhea, and hirsutism. As noted above, the blood level of prolactin rises immediately after seizures, sometimes 4–5-fold from preictal levels, and stays elevated for about 1 hour postictally [20]. Herzog demonstrated that small prolactin surges can occur as the result of interictal discharges in the case of temporal lobe epilepsy [23]. Although theoretically important from a temporolimbic interaction perspective, hyperprolactinemia from a clinical standpoint may be rare in WWE. An evaluation of reproductive disorders in WWE disclosed that out of 238 Finnish women being treated for epilepsy, none had hyperprolactinemia [25].

Premature menopause

Premature menopause (primary gonadal failure with amenorrhea and high gonadotropin levels at age <40) may occur earlier in WWE than in the general population. The highest rate of premature menopause was seen in a study of 50 WWE whose rate of 14% stood far above the control rate of 4% [26]. In their study of the distribution of reproductive disorders in temporal lobe epilepsy, Herzog et al. found that 4% had early menopause compared with an expected general rate of about 1% [24]. A Finnish cohort, however, only found a rate of premature menopause in 1.4% [25].

Effects of chronic epilepsy and acute seizures

The physiologic means by which the HPG-axis may be affected by the epileptic lesion are discussed below. Both interictal and ictal discharges affect function of the HPG-axis at the hypothalamic level [19, 20]. In a study of HPG function in men with temporal lobe epilepsy (in this case used as a "model" for WWE not susceptible to menstrual effects), Quigg et al. evaluated the pattern of pulsatile luteinizing hormone (LH) secretion for 24-hour periods with two comparisons [20]. First, to evaluate the effects of interictal dysfunction (the effect of the chronic epileptic lesion), interictal LH secretion of men with temporal lobe epilepsy was compared to age-matched healthy controls. Second, to evaluate postictal effects, LH secretion patterns from the first 24 hours after a seizure were matched with each patient's interictal sample. Chronic epilepsy, or interictal function in epilepsy compared to healthy controls, was associated with changes in LH pulse frequency, amplitude, and amount per pulse. Acute seizures induced timing irregularity—a degradation in pulse rhythm—in LH secretion. Clinical effects, however, were not measured in this study.

Herzog et al. forged clear links between the clinical phenotype of sexual dysfunction and the epileptic state [19]. A quantitative sexual rating scale and reproductive hormone measures evaluated sexual dysfunction in women with mesial temporal lobe epilepsy. Sexual dysfunction scores were higher in WWE, and sexual dysfunction affected substantially more women with epilepsy than controls. There was a significant inverse correlation between sexual dysfunction and bioactive testosterone levels in women with epilepsy as well as in controls. A study by Morrell et al. with similar intention and findings, but focused more on sexual desire and libido, was discussed above. Certainly, impaired libido associated with active epilepsy can also be seen as a physiologic impairment or disorder [17].

Laterality of the epileptic lesion

Another example of the direct effects of the epileptic lesion on the HPG-axis, and by extension, fertility, is on the unexpected findings of epileptic laterality on HPG dysfunction. Quigg et al.'s study of male LH secretion found that the rate of pulses of LH was faster in men with right-sided temporal foci than in those with left-sided foci. Lateralization of LH pulsatile secretion was also seen in women with temporal lobe epilepsy [27]. Herzog et al. linked physiologic lateralization to clinical phenotype, noting that sexual dysfunction scores, and accompanying low testosterone levels, were more often present in women with right-sided rather than left-sided temporal lobe epilepsy [19]. Furthermore, reproductive disorders aggregated by side of the epileptic lesion; those with PCOS tended to have left-sided epileptic foci, and those with hypogonadotropic hypogonadism, right-sided.

Epilepsy surgery

The argument for the direct effects of epilepsy on HPG-axis function has been investigated in studies of WWE after epilepsy surgery. Bauer et al. [22] assessed menstrual function before and 1 year after either temporal lobectomy or selective amygdala hippocampectomy for 16 women. Eight of the patients achieved seizure remission, and all remained on their AEDs. Documentation of menstrual cycles in addition to laboratory parameters revealed post-surgical changes of the menstrual cycle in eight patients. Four patients had a change in menstrual periodicity. In contrast to cycle changes, no definitive changes were seen in post-surgical concentrations of testosterone, prolactin, dehydroepiandrosterone sulfate, growth hormone, cortisol, and sex hormone-binding globulin. There was, however, a significant increase in serum androstenedione concentration 6 months post-surgically, mainly in those patients achieving seizure remission. The authors interpreted the study as demonstrating that successful epilepsy surgery can alter menstrual cycle function. Although no gross serum changes in sex hormones occurred, one can hypothesize that other physiologic changes—such as in the pulsatile secretion patterns outlined above—may have occurred after surgery and seizure remission.

In summary, some epidemiological studies and a host of neuroendocrine studies suggest that epileptic seizures and the chronic epileptic lesion affect fertility by direct effects upon hypothalamic function.

Antiepileptic drugs (AEDs)

The studies from India [12], Finland [9], and Iceland [10] emphasize that comorbidities of epilepsy play a role in infertility, some of which may be conferred by AED use. In fact, in the Indian prospective study of WWE that compared those who bore children and those who did not, AED exposure was the most important factor in infertility. The proportion of infertile women was highest (60%) for those on three or more AEDs and decreased with the number of AEDs (2 AEDs–41%; 1 AED–32%).

AEDs have been implicated as an important cause, or at least a contributor, to infertility and reproductive disorders in WWE. Potential interactions between AEDs and fertility could arise from the effects of AEDs on gonadal function, the effects of AEDs on hormonal metabolism or serum binding (which in turn may induce changes in hypothalamic regulation/feedback), and in secondary interactions of AEDs with weight/appetite regulation or insulin sensitivity. Isojärvi has written an excellent summary of individual effects of AEDs on HPG function [28]. Some highlights are below.

Of the AEDs, valproate (VPA) has acquired the most evidence in direct alteration of HPG-axis function usually in provocation of PCOS. Isojärvi et al. [25] described the reproductive phenotypes of 238 WWE taking different AED combinations, with 12% on VPA monotherapy, 50% taking carbamazepine (CBZ) monotherapy, 31% on combination or other monotherapy, and 6% untreated. They evaluated ovary status with ultrasound, menstrual cycles, and hormonal levels. Whereas 45% of the women taking VPA had menstrual disturbances and 43% had polycystic ovaries (note: polycystic ovaries are only one component of PCOS), patients on other AEDs had less than one-half the rate of menstrual problems or polycystic ovaries. Some patients on VPA had no polycystic ovaries, but did have hyperandrogenism. Overall, 60% of women on VPA had polycystic ovaries and hyperandrogenism, and if VPA was started before the age of 20 years, 80%.

In a related study, Isojärvi et al. re-evaluated HPG-axis function after changing AED therapy from VPA to lamotrigine (which has not been shown to have direct gonadal effects) in twelve WWE who had PCOS [29]. Once on lamotrigine, high testosterone levels returned to normal within 2 months of VPA discontinuation, and levels remained normal thereafter. Similarly, menstrual disorders and ultrasounds demonstrating polycystic ovaries normalized.

The enzyme-inducing AEDs—phenytoin (PHY), phenobarbital (PB), and CBZ—have earned a reputation for being the most active in interfering with normal function of sex steroid-binding proteins, which in turn reduce the amount of available sex steroids in serum. Although the hypothalamus, via feedback mechanisms, should sense a drop in available sex steroid (Figure 9.1), enzyme-inducing AEDs may also promote the elevation of estradiol [18]. Although estradiol constitutes a small portion of circulating sex steroid, it packs a disproportionately heavy effect in feedback suppression of compensatory gonadotropin secretion. By both sequestration of circulating sex steroid through increased binding and via impaired compensatory feedback, enzyme-inducing AEDs render WWE effectively hypogonadal.

Accordingly, switching AEDs to those with less impact on neuroendocrine function should reverse AED-associated HPG-axis dysfunction. Isojärvi et al. demonstrated this relationship by changing therapy from CBZ to oxcarbazepine in a sample of WWE who had PCOS [28]. Within a year of the change, both free testosterone and the incidence of polycystic ovaries decreased. Although a drop in testosterone with treatment of epilepsy with CBZ in this instance appears to be a "benefit," as noted above, low testosterone associated with use of enzyme-inducing AEDs may cause depressed libido [17, 18].

The effects of AEDs, especially VPA, may result from either direct disruption of the HPG-axis or from secondary effects. For an example of the latter, PCOS is associated with obesity. In turn, excess adipose tissue sequesters steroids and alters the balance of steroid subtype production; therefore obesity is thought to be a main cause of PCOS rather than an effect. Accordingly, AED-induced obesity may contribute to the multifactorial causes of infertility in WWE. Certain AEDs have associations with obesity; VPA is the most notorious. About 50% of women treated with VPA experience weight gain from pretreatment baselines, and fortunately, can lose weight if VPA is changed [29] (to lamotrigine in this study). In this author's experience, every AED, at one time or another, has been blamed for weight gain in both women and men with epilepsy. However, VPA, along with CBZ, gabapentin, and vigabatrin stand out [30]. Interestingly, there are other AEDs that are known for weight loss, namely, topiramate, zonisamide, and felbamate. These have not been studied in the setting of PCOS to evaluate if AED-induced weight loss can improve neuroendocrine function.

Mechanisms for AED-obesity remain controversial. Isojärvi et al., in his study of WWE and PCOS who were switched from VPA to lamotrigine, observed that after the switch the body mass index and fasting insulin both decreased in concert with decreases in testosterone [29]. Hypotheses of mechanisms to account for VPA-induced insulin resistance or hyperinsulinemia are that: (1) lowered blood glucose may stimulate eating through an effect on the hypothalamus; (2) competitive binding of VPA and long chain fatty acids (increased availability of long chain fatty acids stimulates insulin production and lowers glucose) may alter feedback control; and (3) VPA may interact with carnitine, thus reducing fatty acid metabolism and increasing glucose consumption [30].

Evaluation and treatment
Signs and differential diagnosis

An expert panel summarized recommendations for the evaluation and treatment of WWE in regards to reproductive disorders and infertility in 2002 [31].

An important feature in evaluating infertility in WWE is that the factors associated with epilepsy—from social to biological—occur in the context of reproductive health in general. In other words, WWE who are infertile may have the same reproductive problems as women without epilepsy. For example, an epidemiology study from a French population of 1,850,000 people found that 1,686 couples were infertile, for an incidence of 14% (i.e. 1 out 7 French women in this population sought medical help for infertility at some point in their reproductive life) [3]. Female infertility accounted for 37% of infertile couples. The six most common identifiable causes of female infertility were: ovulatory disorders (25%), endometriosis (15%), pelvic adhesions (11%), tubal blockage (11%), other tubal abnormalities (11%), and hyperprolactinemia (7%). Except for ovulatory disorders, the other causes have no particular association with epilepsy, but certainly may occur in WWE.

In a practical sense, most epileptologists or general neurologists will defer some or all investigations of reproductive dysfunction to gynecologists or fertility specialists; however, knowledge of the general outline is recommended for education and patient counseling.

Important clinical signs (and their definitions) associated with reproductive disorders are detailed in Table 9.2. Most of these signs are seen in PCOS, the disorder most often linked directly to epilepsy. However, signs such as menstrual irregularity, of course, are not limited to "epileptic" infertility. WWE can also have dysfunction of components of the HPG-axis unrelated to epilepsy, with differential diagnoses as diverse as functional "lesions" such as stress, older age, or over-exercise, to structural lesions such as hypothalamic hamartomas or hormonally active pituitary adenomas. Another important point is that the HPG-axis does not act in isolation. Interactions with abnormalities outside the HPG-axis—hyper- or hypothyroidism, hypercortisolism (Cushing's), or other endocrine abnormalities—can interfere with normal HPG-axis regulation to an extent to cause infertility.

Table 9.3 shows the typical components of a neuroendocrine and pelvic imaging evaluation for infertility in WWE as recommended by the expert panel [31]. Neuroimaging—an MRI with appropriate fine cuts through the pituitary—also plays an important role depending on examination and findings. An important aspect of reproductive hormone measurement is the circadian and menstrual cycle timing of samples, with most laboratories and ultrasounds taken within the early follicular phase of the menstrual cycle to avoid the

Table 9.2: Symptoms and signs of reproductive disorders in women with epilepsy [31]

Signs	Definition
Infertility	Inability to become pregnant after >12 months unprotected sex, male infertility excluded
Menstrual irregularity	Cycles between 23–35 days • amenorrhea: absence of cycles • oligomenorrhea: cycles >35 days • polymenorrhea: cycles <23 days
Obesity	BMI >25
Hirsutism	Male escutcheon (extension of pubic hair above the pubis symphysis)
Galactorrhea	Expression of milk in non-postpartum women

ovulatory surges in gonadotropins and sex hormones. Samples should also not be taken shortly after a seizure, to avoid postictal changes.

Not listed in the panel's recommendations are the typical "first step" issues common in reproductive medicine [32]. Often, the most common cause of amenorrhea is pregnancy, so appropriate pregnancy testing should always be considered in first presentation. Second, male fertility can be easily checked and potentially treated (i.e., artificial insemination with partner or donor sperm), so a semen sample to evaluate sperm concentration, morphology, and motility is recommended before embarking on causes of female infertility.

AED selection

The selection of AEDs for WWE of childbearing age must not only take into account the issues of fertility discussed in this review but also teratogenic and other intrauterine effects of AEDs on fetal health (for those who wish to become pregnant) and on effectiveness of birth control (for those who do not).

Of utmost priority, a neurologist attempts to render to a woman with epilepsy a correct diagnosis and complete seizure control. Within these primary goals, no particular AED can be recommended over others or labeled with a contraindication for WWE. Although most evidence implicates VPA and enzyme-inducing AEDs with the most interactions with the HPG-axis, newer AEDs may not have yet accumulated the person-years required to fully evaluate issues with reproductive and fetal health. Nevertheless, WWE treated with: (1) VPA, (2) enzyme-inducing AEDs, or (3) those who are obese or experience significant weight gain, may need AED changes in the process of deciding and trying to become pregnant.

The regular monitoring of reproductive function should be a regular feature of clinic visits for WWE, a task recommended as one of the eight "pay-for-performance" screening measures recently recommended by an expert panel on the epilepsy component of the US national Physician Consortium for Performance Improvement (PCPI) [33]. According to the PCPI panel, the screening requirement is: "All female patients of childbearing potential (12–44 years old) diagnosed with epilepsy were counseled about epilepsy and how its treatment may affect contraception and pregnancy at least once per year." The screening included eliciting the symptoms/signs of reproductive function listed in Table 9.2. If a reproductive endocrine disorder is suspected or found, antiepileptic drug treatment should

Table 9.3: Hormone testing and imaging in evaluation of infertility in WWE [31]

Study	Sample window	Abnormalities	Interpretation
LH, FSH	Cycle day 3–6	LH/FSH ratio >2	PCOS
Prolactin	Morning (no cycle dependency)	FSH >35 IU/l; LH >11 IU/l;	Menopause
		LH <7 IU/ml >20 µg/l	Hypothalamic amenorrhea Epilepsy, AED, hypothyroidism, pituitary tumor
Progesterone	Midluteal phase of cycle	<6 nmol/l	Anovulation; common cause: PCOS, hypophyseal adenoma, hyperprolactinemia
Testosterone	Cycle day 3–6	>2.5 nmol/l	PCOS, VPA; non-classical adrenal hyperplasia may cause modest elevation of testosterone
		>4.0 nmol/l	Adrenal/ovarian tumor
Androstenedione	-	>10.0 nmol/l	Non-classical congenital adrenal hyperplasia
Dehydroepiandrosterone sulphate (DHEAS)	-	Age 20–29 >3800 ng/ml Age 30–39 >2700 ng/ml	Non-classical adrenal hyperplasia
Glucose/insulin	Fasting, morning levels	Fasting glucose >7.8 mmol/l	Diabetes
		Glucose/insulin ratio >4	Reduced insulin sensitivity; associated with obesity and PCOS
Pelvic ultrasound	Transvaginal or transabdominal (Cycle day 3–9)	>10 peripheral cysts, 2–8 mm diameter in one ultrasound plane, thickening of ovarian stroma	Polycystic ovaries; associated with PCOS
		Other structural abnormalities of ovaries	Tumours, atrophy, multifollicular ovaries, etc.

PCOS = polycystic ovary syndrome; VPA = valproate; AED = antiepileptic drug; LH = luteinizing hormone; FSH = follicle-stimulating hormone

be reviewed to ensure that it is appropriate for the particular epilepsy syndrome and that it is not contributing to the endocrine problem. Of course, the possible benefits of a change of AED must be balanced against seizure control and potential side effects of other AEDs.

One effective treatment for infertile women in the general population is clomiphene. Clomiphene works by inhibiting negative feedback upon the hypothalamus, thus increasing gonadotropin production, which in turn promotes gonadal function. There is no data on the use of clomiphene for the purposes of infertility treatment in WWE. However, Herzog, in a uncontrolled case series, treated twelve WWE who also had menstrual cycle abnormalities [34]. Ten of twelve experienced improvement in seizure frequency. Furthermore, the ten with improvements also noted a return to normal menstrual cycles. Of note, one patient experienced an unplanned pregnancy during the trial.

Conclusion

WWE have reproductive dysfunction and infertility at rates higher than the general population. Possible explanations for the reduction in fertility among WWE may include social factors that may make WWE less competitive in the pool of potential mates. Such factors include low rates of marriage, marriage at older, less fertile, ages, social isolation and stigma, and cognitive and psychiatric comorbidities. Potential biological factors include the effect of the epileptic lesion, seizures, or AEDs upon the female neuroendocrine system. Although some studies emphasize one factor or another, none of these are mutually exclusive, and infertility in WWE probably is multifactorial. Reproductive function should be screened regularly for infertility, menstrual disorders, obesity/weight gain, hirsutism, and galactorrhea. Symptoms and signs of neuroendocrine causes of infertility should be evaluated with appropriate hormonal testing and imaging, or referred to appropriate specialists. AED selection, with special attention to VPA, enzyme-inducing AEDs, or to untoward weight gain on any AED, should be part of overall planning and management of WWE who wish to or may become pregnant.

References

1. Fritz MA, Ory SJ, Barnhart K, et al. Practice Committee of the American Society for Reproductive Medicine: definitions of infertility and recurrent pregnancy loss. *Fertil Steril* 2008; 89:1603.

2. Unuane D, Tournaye H, Velkeniers B, et al. Endocrine disorders & female infertility. *Best Pract Res Clin Endocrinol Metab* 2011; 25:861–73.

3. Thonneau P, Marchand S, Tallec A, et al. Incidence and main causes of infertility in a resident population (1,850,000) of three French regions (1988–1989). *Hum Reprod* 1991; 6(6):811–6.

4. WHO. Epilepsy: social consequences and economic aspects; fact sheet 166. 2001.

5. D'Souza C. Epilepsy and discrimination in India. *Neur Asia* 2004; 9:53–4.

6. Webber MP, Hauser WA, Ottman R, et al. Fertility in persons with epilepsy: 1935–1974. *Epilepsia* 1986; 27(6):746–52.

7. Wallace H, Shorvon S and Tallis R. Age-specific incidence and prevalence rates of treated epilepsy in an unselected population of 2,052,922 and age-specific fertility rates of women with epilepsy. *Lancet* 1998; 352 (9145):1970–3.

8. Artama M, Isojärvi JI, Raitanen J, et al. Birth rate among patients with epilepsy: a nationwide population-based cohort study in Finland. *Am J Epidemiol* 2004; 159(11):1057–63.

9. Viinikainen K, Heinonen S, Eriksson K, et al. Fertility in women with active epilepsy. *Neurology* 2007; 69(22):2107–8.

10. Olafsson E, Hauser WA and Gudmundsson G. Fertility in patients with epilepsy: a population-based study. *Neurology* 1998; 51 (1):71–3.

11. Schupf N and Ottman R. Reproduction among individuals with idiopathic/ cryptogenic epilepsy: risk factors for reduced fertility in marriage. *Epilepsia* 1996; 37(9):833–40.

12. Sukumaran SC, Sarma PS and Thomas SV. Polytherapy increases the risk of infertility in women with epilepsy. *Neurology* 2010; 75(15):1351–5.

13. Jalava M and Sillanpaa M. Reproductive activity and offspring health of young adults with childhood-onset epilepsy:

a controlled study. *Epilepsia* 1997; 38(5):532–40.

14. Pal SK, Sharma K, Prabhakar S, et al. Psychosocial, demographic, and treatment-seeking strategic behavior, including faith healing practices, among patients with epilepsy in northwest India. *Epilepsy Behav* 2008; 13(2):323–32.

15. Dansky LV, Andermann E and Andermann F. Marriage and fertility in epileptic patients. *Epilepsia* 1980; 21(3):261–71.

16. Fong CY and Hung A. Public awareness, attitude, and understanding of epilepsy in Hong Kong Special Administrative Region, China. *Epilepsia* 2002; 43:311–6.

17. Morrell MJ, Flynn KL, Done S, et al. Sexual dysfunction, sex steroid hormone abnormalities, and depression in women with epilepsy treated with antiepileptic drugs. *Epilepsy Behav* 2005; 6(3):360–5.

18. Herzog AG, Drislane FW, Schomer DL, et al. Differential effects of antiepileptic drugs on sexual function and hormones in men with epilepsy. *Neurology* 2005; 65(7):1016–20.

19. Herzog AG, Coleman AE, Jacobs AR, et al. Relationship of sexual dysfunction to epilepsy laterality and reproductive hormone levels in women. *Epilepsy Behav* 2003; 4(4):407–13.

20. Quigg M, Kiely JM, Shneker B, et al. Interictal and postictal alterations of pulsatile secretions of luteinizing hormone in temporal lobe epilepsy in men. *Ann Neurol* 2002; 51(5):559–66.

21. Chen DK, So YT and Fisher RS. Use of serum prolactin in diagnosing epileptic seizures: report of the Therapeutics and Technology Assessment Subcommittee of the American Academy of Neurology. *Neurology* 2005; 65(5):668–75.

22. Bauer J, Stoffel-Wagner B, Flugel D, et al. The impact of epilepsy surgery on sex hormones and the menstrual cycle in female patients. *Seizure* 2000; 9(6):389–93.

23. Herzog AG. Disorders of reproduction in patients with epilepsy: primary

neurological mechanisms. *Seizure* 2008; 17(2):101–10.

24. Herzog AG, Seibel MM, Schomer DL, et al. Reproductive endocrine disorders in women with partial seizures of temporal lobe origin. *Arch Neurol* 1986; 43(4):341–6.

25. Isojärvi JI, Laatikainen TJ, Pakarinen AJ, et al. Polycystic ovaries and hyperandrogenism in women taking valproate for epilepsy. *N Engl J Med* 1993; 329(19):1383–8.

26. Klein P, Serje A and Pezzullo JC. Premature ovarian failure in women with epilepsy. *Epilepsia* 2001; 42(12):1584–9.

27. Drislane FW, Coleman AE, Schomer DL, et al. Altered pulsatile secretion of luteinizing hormone in women with epilepsy. *Neurology* 1994; 44(2):306–10.

28. Isojärvi J. Disorders of reproduction in patients with epilepsy: antiepileptic drug related mechanisms. *Seizure* 2008; 17(2):111–9.

29. Isojärvi JI, Rattya J, Myllyla VV, et al. Valproate, lamotrigine, and insulin-mediated risks in women with epilepsy. *Ann Neurol* 1998; 43(4):446–51.

30. Jallon P and Picard F. Bodyweight gain and anticonvulsants: a comparative review. *Drug Saf* 2001; 24(13):969–78.

31. Bauer J, Isojärvi JI, Herzog AG, et al. Reproductive dysfunction in women with epilepsy: recommendations for evaluation and management. *J Neurol Neurosurg Psychiatry* 2002; 73(2):121–5.

32. Hataska H. An efficient infertility evaluation. *Clin Obstet Gynecol* 2011; 54:644–55.

33. Fountain NB, Van Ness PC, Swain-Eng R, et al. Quality improvement in neurology: AAN epilepsy quality measures: Report of the Quality Measurement and Reporting Subcommittee of the American Academy of Neurology. *Neurology* 2011; 76(1):94–9.

34. Herzog AG. Clomiphene therapy in epileptic women with menstrual disorders. *Neurology* 1988; 38(3):432–4.

Selecting contraception for women with epilepsy

Page B. Pennell and Anne Davis

Key points:

- 50% of pregnancies among women with epilepsy (WWE) are unplanned, similar to the general population
- Enzyme-inducing antiepileptic drugs (EIAEDs), such as phenytoin, carbamazepine, oxcarbazepine, and phenobarbital, induce the hepatic P450 enzyme system and accelerate metabolism of contraceptive steroid hormones which, in turn, may decrease contraceptive efficacy
- The intrauterine device (IUD) is the first line contraceptive choice for all WWE, including nulliparous women. For WWE taking EIAEDs the IUD and depot-medroxy progesterone acetate (DMPA) provide reversible, highly effective contraception. DMPA effects on bone health should be considered
- Hormonal contraception with estrogenic components induces the metabolism of lamotrigine, valproate, and likely oxcarbazepine, via induction of glucuronidation pathways
- Hormonal contraceptives may be considered as a therapeutic option in catamenial epilepsy

Introduction

Effective and safe contraceptive options are important for all women, but are arguably even more essential, and more complicated, for WWE. Avoiding unplanned pregnancies is a key cornerstone to improving outcomes for children born to women with epilepsy. Using an antiepileptic drug (AED) with a favorable risk profile for structural and neurodevelopmental teratogenicity, at the lowest effective dose for that patient, good seizure control for the prior 9 months, and use of periconceptional supplemental folic acid optimize pregnancy outcomes [1–3]. When a pregnancy is unplanned, WWE can miss the opportunity to benefit from these modifiable aspects of care.

The average woman, assuming she has two children, will require some form of contraception for about three decades during her childbearing years. In the USA, of the 43 million fertile and sexually active women not seeking pregnancy, 89% use contraception [4]. Nationally representative surveys in the USA show that 63% of those who use contraception rely on reversible methods, most often the oral contraceptive pill and male condom, whereas 37% rely on the permanent methods of tubal sterilization or vasectomy [4].

Notably, use of long-acting reversible methods in the USA (IUD or implant) increased to 8.5% by 2009, but remains relatively uncommon compared to European countries where sterilization is much less common and use of the IUD is widespread.

Contraceptive use in women with epilepsy

Data from existing, large contraception surveys cannot be used to estimate contraception use among WWE because such surveys do not collect information on co-existent chronic illness. Data from small samples of women suggest contraception remains a challenge for WWE, despite published guidelines [5]. One questionnaire study at an urban medical center queried 145 WWE regarding current sexual activity and contraception use [6]. Only 53% of those at risk of unplanned pregnancy used methods with typical pregnancy rates of ≤10% in the first year of use; most often sterilization or oral contraceptives. The rest relied on condoms, spermicide, natural family planning (timed intercourse), or withdrawal, alone or in combination. These methods have typical failure rates between 10% and 20% per year. Not surprisingly, half of their 181 pregnancies were unplanned. Poor, Hispanic WWE were more vulnerable; they experienced more unplanned pregnancies than Caucasian women of higher socioeconomic status. This disparity mirrors the US population overall.

Healthy women face barriers to access effective contraception, including prohibitive cost and misperceptions regarding efficacy and safety. WWE face another barrier; physicians responsible for contraceptive counseling are often not adequately knowledgeable about this complicated topic. Although performed almost two decades ago, a national survey of US obstetricians and neurologists highlighted this gap in the treating physicians' knowledge. The 1996 survey queried US obstetricians and neurologists about interactions between oral contraceptives and AEDS [7]. Approximately a quarter in both groups reported awareness of contraceptive failures in their patients taking AEDs and oral contraceptives (OCs). They were asked if they knew the interactions between OCs and the six most common AEDs at that time (phenytoin, carbamazepine, valproic acid, phenobarbital, primidone, and ethosuximide). The average percentage correct for the neurologists' knowledge of OC interactions was $61 \pm 2.2\%$, and for obstetricians' knowledge was $37.8 \pm 1.9\%$. Only 4% of the neurologists and none of the obstetricians answered correctly for all six AEDs. Since this survey was published, the subject has gotten even more complicated with new AEDs and contraceptives. Like many health care providers, WWE also experience confusion about AEDs and contraception. In their questionnaire study of WWE, Pack and Davis found that among the 66 women currently using EIAEDs, 65% did not know whether or not their AED changed the effectiveness of OCs [8].

Contraception methods

For WWE, and women in general, efficacy and safety are primary considerations when selecting a contraceptive method. Pregnancy rates are less than 1% per year for highly effective methods and these should be considered first line, or top-tier (Table 10.1). Highly effective methods include permanent contraception via tubal ligation or vasectomy and long-acting reversible contraceptive (LARC) methods of IUD and the single-rod, three-year contraceptive implant. A recent large, prospective cohort study demonstrated that unplanned pregnancy was 20 times more likely among users of short-term hormonal methods such as OCs compared to LARC [9].

Table 10.1: Contraceptives available in the USA

Method	Efficacy*	Reversibility	Menstrual bleeding	Duration of use	Ovulation inhibition
Oral contraceptive pill	88–94%	Immediate	Decreased, regular	Daily	Yes
Transdermal patch	88–94%	Immediate	Decreased, regular	Weekly	Yes
Vaginal ring	88–94%	Immediate	Decreased, regular	Monthly	Yes
Depot-medroxyprogesterone acetate (DMPA)	88–94%	Delayed†	Initially irregular, amenorrhea likely with continuation	Every 3 months	Yes
Subdermal implant	>99%	Immediate	Decreased, irregular	3 years	Yes
Levonorgestrel IUD	>99%	Immediate	Decreased, initially irregular	5 years	Sometimes
Copper IUD	>99%	Immediate	Sometimes increased, regular	10 years	No

* With typical use, per year, assuming no drug interaction present
† Median return to ovulation >6 months from time of last injection

Long-acting reversible contraception

The progestin (levonorgestrel (LNG))-releasing and the copper T 380A IUDs are widely used around the world (Figures 10.1 and 10.2). The LNG IUD is approved for 5 years of use by the US FDA; the non-hormonal copper device for 10 years. Both IUDs primarily prevent pregnancy by pre-fertilization mechanisms of interference with sperm transport and function [10]. The IUD is an appropriate choice for women and adolescents who have never been pregnant as well as women who have children [11]. Recent data clearly demonstrates excellent safety and efficacy for nulliparous women [9]. Neither IUD increases rates of pelvic infection or associated infertility. Both IUDs are completely reversible; fertility quickly and completely returns after removal.

The contraceptive implant is a 3 cm soft, flexible single rod placed subdermally in the upper arm (Figure 10.3). The device continuously elutes the contraceptive progestin etonogestrel and is approved for 3 years of use. A trained provider can place the implant in a few minutes after administering a small amount of local anesthesia. Implant use may be complicated by difficult removal due to deep insertion. Implant use is not associated with weight gain. Neither IUD nor the implant contain estrogenic components and therefore do not increase the risk of thrombosis.

Long-acting reversible methods have different effects on menstrual bleeding. Copper IUD users experience no change in cycle length; however, menstrual flow and cramping may increase. The LNG IUD causes irregular bleeding during the first months after insertion. Thereafter, menstrual bleeding becomes regular and decreases markedly for most women; 20% develop amenorrhea after 1 year. The LNG IUD is approved for the

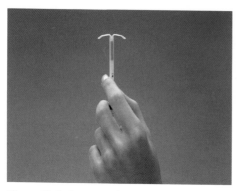

Figure 10.1: Progestin-releasing intrauterine device, containing levonorgestrel.

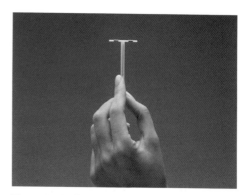

Figure 10.2: Copper T 380A intrauterine device.

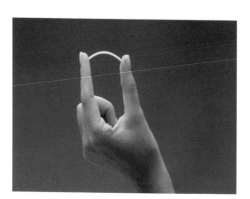

Figure 10.3: The contraceptive implant elutes etonogestrel. Images courtesy of Association of Reproductive Health Professionals (AHRP).

treatment of heavy menstrual bleeding in the USA. Bleeding is irregular during use of the contraceptive implant, users may experience more or fewer episodes of bleeding than during spontaneous menstrual cycles. The implant is the only top-tier method which reliably inhibits ovulation.

Intramuscular DMPA is also a highly effective method, with a failure rate comparable to the IUD or implant. Unlike those methods, however, the high efficacy of DMPA depends on re-injection every three months. Like the contraceptive implant, DMPA reliably inhibits ovulation. Bleeding with DMPA is irregular but decreases greatly over time. After 1 year, 75% of users experience amenorrhea. Unlike the IUD and all other hormonal methods, DMPA is not immediately reversible. Return to full fertility may be delayed up to 18 months. Overall, intramuscular DMPA is relatively safe; like other progestin-only methods, DMPA does not increase the risk of thrombosis. However, DMPA does cause modest decreases in bone mineral density. Compared to the contraceptive implant, DMPA has more profound inhibition of the hypothalamic-pituitary-ovarian axis. The stronger inhibition of follicle-stimulating hormone (FSH) production reduces endogenous estradiol production, leading to bone changes. With the contraceptive implant, FSH is produced and endogenous estradiol levels remain in the physiologic range. In healthy women receiving DMPA, these bone mineral density changes are reversible and do not appear to increase the risk of fracture in the short or long term [12]; therefore, no routine bone density screening is recommended. The US Center for Disease Control's Medical Eligibility Criteria (CDC MEC) guidelines for contraception recommend caution (risk may outweigh benefits) when using DMPA in women with other risk factors for osteoporosis such as chronic steroid use [13]. Since some AEDs may decrease bone density as discussed in Chapter 22, use of DMPA with these AEDs should be individualized.

Oral contraceptives

Many OCs are available. Combined oral contraceptives (COCs) contain an estrogen (usually ethinyl estradiol) and a synthetic progestin, which differs from natural progesterone. Early progestins include norethindrone and levonorgestrel, whereas newer progestins include desogestrel, norgestimate, and drospirenone. The progestins differ in half-life, potency, and bioavailability. Norethindrone has the shortest half-life, drospirenone the longest. In one large study, pregnancy rates were lower among women using an ethinyl estradiol and drospirenone-containing OC than among users of a pill with a comparable ethinyl estradiol dose and a shorter-acting progestin. The majority of available OCs contain ethinyl estradiol as the estrogenic component, some newer formulations have estradiol valerate. For non-contraceptive indications, most of these differences do not directly impact choice of an OC because few head-to-head comparisons guide pill choice. Acne and heavy menstrual bleeding are expected to improve on all combined OCs; some OCs have FDA approval for those indications. When choosing a pill for a WWE treated with a strong inducer, a pill with highest doses should be chosen. A formulation with 50 micrograms of ethinyl estradiol and relatively high doses of progestin is best; however, these pills are not widely available. While practical and often suggested in the clinical literature, this strategy is unsupported by data proving efficacy. Any woman treated with a strong inducer using an OC should use another method, such as condoms, as well.

The progestin-only pill (POP) formulation available in the USA is a very low dose pill; it is taken continuously and does not reliably inhibit ovulation. Its primary mechanism is thickening of cervical mucous. Additionally, it is difficult to use, as it must be taken at the same time of day since the progestin dose is low and has a short half-life. Prescription of the progestin-only pill in the USA is generally limited to women who are breastfeeding or have other contraindications to the use of ethinyl estradiol. Higher dose progestin-only OCs are available in other parts of the world.

In addition to COCs, which are taken daily, other combined methods include a transdermal patch and a vaginal ring. These are administered weekly and for 4 weeks, respectively. These methods inhibit ovulation and have non-contraceptive benefits of regular and decreased menstrual bleeding. Oral contraceptive use improves acne and prevents ovarian cysts and, if sustained, greatly decreases the risk of ovarian cancer and uterine cancer. The estrogenic component of combined methods is associated with an increased risk for thrombosis; however, the absolute risk of venous thrombosis for a healthy woman using these methods is very low, about 1 in 1,000 users. Women with risk factors for thrombosis, stroke, or myocardial infarction should not use combined hormonal contraception, including migraine with aura and even migraine without aura if the woman is >35 years old. For smokers over age 35, OC use is contraindicated because of an increased risk of myocardial infarction and stroke [13].

Traditional OC formulations as well as the patch and ring are used for 3 weeks then stopped for 1 week to allow for a menstrual withdrawal bleed. Newer OC formulations shorten the time off (pill-free interval) to 4 days monthly, or 1 week every 3 months, or eliminate the pill-free interval completely. Some of these methods result in very short, infrequent menses or induce complete amenorrhea. This is safe for women; the amenorrhea is due to reversible endometrial thinning and does not impact fertility after discontinuation. Breakthrough bleeding may occur with these extended regimens. Studies of continuous OC use show excellent safety and return to fertility up to 1 year. Longer studies are lacking, but data from long-term use of traditionally administered OCs are reassuring.

Dual method contraception

The term dual method use usually refers to a male barrier method combined with some other method. Most often, in healthy women this strategy is recommended for pregnancy prevention and sexually transmitted infection (STI) prevention, especially for adolescents. In the context of WWE, the usual STI prevention recommendations would apply for those at risk, but condoms could also be recommended as a "back-up" method to reduce the risk of pregnancy in the context of a drug interaction. If STI prevention is not a concern, dual method use is not a first choice strategy for contraception because adherence becomes more complex. Dual method use would be recommended for strong inducer AEDs co-administered with oral contraceptives, ring, patch, or implant. Dual method use would not improve efficacy in a clinically meaningful way for either IUD or DMPA.

Bidirectional interactions of hormonal contraceptives and AEDs
Effects of antiepileptic drugs on reproductive hormones

Oral contraceptives were the first effective reversible method of contraception and became available in the 1960s. Shortly after their introduction, clinicians caring for WWE observed pregnancies during co-administration of certain AEDS, despite the high doses of contraceptive steroids in these early formulations [14]. Since those early observations, AEDS have been systematically studied for how they impact the pharmacokinetic properties of ethinyl estradiol and various contraceptive ingredients and grouped as enzyme-inducing or non-enzyme-inducing. Unfortunately, these groupings based on pharmacokinetic changes do not clearly and directly relate to the risk of ovulation or pregnancy.

Antiepileptic drugs may impact contraceptive pharmacokinetics by several mechanisms. Some induce the hepatic cytochrome P450 system, and specifically CYP3A4, the primary metabolic pathway of ethinyl estradiol and progestins. Some AEDs also enhance glucuronidation, another hepatic elimination pathway for these sex steroid hormones. More rapid clearance of the sex steroid hormones may allow ovulation in women using hormonal contraceptive agents [15]. In general, AEDs that induce hepatic metabolic enzymes are labeled EIAEDs, and directly alter reproductive hormone levels (Table 10.2). These AEDs also induce production of sex hormone-binding globulin (SHBG), thereby reducing biologically active (free) reproductive hormone serum levels [16].

Hormonal contraceptives work by inhibiting ovulation and changes in cervical mucous. Ovulation inhibition depends largely on the contraceptive progestin, via inhibition of

Table 10.2: Antiepileptic drugs: degree of induction of metabolism of hormonal contraceptive agents

Strong inducers*	Weak inducers*	Non-inducers
Phenobarbital	Topiramate	Ethosuximide
Phenytoin	Lamotrigine	Valproate
Carbamazepine	Felbamate	Gabapentin
Primidone	Rufinamide	Clonazepam
Oxcarbazepine		Tiagabine
Clobazam		Levetiracetam
		Zonisamide
		Pregabalin
		Vigabatrin
		Lacosamide
		Ezogabine

* Avoid concomitant use with the lowest dose oral contraceptive pills

luteinizing hormone (LH) production. This is a threshold effect. If the progestin component remains above the level at which ovulation is inhibited, the contraceptive effect should be preserved even if enzyme induction occurs. Prescribers of hormonal contraception for WWE should be aware that efficacy also depends on adherence. Missed pills, late patches or rings decrease contraceptive effectiveness. These adherence problems are very common in typical users of short-acting hormonal contraception.

Pharmacokinetic (PK) studies have been performed with many specific AEDs and various formulations of hormonal contraceptives. No clear data identify which pharmacokinetic parameters relate to pregnancy risk; trough progestin levels are likely to be critical (see above). Only one study has extended PK changes to a true pharmacodynamics study of pregnancy risk, and this study was for the commonly prescribed AED carbamazepine [17].

Categorization of the AEDs and recommendations in this chapter were developed with the best available information at this time despite the limitations of the study designs and the data available.

Older AEDs

Phenobarbital: A prospective study of the effect of phenobarbital (PB) on OC hormonal levels was performed in four women [18]. In this very small study, all four women used an OC with 50 micrograms of ethinyl estradiol, in three cases with norethindrone and in one case norgestrel. Hormone levels were measured for one cycle prior to PB administration, and then for 2 months with PB 30 mg BID. Significant falls in the peak plasma ethinyl estradiol concentrations occurred in two women (from 104.8 +/-13.4 to 37.7 +/-2.0 pg/ml and from 125.6 +/-23.8 to 34.8 +/-6.7 pg/ml), and they experienced breakthrough bleeding. No changes occurred in progesterone, norethindrone, norgestrel, or follicle-stimulating hormone levels. A significant increase in sex hormone-binding globulin capacity occurred (100.7 +/-5.8 to 133.3 +/-1.2 nmoles/l).

Primidone: Primidone (PMD) is metabolized to PB, and therefore the same principles should be applied for interactions with hormonal contraceptives. Previous reports included primidone as polytherapy and unexpected pregnancies occurred.

Phenytoin and carbamazepine: An early study directly examined the effects of phenytoin (PHT) (n = 6) and carbamazepine (CBZ) (n = 4) on the pharmacokinetic parameters of a single dose of a combined oral contraceptive containing 50 ug of ethinyl estradiol and 250 ug of levonorgestrel [19]. Initial evaluation was prior to beginning the AED and compared to findings of the single dose study after 8–12 weeks of treatment of PHT or CBZ. The area under the plasma concentration-time curve (AUC) was measured over a 24-hour period. Significant reductions were seen with both AEDs. With chronic PHT use, the AUC for ethinyl estradiol was reduced from 806 ± 50 (mean $\pm$ s.d.) to 411 ± 132 pg/ml-' h (p<0.05), and for levonorgestrel from 33.6 ± 7.8 to 19.5 ± 3.8 ng/ml-' h (p<0.05). With chronic CBZ use, the AUC for ethinyl estradiol was reduced from 1163 ± 466 to 672 ± 211 pg/ml-' h (p<0.05), and for levonorgestrel from 22.9 ± 9.4 to 13.8 ± 5.8 ng/ml-' h (p<0.05).

Carbamazepine: Only one enzyme-inducing AED, CBZ, has been adequately studied to determine if changes in ethinyl estradiol (EE) and the progestin levonorgestrel permitted ovulation [17]. In that study, 10 healthy women took 600 mg of CBZ or a placebo daily for 2 months with a low-dose oral contraceptive (EE 20 ug and LNG 150 ug). Ovulation was detected by twice weekly sonography to identify developing dominant follicles and repeated progesterone assays. Compared to placebo, dramatic changes in EE and LNG occurred during CBZ use. Importantly, the trough level of LNG during CBZ use was very low, even undetectable. This large decrease in progestin levels was associated with ovulation in half of the CBZ cycles and an increase in breakthrough bleeding. Results demonstrate clearly that CBZ at 600 mg daily can lead to low-dose OC failure.

Newer AEDs

Reports and recommendations regarding many of the second generation AEDs have been conflicting and incongruous.

Oxcarbazepine: A randomized, double blind cross over study of oxcarbazepine (OXC) (1200 mg/day) in 16 healthy women, and on an OC with 50 meg of EE and 250 mcg of LNG, demonstrated a decrease in EE AUC by 47%, Cmax by 35%, and LNG AUC by 46% and Cmax by 24%, compared with the cycle with no OXC intake [20]. Many experts now include OXC in the strong-inducer category for effects on hormonal contraceptive agents [19].

Felbamate: A randomized, placebo-controlled trial of 30 healthy women reported that with felbamate and a low-dose OC, there was minor (13%) decline in EE AUC, but a larger decline in the progestin gestodene AUC by 42%, compared with placebo. Despite this, there was no evidence of ovulation in either group by progesterone and LH levels [21]. Felbamate is considered a weak inducer (Table 10.2).

Topiramate: A study of 12 WWE with topiramate (TPM) 200–800 mg/day and OCs (35 mcg EE/1 mg norethisterone) demonstrated that EE mean AUC values significantly declined (18–30%) compared to baseline, in a dose-dependent manner. However, no changes in norethisterone occurred [22]. A randomized trial in healthy women using lower doses of TPM and low-dose OCs showed non-significant minor changes (<12%) in PK parameters, with TPM 50–200 mg/day [23]. Therefore, TPM is considered a weak inducer, with induction impacting EE but not progestins (Table 10.2).

Lamotrigine: Lamotrigine (LTG) is considered a weak inducer of contraceptive progestins. A cross over study in 16 healthy women on a medium dose OC (30 mcg EE/150 mcg LNG) and moderate dose of LTG (300 mg/day) demonstrated that EE pharmacokinetics were unchanged. The Cmax, AUC, and trough levels of LNG, however, decreased about 20% with co-administration of LTG. FSH and LH concentrations were increased by 3.4–4.7-fold, and ovulation was not detected by single progesterone measurements. Intermenstrual bleeding was reported by 32% of subjects [24].

Rufinamide: Co-administration of rufinamide (800 mg BID for 14 days) and a COC (35 mcg EE/1 mg norethindrone) resulted in a mean decrease in the EE AUC_{0-24} of 22% and Cmax by 31%, and norethindrone AUC_{0-24} by 14% and Cmax by 18% [25]. Rufinamide should be considered a weak inducer.

Clobazam: Clobazam and N-desmethylclobazam induce CYP3A4 activity in a concentration-dependent manner. There are no specific pharmacokinetic studies published with COCs, but the manufacturer recommends that additional non-hormonal forms of contraception should be used [26]. Data is lacking to categorize clobazam as a strong or weak inducer, and the more conservative approach is it to include it in the strong-inducer category.

Non-inducers

Non-inducers: Pharmacokinetic interaction studies have been performed with the other AEDs and various formulations of hormonal contraceptives and reported in journal articles and package inserts. Findings support lack of significant induction of metabolism of hormonal contraceptive agents with both older and newer AEDs: ethosuximide, valproate, gabapentin, clonazepam, tiagabine, levetiracetam, zonisamide, pregabalin, vigabatrin, lacosamide, and ezogabine (Table 10.2) [15].

Recommendations

Many authors have recommended "high-dose" OCs ($\geq$50 µg ethinyl estradiol) with enzyme-inducing AEDs, assuming enzyme induction will lower levels to what occurs with an effective lower dose OC [5]. A few OCs with higher doses of EE and progestin remain available but are infrequently used in practice for healthy women. While reasonable in the context of EIAEDs, no direct evidence supports efficacy in this situation. The CDC Medical Eligibility Criteria for contraception classified certain AEDs (PHT, CBZ, PB, PMD, TPM, and OXC) as a Category 3: the risks generally outweigh the benefits. In this category, the risk refers to birth control failure. The authors clarify that although the interaction of certain AEDs with COCs, POP, or the vaginal ring is not harmful to women, it is likely to reduce the effectiveness. The authors further state that if a COC is chosen, a preparation containing a minimum of 30 µg EE should be used [13].

Oral contraceptives, as well as patches, rings, and the implant, are not first line contraceptive methods for WWE who use EIAEDs known to cause substantial changes in progestin levels (Table 10.2). For these women, the copper or LNG IUD are excellent choices. One caution with the copper IUD is that some radiology departments are not willing to perform a 3Tesla (or higher) brain MRI on women with a copper IUD in place, potentially compromising the evaluation of WWE. The LNG IUD prevents pregnancy by local hormonally mediated changes in cervical mucous which are not likely to be impacted by hepatic changes in P450 enzyme induction. One reassuring prospective registry study in the UK demonstrated a pregnancy rate of 1.1 per 100 women-years for 56 women using the LNG IUD with enzyme-inducing AEDs, a rate slightly higher than expected but still very low compared to other contraceptive methods available [27]. DMPA is another choice with enzyme-inducing AEDs. No direct evidence examines how DMPA metabolism is impacted by enzyme-inducing AEDs; however, the dose of DMPA even at 12 weeks significantly exceeds the level needed for ovulation inhibition. Use of DMPA has to be considered in light of side effects discussed in this chapter.

Effects of hormonal contraceptives on AEDs

Earlier studies highlighted the finding that lamotrigine clearance is markedly enhanced during pregnancy. This observation prompted specific investigations of the effects of hormonal contraceptives. An early retrospective comparative study in WWE on LTG, ages 15–30 years old, enrolled 22 COC users and 39 non-users. The authors reported that LTG clearance (LTG dose/body weight/plasma concentration] was over 2-fold higher in the COC group compared to the non-user group [28]. A study investigating the mechanism of the enhanced clearance measured the main metabolite, lamotrigine-2-N-glucuronide, in WWE taking COC ($n = 31$), in WWE with the LNG IUD ($n = 12$), and in WWE on no contraceptive ($n = 20$) [29]. Compared to controls, the LTG dose/concentration ratio was 56% higher in the COC group, and the N-2-glucuronide/LTG ratio was 82% higher ($p < 0.01$ in both). There were no differences between the control and the IUD group. Findings indicate that the enhanced metabolism of LTG is primarily by induction of the N-2-glucuronide pathway. Another study demonstrated increased LTG clearance in women on COC but a lack of difference in LTG clearance between non-hormonal users and those using POP, DMPA, progestin implant, or the LNG IUD, further supporting the theory that the enhanced glucuronidation is due to the estrogenic component [30]. A small study of seven women also reported lower plasma concentrations with COC use, but added information about the time course; baseline LTG levels were reached at an average of 8.0 (s.d. 3.69) days after the starts of COCs. Two of the seven women experienced seizure worsening that correlated with reduced LTG concentrations [31].

The CDC Medical Eligibility Criteria specifically labels lamotrigine monotherapy as category 3 (risks generally outweigh the benefits) for use with COC, given that pharmacokinetic studies have shown not only decreased LTG levels but also associated increased seizures [13].

Valproate (VPA) and oxcarbazepine (OXC) also undergo hepatic glucuronidation as a major elimination pathway. Similar pharmacokinetic interaction principles likely apply with estrogens decreasing AED concentrations, although surprisingly, this is not reported with

Table 10.3: Antiepileptic drugs with increased clearance with concomitant use of a combined oral contraceptive

Antiepileptic Drugs
Lamotrigine
Valproate
Oxcarbazepine*

* Reports in the literature are lacking, but increased clearance is probable given that hepatic glucuronidation is the major route of elimination

OXC in the literature. Enhanced clearance of OXC during pregnancy is reported, however. A later study investigated the effects of OCs on VPA as well as LTG serum concentrations [32]. They enrolled four groups of WWE, with twelve women in each group: VPA, VPA plus OC, LTG, and LTG plus COC. VPA concentrations were lower in the VPA plus COC group than the VPA-only group, with a median decrease of 23.4%. LTG concentrations were 32.6% lower in the LTG plus COC group compared to the LTG-only group (Table 10.3).

Potential of contraceptives as a therapeutic tool for seizure control

Catamenial epilepsy is the term used for the pattern of seizure worsening associated with different menstrual phases. Some women with epilepsy tend to have seizure worsening during certain phases of their menstrual cycles: perimenstrual, periovulatory, or during the second half of anovulatory cycles. Approximately one-third of reproductive-aged women with focal epilepsy and on no exogenous hormones will meet criteria for at least one catamenial pattern [33]. Animal models and a few human studies suggest that the enhanced seizure susceptibility is related to premenstrual withdrawal of the anticonvulsant effects of progesterone and its neurosteroid metabolite, allopregnanolone, the sudden estrogen peak in the day prior to ovulation, and increased frequency of anovulatory cycles and consequent low progesterone luteal phases [34].

Hormonal contraceptives could potentially be used as a therapeutic tool in women with a catamenial pattern to their epilepsy, by providing continuous levels of sex steroid hormones, as opposed to variable levels of estrogen peaks and progesterone withdrawal, or unopposed estrogen during the second phase of an anovulatory cycle. However, synthetic progestins are not metabolized to allopregnanolone, and therefore, there is no binding to the GABA-A-benzodiazepine receptor at the neurosteroid site and likely no direct benefit. There is no clear evidence that hormonal contraceptives worsen seizure control in WWE, although rare anecdotal reports exist. The exception can occur when the hormonal contraceptive lowers the AED concentration as discussed in the previous section.

DMPA is a synthetic progestin not metabolized to allopregnanolone. It is a powerful suppressor of the hypothalamic-pituitary axis and completely inhibits ovulation, which may be beneficial in cases when seizures worsen with peaks of estrogen or progesterone withdrawal in spontaneous cycles. Two small cohorts were enrolled in a pilot study nearly 30 years ago to investigate the use of medroxyprogesterone acetate for "intractable" epilepsy (n = 14 and n = 19) [35]. In this study, participants received both oral and intramuscular MPA in variable doses at variable intervals. Seizure frequency was significantly reduced in both cohorts, with average reductions of 30% and 39%. AED levels did not change. Some women discontinued because of side effects. These findings have not been duplicated since this report. A more rigorous controlled study is needed to investigate whether intramuscular DMPA affects seizure control. Additionally, after cessation of use, the transition period with erratic endogenous hormone cycling could theoretically cause seizure worsening as well as prolonged return to normal fertility. The etonogestrel contraceptive implant reliably inhibits ovulation. As yet, however, no published data document use of progestin implants for catamenial epilepsy. As with the contraceptive implant and DMPA, OC formulations at effective doses cause continuous suppression of ovulation and may theoretically benefit women with epilepsy sensitive to endogenous fluctuations. Some clinicians may preferentially prescribe continuous OC in women with catamenial epilepsy or women on lamotrigine to provide non-fluctuating hormone levels.

However, no published study has yet investigated the use of any OC regimen for seizure control in women with epilepsy.

Cyclic administration of progesterone lozenges during the second half of the menstrual cycle has been studied in a multi center, double blind, placebo-controlled, randomized trial, but results found that adjunctive progesterone was effective only for women with a strong catamenial pattern of seizure worsening during the perimenstrual phase [36]. However, this is not a form of contraception, and its administration can be especially difficult given that the woman cannot be on a hormonal contraceptive and needs to maintain their natural menstrual cycles.

Preconception planning

Transitioning from contraception to preconception planning provides a valuable window of opportunity for the clinician. Not only does it allow the clinician to reassess the type of AED(s) prescribed and reinforce supplemental folic acid and prenatal vitamins but also provides an opportunity to reassess the dose prescribed. This is especially important for the AEDs that undergo glucuronidation as a major metabolic pathway of elimination. Cessation of any hormonal contraceptives that contain an estrogen will result in a rise in the level of these AEDs (LTG, VPA, OXC). If this is not considered, it can result in symptomatic toxicity and unnecessary over-exposure of the fetus to the AED during the critical period of organogenesis. Findings from EURAP demonstrated that for each AED studied (LTG, VPA, PB, and CBZ), the odds ratio for a major congenital malformation increased with the higher dose ranges at the time of conception [2].

The clinician cannot wait until the diagnosis of pregnancy to determine the optimal lowest dose for the individual patient. Nor should they wait until the decision to become pregnant. As in healthy women, many pregnancies in WWE will be unplanned. However, if a patient does decide to stop an estrogen-containing contraceptive, this provides a window of opportunity to lower fetal risk by adjusting the AED dose downward if she is on an AED with a metabolic route that is induced by estrogens (e.g., LTG, VPA, OXC), and to perform a follow-up blood test to determine if the AED concentration is still in the individual target range. The general principle that teratogens act in a dose-dependent manner for major congenital malformations (MCMs) likely holds true for other effects of in utero AED exposure, including fetal brain development.

Summary and conclusions

Effective contraception in women with epilepsy is essential to allow for preconception planning and to implement the measures known to improve pregnancy outcomes. However, concomitant use of AEDs and hormonal contraceptives is complicated because of the bidirectional pharmacokinetic interactions, the pharmacodynamic consequences, and the potential effects on seizure control. In summary, if a woman is on a weak inducer of metabolism of hormonal contraceptive agents, then avoid use of a very low-dose COC or POPs; other hormonal methods are likely to be effective. If she is on a strong inducer, either IUD is a first line method for those who desire pregnancy in the future and sterilization for those who have completed childbearing or do not wish to have children (Tables 10.1 and 10.2). This chapter provides the groundwork necessary for practitioners from neurology, gynecology, and primary care to counsel this vulnerable patient population appropriately and to make informed prescribing choices.

References

1. Harden CL, Meador KJ, Pennell PB, et al. American Academy of Neurology; American Epilepsy Society. Practice parameter update: management issues for women with epilepsy–focus on pregnancy (an evidence-based review): teratogenesis and perinatal outcomes: report of the Quality Standards Subcommittee and Therapeutics and Technology Assessment Subcommittee of the American Academy of Neurology and American Epilepsy Society. *Neurology* 2009; 73(2):133–41.

2. Tomson T, Battino D, Bonizzoni E, et al. For the EURAP study group. Dose-dependent risk of malformations with antiepileptic drugs: an analysis of data from the EURAP epilepsy and pregnancy registry. *Lancet Neurol* 2011; 10(7):609–17.

3. Meador KJ, Baker GA, Browning N, et al. Fetal antiepileptic drug exposure and cognitive outcomes at age 6 years (NEAD study): a prospective observational study. *Lancet Neurol* 2013; 12(3):244–52.

4. Mosher WD and Jones J. Use of contraception in the United States: 1982–2008. *Vital 23 Health Stat* 2010; No 29.

5. Practice Parameter. Management issues for women with epilepsy (summary statement). Report of the Quality Standards Subcommittee of the American Academy of Neurology. *Neurology* 1998; 51(4):944–8.

6. Davis AR, Pack AM, Kritzer J, et al. Reproductive history, sexual behavior and use of contraception in women with epilepsy. *Contraception* 2008; 77(6):405–9.

7. Krauss GL, Brandt J, Campbell M, et al. Antiepileptic medication and oral contraceptive interactions: a national survey of neurologists and obstetricians. *Neurology* 1996; 46(6):1534–9.

8. Pack A, Davis AR, Kritzer J, et al. Anti-epileptic drugs: are women aware of interactions with oral contraceptives and potential teratogenicity? *Epilepsy Behav* 2009; 14(4):640–4.

9. Winner B, Peipert JF, Zhao Q, et al. Effectiveness of long-acting reversible contraception. *N Engl J Med* 2012; 366(21):1998–2007.

10. Ortiz ME and Croxatto HB. Copper-T intrauterine device and levonorgestrel intrauterine system: biological bases of their mechanism of action. *Contraception* 2007; 75(6 Suppl):S16–S30.

11. ACOG Committee Opinion no. 539: adolescents and long-acting reversible contraception: implants and intrauterine devices. *Obstet Gynecol* 2012; 120 (4):983–8.

12. Isley MM and Kaunitz AM. Update on hormonal contraception and bone density. *Rev Endocr Metab Disord* 2011; 12(2): 93–106.

13. Centers for Disease Control and Prevention. U. S. Medical Eligibility Criteria for Contraceptive Use, 2010. *MMWR Recomm Rep* 2010; 59(RR-4):1–86.

14. Kenyon IE. Unplanned pregnancy in an epileptic. *Br Med J* 1972; 1:686–7.

15. Gaffield ME, Culwell Kelly R and Lee CR. The use of hormonal contraception among women taking anticonvulsant therapy. *Contraception* 2011; 83:16–29.

16. Stoffel-Wagner B, Bauer J, Flügel D, et al. Serum sex hormones are altered in patients with chronic temporal lobe epilepsy receiving anticonvulsant medication. *Epilepsia* 1998; 39:1164–73.

17. Davis AR, Westhoff CL and Stanczyk FZ. Carbamazepine coadministration with an oral contraceptive: effects on steroid pharmacokinetics, ovulation, and bleeding. *Epilepsia* 2011; 52(2):243–7.

18. Back D, Bates M, Bowden A, et al. The interaction of phenobarbital and other anticonvulsants with oral contraceptive steroid therapy. *Contraception* 1980; 22:495–503.

19. Crawford P, Chadwick DJ, Martin C, et al. The interaction of phenytoin and carbamazepine with combined oral contraceptive steroids. *Br J Clin Pharmacol* 1990; 30:892–6.

20. Fattore C, Cipolla G, Gatti G, et al. Induction of ethinyl estradiol and lovonorgestrel metabolism by oxcarbazepine in healthy women. *Epilepsia* 1999; 40: 783–7.

21. Saano V, Glue P, Banfield CR, et al. Effects of felbamate on the pharmacokinetics of a low-dose combination oral contraceptive. *Clin Pharmacol Ther* 1995; 58:523–31.

22. Rosenfeld WE, Doose DR, Walker SA, et al. Effect of topiramate on the pharmacokinetics of an oral contraceptive containing norethindrone and ethinyl estradiol in patients with epilepsy. *Epilepsia* 1997; 38(3):317–23.

23. Doose DR, Wang SS, Padmanabhan M, et al. Effect of topiramate or carbamazepine on the pharmacokinetics of an oral contraceptive containing norethindrone and ethinyl estradiol in healthy obese and nonobese female subjects. *Epilepsia* 2003; 44(4):540–9.

24. Sidhu J, Job S, Singh S, et al. The pharmacokinetic and pharmacodynamic consequences of the co-administration of lamotrigine and a combined oral contraceptive in healthy female subjects. *Br J Clin Pharmacol* 2006; 61(2):191–9.

25. Rufinamide (Banzel) Package Insert. Eisai Inc. http://dailymed.nlm.nih.gov/dailymed/lookup.cfm?setid=0a3fa925-1abd-458a-bd57-4ae780a1ef2d.

26. Clobazam (Onfi) Package Insert. Lundbeck Inc. http://dailymed.nlm.nih.gov/dailymed/lookup.cfm?setid=de03bd69-2dca-459c-93b4-541fd3e9571c.

27. Bounds W and Guillebaud J. Observational series on women using the contraceptive Mirena concurrently with anti-epileptic and other enzyme-inducing drugs. *J Fam Plann Reprod Health Care* 2002; 28:78–80.

28. Sabers A, Ohman I, Christensen J, et al. Oral contraceptives reduce lamotrigine plasma levels. *Neurology* 2003; 61(4):570–1.

29. Ohman I, Luef G and Tomson T. Effects of pregnancy and contraception on lamotrigine disposition: new insights through analysis of lamotrigine metabolites. *Seizure* 2008; 17:199–202.

30. Reimers A, Helde G and Brodtkorb E. Ethinyl estradiol, not progestogens, reduces lamotrigine serum concentrations. *Epilepsia* 2005; 46(9):1414–17.

31. Wegner I, Edelbroek PM, Bulk S, et al. Lamotrigine kinetics within the menstrual cycle, after menopause, and with oral contraceptives. *Neurology* 2009; 73 (17):1388–93.

32. Herzog AG, Blum AS, Farina EL, et al. Valproate and lamotrigine level variation with menstrual cycle phase and oral contraceptive use. *Neurology* 2009; 72: 911–14.

33. Herzog AG, Harden CL, Liporace J, et al. Frequency of catamenial seizure exacerbation in women with localization-related epilepsy. *Ann Neurol* 2004; 56 (3):431–4.

34. Harden CL and Pennell PB. Neuroendocrine considerations in the treatment of men and women with epilepsy. *Lancet Neurol* 2013; 12(1):72–83.

35. Mattson RH, Cramer J, Caldwell BV, et al. Treatment of seizures with medroxyprogesterone acetate: preliminary report. *Neurology* 1984; 34:1255–8.

36. Herzog AG, Fowler KM, Smithson SD, et al. Progesterone Trial Study Group. Progesterone vs placebo therapy for women with epilepsy: a randomized clinical trial. *Neurology* 2012; 78(24):1959–66.

Chapter 11

Preconception counseling for women with epilepsy

Elizabeth E. Gerard

Key points:

- More than half of women with epilepsy (WWE) do not recall being counseled on antiepileptic drugs (AEDs) and teratogenicity
- Preconception counseling should be started early and revisited frequently for WWE of childbearing age
- The majority of WWE are likely to have a safe pregnancy and a healthy newborn
- Commonly discussed topics include transmission of epilepsy from mother to child, teratogenicity of AEDs, and seizure exacerbation in pregnancy
- Under ideal circumstances, pre-partum optimization of AEDs should be done 9–12 months before a planned pregnancy, as seizure pattern in the year prior to conception is the best predictor of seizure frequency during pregnancy

Introduction

It is critical that WWE receive regular counseling about pregnancy and contraception from their physicians. Both seizures and AEDs pose risks to a pregnancy, which must be carefully discussed with WWE. Additionally, the epilepsy and AED-related risks can be significantly reduced by early and careful planning. Unfortunately, patient surveys demonstrate that less than half of WWE recall being counseled on tetratogenic effects of AEDs or the need to plan pregnancy [1, 2], and many are misinformed [3]. Most patients feel that when the topic is discussed, it is more likely to be raised by the patient herself rather than her physician [4]. Without effective counseling women are liable to either over- or underestimate the risks to a potential pregnancy.

Preconception counseling is not limited to a discussion of pregnancy. It should include all elements of family planning, such as fertility, contraception, pre-partum screening, breastfeeding, and social support (Table 11.1). The length of a typical doctor's visit does not allow for a comprehensive review of all these topics, which makes it all the more important that a physician introduce reproductive health early in the patient–physician relationship and re-visit the topic regularly.

Approach to preconception counseling

While several consensus opinions have agreed upon the importance of preconception counseling for women with epilepsy [5–7], there are no evidence-based guidelines on

Women with Epilepsy, ed. Esther Bui and Autumn Klein. Published by Cambridge University Press.
© Cambridge University Press 2014.

Table 11.1: Key elements of preconception counseling for women with epilepsy

- Contraceptive options and interactions with antiepileptic medications
- Fertility
- Risk of epilepsy in the child
- Risks of antiepileptic medications in pregnancy
- Folic acid supplementation/prenatal vitamins
- Risks of seizures during pregnancy
- Importance of monitoring drug levels
- Risk of obstetrical complications
- Breastfeeding
- Importance of avoiding sleep deprivation
- Seizure safety and importance of social support in taking care of an infant
- Postpartum depression

how to effectively counsel patients [5]. This chapter will present an approach to counseling WWE of reproductive age and summarize the information required to effectively counsel most patients. Some of the essential components to effective counseling in this unique population are listed below:

Start early – Preconception counseling should start as early as possible, often at a woman's first visit. It is important to note that teen pregnancies also can occur among WWE. Deferring counseling until a woman knows she wants to become pregnant is unrealistic as 50% of pregnancies in women with epilepsy are not planned [1, 8], a rate similar to the general population. In addition, most useful interventions take more than 1 year to implement.

Ask – The preconception discussion should be tailored to the patient's personal goals, concerns, and risks. A prior history of irregular menses, miscarriages, or a family history of fetal malformations may affect an individual's risk for complications and certainly their anxiety about pregnancy. It is also important to understand the patient's sexual history as well as her personal goals and timeline.

Listen – In most circumstances, counseling should be an interactive encounter between the patient and her physicians. There is tremendous variability in the concerns which patients find most important to their reproductive decisions.

Reassure – Among WWE, 23–33% report that they would likely refrain from having children on account of their epilepsy [3, 9]. Many women with epilepsy are under the impression that it is unwise or irresponsible for them to become pregnant on account of their seizures or medications. For many patients, advice about the pregnancy and AED-related risks may be frightening. Reassuringly >94% of pregnancies exposed to AEDs and maternal epilepsy are NOT complicated by major congenital malformations. Exposure to AEDs is almost never an indication to terminate a pregnancy. It is important to emphasize that the risks related to AEDs and seizures during pregnancy can be reduced in many circumstances by careful and early planning.

Repeat – Thorough and comprehensive reproductive health counseling frequently need to be reinforced. In one survey of British WWE, Fairgrieve et al. reviewed the medical charts of women who did not recall receiving preconception counseling [1]. The medical records indicated that in 32% of these cases, the patient's physician had documented that counseling had occurred. This indicates that even when physicians attempt to counsel their patients, the initial message does not always get through.

Refer – The responsibility of preconception counseling for women with epilepsy should be shared among all her physicians, including her neurologist, gynecologist, and internist. In practice however, the principal responsibility usually falls on the neurologist who is prescribing the antiepileptic drug. In most cases it is appropriate for a neurologist to refer a patient for an early subspecialty opinion regarding preconception counseling for women with epilepsy.

Common questions encountered

This chapter will provide an overview of most of the topics essential to an effective preconception visit. Since fertility, contraception, and obstetrical concerns are reviewed elsewhere, this chapter will focus on other essential components of counseling for WWE of childbearing age. This will provide the information to answer the most common questions regarding pregnancy and epilepsy, including: "Will my child have epilepsy?"; "Will my medications or seizures hurt my baby?"; and "What will happen to my seizures during pregnancy?".

Heritability of epilepsy

While genetic susceptibility clearly plays a role in most epilepsies, only a few have identifiable genes that can be tested, and even fewer have complete or predictable penetrance. A detailed history of the patient's personal and family epilepsy history is critical to assessing a patient's risk of passing epilepsy to her children. An open discussion about these risks is important as a patient's perception of the risk of passing on epilepsy seems to strongly influence her decision to have children [10].

In general, the risk of a parent with epilepsy having a child with epilepsy is approximately 2.4–4.6% [11]. When compared to a life time incidence in the general population of 1–3%, epilepsy in one parent increases the risk approximately 2-fold. Some studies suggest mothers with epilepsy are more likely than fathers to pass on epilepsy, with an absolute risk of 2.8–8.7% in children born to WWE. Risk may be on the higher end of this spectrum for parents in whom epilepsy began before age 20, while it is exceedingly rare for parents whose epilepsy presents after age 35 to have affected children. Additionally, acquired epilepsies known to be secondary to traumatic brain injury sustained as an adult do not confer increased likelihood of epilepsy in the child [11].

A patient with a first-degree relative with epilepsy should be counseled differently than a patient with no relatives with epilepsy or affected individuals outside of her immediate family. It is important to recognize that there are recently identified focal epilepsies which demonstrate Mendelian inheritance, including autosomal dominant nocturnal frontal lobe epilepsy (ADNFLE) and autosomal dominant partial epilepsy with auditory features (ADPEAF). It is not yet clear whether genetic or prenatal testing should be recommended for these patients [12]. Genetic testing is commercially available only in a handful of countries and prenatal diagnosis is available in only three countries. Overall these autosomal dominant focal epilepsies are uncommon, but patients with a first-degree relative, particularly a parent with a syndrome similar to their own, should be advised that their chances of passing this on to their child is higher than for other patients with epilepsy. For many patients this is not a deterrent to having their own children; however, it certainly merits a detailed discussion and referral to genetic counseling.

Finally, patients whose epilepsy is symptomatic of an underlying condition also deserve closer evaluation and counseling. This includes, but is not limited to, patients with heritable syndromes such as tuberous sclerosis, progressive myoclonic epilepsy, and mitochondrial disease, including MELAS and MERRF. It is also important to recognize particular malformations of cortical development associated with epilepsy in women which have very specific genetic counseling implications. For example, bilateral periventricular nodular heterotopia (a subtle imaging finding that is often missed on routine MRIs) may be associated with an X-linked filamin A mutation which is typically lethal in males. Similarly, subcortical band heterotopia can be associated with an X-linked doublecortin gene, which cause a mild phenotype in females, but may cause lissencenphaly in a male child [13].

Risk of antiepileptic drugs in pregnancy

Antiepileptic drugs and major congenital malformations

Pre-partum counseling for WWE has changed significantly in the past decade on account of data from several international antiepileptic drug pregnancy registries (see Table 11.2). It is important that patients are provided with a basic understanding of how registry data is acquired and what it means in order to correctly interpret the risks presented and apply them to their own situation appropriately. Obviously the explanation needs to be tailored to the sophistication of the patient, though every patient should be encouraged to enroll in the appropriate registry.

There are no placebo-controlled studies of AEDs in pregnancy. The registries are predominantly prospective, observational studies which enroll WWE early in their pregnancies. The primary endpoint of most registries is risk of major congenital malformations (MCMs) associated with each antiepileptic drug. The patient being counseled should understand that MCMs are defined as structural malformations of development that have functional or cosmetic significance and typically require surgical repair. They range from neural tube defects to hypospadias. Other MCMs associated with AEDs include heart defects and cleft lip/cleft palate. MCMs occur typically before the 8–10th week of pregnancy. This underscores the need for early preconception counseling and planning. There is an increased risk of MCMs in WWE which seem to be a consequence of the medication(s) and not epilepsy itself [14]. The baseline risk of MCMs among the general population is 1.5–3%, but varies by country and study. In general, the risk associated with any AED therapy in pregnancy has been reported to be approximately 4–5% [15, 16]. When possible, this information should be tailored to the patient, addressing their personal risk factors and the medication she is taking. When discussing MCM risk for a given AED, it is reasonable to summarize the absolute risk data from multiple registries, which have for the most part been congruent (see Table 11.3). However, it is important to recognize the strength of the data for each AED; clearly 0% risk of MCMs among 50 pregnancies is much less informative than a 3–6% risk among 5,000 enrolled pregnancies (see Figure 11.1).

Table 11.2: Antiepileptic drug and pregnancy registries

North American Antiepileptic Drug Pregnancy Registry
www.aedpregnancyregistry.org
001 888 233 2334
International Register of Antiepileptic Drugs and Pregnancy (EURAP)
www.eurapinternational.org
Australian Epilepsy Pregnancy Register
www.apr.org.au
0061 1800 069 722
UK Epilepsy and Pregnancy Register
www.epilepsyandpregnancy.co.uk
0800 389 1248
Neurodevelopmental Effects of Antiepileptic Drugs (NEAD)
www.web.emmes.com/study/nead/index.htm

Table 11.3: Rate of major congenital malformations with individual AEDs as monotherapy published in six international pregnancy registries and one commercial registry (GSK lamotrigine registry). This data provides absolute rates of MCMs reported and does not represent relative risk, which differed by study depending on the control group used.

Registry	Study	Rate of major congenital malformations with individual AEDs as monotherapy								
		CBZ	GBN	LTG	LEV	OXC	PHB	PHT	TPM	VPA
UK Pregnancy Registry	Morrow [15] Hunt [51] Hunt [52]	2.2% (927)	3.2% (32)	3.1% (684)	0.7% (304)			3.7% (82)	9% (203)	6.2% (715)
North American AED Pregnancy Registry	Hernandez [17]	3.0% (1,033)	0.7% (145)	2.0% (1,562)	2.4% (450)	2.2% (182)	5.5% (199)	2.9% (416)	4.2% (359)	9.3% (323)
Australian Pregnancy Registry	Vajda [25] Vajda [19]	6.3% (301)	0% (11)	5.2% (231)	0% (22)			2.9% (35)	3.2% (31)	16.3% (215)
Finland National Birth Registry	Artama [16]	2.7% (805)								10.7% (263)
Swedish Medical Birth Registry	Wide [20]	3.9% (703)	0% (18)	4.4% (90)			14% (7)	6.7% (103)		9.7% (268)
GSK Lamotrigine Registry	Cunnington [22]			2.2% (1,558)						
Danish Registry	Molgaard [21]		1.7% (59)	3.7% (1,019)	0% (58)	2.8% (393)			4.6% (108)	
EURAP	Tomson [18]	5.6% (1,402)		2.9% (1,280)	1.6% (126)	3.3% (184)	7.4% (217)	6% (103)	6.8% (73)	9.8% (1,010)

AED = antiepileptic drug; CBZ = carbamazepine; EURAP = International Registry of Antiepileptic Drugs and Pregnancy; GBN = gabapentin; GSK = GlaxoSmithKline; LEV = levetiracetam; LTG = lamotrigine; OXC = oxcarbazepine; PHB = phenobarbital; PHT = phenytoin; TPM = topiramate; VPA = valproic acid.

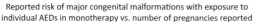

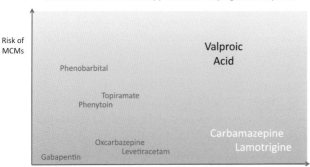

Reported risk of major congenital malformations with exposure to individual AEDs in monotherapy vs. number of pregnancies reported   **Figure 11.1**

The most consistent finding across all antiepileptic drug registries is that valproate significantly increases the risk of major congenital malformations. The absolute risk of MCM with valproate monotherapy has been reported to range from 6.2% to 16.3% in six registries and over 2,000 pregnancies [15–20, 25]. Drugs with a favorable risk profile include carbamazepine and lamotrigine, both of which have over 5,000 pregnancies reported. Rates of congenital malformations for these drugs range from 2.2% to 6.3% for carbamazepine and 2–5.2% for lamotrigine [15–21, 25], with some publications finding no statistically significant difference between the rate of MCMs with these drugs when compared with the control group [15, 17]. Preliminary data on levetiracetam is also reassuring, though most studies have included only small samples. The largest study of levetiracetam monotherapy included 450 pregnancies with a malformation rate of 2.4% [17].

The remaining antiepileptic drugs require further study, and the ability to summarize their absolute or relative risk is limited. Preliminary data for both topiramate and phenobarbital suggest that they should be used with caution in women of childbearing age. Phenobarbital has been specifically associated with a risk of congenital heart malformations [23] and the US FDA has recently listed topiramate as a category D drug on account of a significant, 20-fold increase in the risk of cleft lip and/or cleft palate [24].

Major congenital malformations: effect of AED dose

It has been known for some time that the adverse effects of valproate are clearly dose-related, with a greater risk of malformations at doses of more than 700–1,000 mg a day [16, 17, 19, 25]. A similar dose-related effect has been shown in some, but not all, studies of lamotrigine [15, 19, 22]. A recent publication by the International Antiepileptic Drug and Pregnancy Registry (EURAP) assessed the rates of MCM in close to 4,000 pregnancies with monotherapy exposures to carbamazepine, lamotrigine, valproate, or phenobarbital. The authors found that for each of these AEDs, higher doses at the time of conception were associated with a higher rate for major congenital malformations [18]. Future studies will need to look at the association between MCM and AED levels, which can vary greatly by individual and may be more likely to influence the effect of the drug on the fetus.

Antiepileptic drugs and cognitive teratogenesis

Data on the effects of antiepileptic drugs on cognition have been conflicting, which may be due in large part to differences in study design and incomplete control of important variables [23]. Studies of WWE not taking antiepileptic drugs have not shown any significant decrease in the cognitive abilities of their children, suggesting that epilepsy itself does not complicate cognitive development (though this is somewhat confounded by the presumably milder epilepsy syndromes in these patients). On the other hand, several studies have suggested that AEDs can adversely affect developmental outcomes [26]. Despite discrepancies between studies, most have consistently demonstrated an adverse effect of valproate on cognitive development, and two studies have implicated it in behavioral abnormalities and autism spectrum disorder [23, 26–28].

The Neurodevelopmental Effects of Antiepileptic Drugs (NEAD) study is a multicenter prospective, observational study of children born to WWE taking AEDs. It has demonstrated a dose-related effect of valproate on cognitive development. When adjusted for maternal IQ and gestational age, the average IQ of children exposed to valproate was 10 points lower than that of children exposed to phenytoin, lamotrigine, or carbamazepine. This study has also demonstrated that while maternal IQ is a strong predictor of a child's IQ, this correlation is not significant in children exposed to valproate [29]. Several early studies demonstrated potential adverse effects of phenytoin and phenobarbital on cognition, though the phenytoin effect was not substantiated by the NEAD study. Data on carbamazepine has been conflicting, but as of 2009, the American Academy of Neurology's Practice Parameter concluded that carbamazepine "probably does not increase poor cognitive outcomes," and a recent meta-analysis drew a similar conclusion [26, 28]. One study has addressed the effects of levetiracetam exposure on cognitive function of 51 children and did not find a significant difference in the IQ of exposed children when compared to a control population [27].

Polytherapy vs. monotherapy

Early studies presented consistent evidence that polytherapy was associated with a greater risk of MCM compared with monotherapy [26, 30]. A recent paper from the North American AED Pregnancy Registry, however, suggests that risks related to polytherapy may have been largely driven by the inclusion of valproate in these polytherapy combinations [31]. In this study, pregnancies exposed to lamotrigine and valproate had a 9% rate of MCMs, while combinations of lamotrigine with other AEDs were associated with a rate of 3%. Similarly, carbamazepine and valproate together resulted in a 15% rate of MCMs, while carbamazepine and other AEDs in polytherapy were associated with a 2% risk. Other registries have also found that valproate was largely responsible for the increased risk of MCMs in polytherapy [15, 16]. This data needs to be replicated in other prospective studies but, if substantiated, it poses an interesting challenge the prior dogma that monotherapy should be a paramount objective in managing young WWE. Given the established correlation between antiepileptic drug doses and MCMs, perhaps combinations of two drugs at lower doses may prove to be a better strategy for minimizing the risks related to AEDs in pregnancy in some patients who otherwise require high doses of a single agent. An important caveat, however, is that in limited studies, AED polytherapy has also increased the risk of adverse cognitive outcomes [26]. Thus future studies on the effect of AED combinations and cognition will also be needed to determine if this approach is reasonable.

Folic acid supplementation

Folic acid supplementation is typically recommended for all women of childbearing age taking AEDs. Historically, the recommendation of folic acid supplementation for WWE is largely extrapolated from studies demonstrating that it is associated with a lower risk of neural tube defects in the general population and in women at risk due to a previously affected pregnancy [32, 33]. Low first-trimester serum folic acid levels have also been associated with an increased risk for congenital malformations in WWE taking certain AEDs [34]. It is not yet clear if folic acid depletion is one of the mechanisms by which antiepileptic medications lead to fetal malformations. Only a few studies have detected a protective effect of folic acid on MCM rates in women taking AEDs [35]. One study demonstrated a decrease in spontaneous abortions in WWE taking folic acid, particularly those treated with valproate [36]. The majority of studies, however, have not been able to demonstrate a significant effect of folic acid on malformation rates in AED-exposed pregnancies. The American Academy of Neurology's 2009 Practice Parameter update on pregnancy in epilepsy concluded that these studies were not sufficiently powered to exclude a beneficial effect of folic acid supplementation. The committee concluded that the risk of malformation is "possibly decreased by folic acid supplementation" and "preconceptional folic acid supplementation in WWE may be considered to reduce the risk of MCMs" [37].

An interesting new finding is that folic acid may be beneficial for cognitive development: the NEAD study found that preconception folic acid supplementation was associated with higher IQ scores, particularly verbal IQ scores, in children born to women with epilepsy [38]. While it is not clear if this is an effect specific to WWE, it provides on additional rationale for folic acid supplementation.

Large epidemiological studies will be needed to thoroughly evaluate the effect of folic acid supplementation on AED-exposed pregnancies. In the meantime, most clinicians and guidelines agree that folic acid supplementation is an important part of preconception planning for women with epilepsy. There are wide variations in the recommended dose, with 0.4–4 mg recommended in the USA and 5 mg recommended in the UK, Europe, and Canada [7, 35, 39]. Most women's multivitamins include 0.4 mg of folic acid, whereas prenatal vitamins include 0.8 mg. In the USA, folic acid comes in a 1 mg pill by prescription, whereas it is available as a 5 mg pill in most other countries. In the USA, a common practice is to start all WWE on 0.4–1 mg of folic acid and increase the dose to 4–5 mg (3–4 mg by prescription plus a prenatal vitamin) when the patient is actively trying to conceive. These higher doses should also be considered in women who are at risk for an unplanned pregnancy.

Risk of seizures during pregnancy

Seizure frequency during pregnancy

The best predictor of seizure occurrence and frequency during pregnancy is a patient's seizure pattern prior to pregnancy [7, 23, 40]. Most studies of WWE demonstrate that seizure frequency typically remains unchanged in the majority of women when compared to their individual pre-pregnancy baseline (54–80%). It tends to increase in less than a third (17–32%), and decreases in the remainder of cases (3–24%). Rates of status epilepticus during pregnancy in WWE range from 0% to 1.8%. Seizure freedom for 9 months prior to conception is associated with an 84–92% likelihood of seizure freedom throughout the pregnancy [40]. Monitoring AED levels and appropriately adjusting doses during pregnancy is critical to seizure control. This applies to all AEDs, but most is best illustrated by lamotrigine, which often needs to be increased by 2 to 3-fold over the course of a pregnancy [41, 42].

Risks related to seizures during pregnancy

It is generally accepted that the risks of seizures, particularly tonic-clonic seizures, during pregnancy outweigh the risk of the medications. Seizures can put the patient (and thus her unborn child) at risk for falls and other accidental injuries. Tonic-clonic seizures and complex partial seizures can result in maternal hypoxia and arrhythmias, as well as put her at risk for sudden unexpected death in epilepsy (SUDEP). Case reports have documented fetal and maternal deaths with status epilepticus, and fetal intracranial hemorrhage and bradycardia in association with convulsions. One report of a complex partial seizure during pregnancy also documented fetal heart rate changes and prolonged contractions [43]. A study of cognitive development associated the presence of tonic-clonic seizures in pregnancy with lower verbal IQ in exposed children [44]. More recently, the EURAP study evaluated seizure frequency and outcomes among 406 women with epilepsy. In this cohort there were no stillbirths, miscarriages, or maternal deaths associated with isolated convulsions or nonconvulsive seizures. Among twelve cases of status epilepticus, there was one stillbirth and no cases of maternal death [45]. One study from Taiwan and another from Austria demonstrated an association between generalized tonic-clonic seizures during pregnancy and pre-term birth [46, 47]. On the whole, the risks of individual seizures to a given pregnancy are not clear. For now, advice about seizure control during pregnancy needs to be practical and cautious, emphasizing the risks of abruptly stopping seizure medications in most patients.

Breastfeeding

Most WWE should be encouraged to breastfeed, as it is largely felt that the important health benefits of breastfeeding outweigh any real or theoretical effects of AED exposure in the baby. Highly protein-bound AEDs such as phenytoin, carbamazepine, and valproate are expressed in breast milk at very low levels that are unlikely to affect an infant. Lamotrigine does pass to breast milk but has not been shown to have significant adverse effects [48]. The NEAD study evaluated the cognitive development of breastfed infants exposed to lamotrigine, valproate, phenytoin, and carbamazepine and found no difference in their IQs when compared to children with in utero exposures who did not breastfeed [49]. Levetiracetam and topiramate also pass to breast milk but are metabolized quickly with

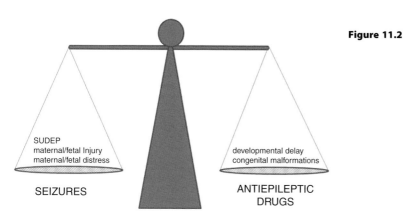

Figure 11.2

SUDEP
maternal/fetal Injury
maternal/fetal distress

SEIZURES

developmental delay
congenital malformations

ANTIEPILEPTIC
DRUGS

low levels in the infant. Most women are very surprised to learn they can breastfeed. It is often helpful to point out that in most cases the baby has been exposed to the medication in utero, albeit with the drug(s) metabolized by the mother.

Putting it all together: balancing the risks of seizure and medications before and during pregnancy

A patient and her physician must balance the potential risks of antiepileptic drugs with her personal risk for seizures. This often requires a highly individualized treatment plan. For example, valproate, despite its known risks for teratogenicity may be the most effective medication for the patient (especially in cases of juvenile myoclonic epilepsy (JME)). However, since the majority of patients with JME may also respond favorably to another broad-spectrum drug such as lamotrigine or levetiracetam, a young woman with newly diagnosed JME should not be started on valproate as a first line agent. If, however, the same patient proves refractory to several broad-spectrum antiepileptic medications at reasonable doses, it may be reasonable to use valproate at the lowest dose that controls seizures instead of continuing high doses of multiple other agents that have been ineffective. This should be done with very careful counseling of the patient as to all potential risks.

In choosing a first line antiepileptic medication for a WWE it makes sense to start with carbamazepine (for focal epilepsies), lamotrigine, or levetiracetam. Deciding whether to switch a patient who is already controlled on a different single agent depends on several factors, including the risks related to the present medication and the patient's personal preference and timeline. Some patients who have been seizure-free for 2–4 years can also consider weaning AEDs completely as they have a reasonable chance of staying seizure-free [50]. Whenever possible, it is best to make attempts to optimize therapy for pregnancy >9–12 months before the patient plans to conceive, as it is seizure frequency in the ensuing year that will best predict her pattern in pregnancy. Making medication changes in a patient who is currently pregnant should be done only in exceptional cases where benefits clearly outweigh risks, as changes in medications during pregnancy expose the patient and her fetus to polytherapy and the possibility of worsening seizures. Similar caution is advised in making changes in women who are actively trying to conceive or are not using contraception. There are, however, cases in which these late changes may be merited, such as women on valproate when it is not clearly needed. In these patients referral to an epileptologist with expertise in the area is highly recommended.

In a woman whose epilepsy has been well controlled, it is reasonable to consider tapering the dose of her medications well in advance of her pregnancy to determine her minimal therapeutic drug level. For this reason it is important to check AED levels regularly in WWE as part of their routine care, both when they are doing well and in the event of a seizure. Checking drug levels on a regular basis establishes the patient's individual therapeutic window, which is critical in planning pregnancy and managing AEDs during the pregnancy. For example, in a patient who was controlled for many years on 400 mg of lamotrigine and birth control pills should be able to substantially reduce her lamotrigine dose once she discontinues her oral contraceptive pills (OCPs) and still maintain her previous levels, as the OCPs effect on glucouronidation will be reversed (see Chapter 10).

Table 11.4: Timeline: management of women with epilepsy from diagnosis to conception

At diagnosis	• Take a careful history including all seizure types, frequency, risk factors, family history of epilepsy • Take sexual and reproductive history, including family history of fetal malformations • Perform basic epilepsy evaluation, including MRI and EEG • Consider inpatient monitoring prior to AEDs in patients with atypical histories • Start an AED most appropriate for patient AND with low risk of teratogenesis • Discuss available data on tertatogenic risk and the AED chosen • Discuss risks of seizures and AED noncompliance in general and in regards to pregnancy • Start folic acid 0.4–5 mg • Ensure adequate contraception • Consider discussion of fertility in epilepsy, social support, and breastfeeding

>1 year preconception	• Recommend inpatient monitoring if seizures have not responded to AEDs
	• Consider epilepsy surgery in appropriate patients
	• Consider medication change in patients taking:
	  • AEDs associated with higher rates of teratogenicity
	  • AEDs that are not controlling seizures
	• Consider trial of AED withdrawal in patients who have been seizure-free for >2–4 years
	• Decrease dose of AEDs in patients whose seizures have been well controlled
	• Establish therapeutic drug levels (ideally troughs) at least twice a year
	• Discuss balancing risks of AEDs and risks of seizures during pregnancy
	• Continue folic acid 0.4–5 mg

<1 year preconception	• Recommend inpatient monitoring if seizures have not responded to AEDs
	• Consider cautious AED adjustment in appropriate patients who are not trying to conceive
	• Check AED levels (ideally troughs) 3–4 times a year and establish target level for pregnancy
	• Discuss genetic screening/counseling with appropriate patients
	• Establish a pregnancy plan with patient:
	  • Patient should notify doctors at first sign of pregnancy
	  • AED levels should be checked more frequently, at least every 4 weeks
	  • Decide which seizure types and/or AED levels will prompt medication adjustment
	• Increase folic acid to 3–5 mg and start prenatal vitamin
	• Discuss social support, seizure safety in caring for infants, and need to avoid sleep deprivation
	• Discuss breastfeeding

Table 11.4: *(cont.)*

Peri- and post-conception	• Confirm patient is taking pre natal vitamin and supplemental folic acid (total 4–5 mg)
	• Establish/review pregnancy plan
	• Adjust or lower AEDs only in exceptional cases where benefits clearly outweigh risks
	• Discuss appropriate prenatal screening with patient and other physicians:
	  • Genetic counseling in appropriate patients
	  • Targeted anatomic ultrasound at 18–20 weeks
	• Discuss social support, seizure safety, sleep deprivation, and breastfeeding

Recognizing this important interaction and adjusting her dose appropriately may reduce the risk of MCM.

One of the most challenging issues in counseling and managing WWE during pregnancy is deciding how aggressively to adjust medications. In an ideal situation all patients can be kept seizure-free throughout pregnancy on a low dose of medications. For many patients, however, this is not realistic. Deciding on a "pregnancy plan" that includes which seizures to target is an important part of preconception counseling. For example, a patient who only has convulsions without any warning when her AED levels fall will be managed very differently from a patient who always has several days of subjective auras before any seizures involving loss of consciousness. In the first scenario, levels need to be monitored closely and adjusted in anticipation of any significant fall. In the case of the second patient, it may be reasonable to keep AED levels relatively low in the first trimester, increasing the dose when auras become frequent. Other important considerations are the patient's need to drive during pregnancy and her feelings about recurrent seizures.

Safety and social support

In explaining and managing all the important risks related to AEDs and seizures in pregnancy, it is easy to lose sight of some of the most important considerations, which include the patient's home life and ability to take care of their infant. WWE are at increased risk for seizures in the postpartum period due to hormone and AED fluctuations, as well as sleep deprivation. Even a woman with rare seizures needs to think practically how one of her typical seizures might affect the safety of her child. Worthwhile tips include changing the baby or feeding the baby on the floor, using a stroller around the house, and not bathing the baby alone. While breastfeeding is strongly encouraged, new mothers need to consider asking for help with night feeding from their partners and/or family to minimize sleep deprivation. In addition, patients should be aware that postpartum depression in women is common and WWE are at even great risk, with 25–29% reporting significant symptoms. These considerations and a patient's social support should be discussed within preconception counseling and re-visited during the pregnancy [48].

Conclusions

Preconception counseling for women with epilepsy should begin as early as possible, usually at the time of initiating an antiepileptic drug in a woman of childbearing age, or near puberty in an adolescent taking seizure medication. While counseling should be tailored to the patient's sophistication and personal timeline, it should be repeated at regular intervals, no less than yearly, allowing the patient to ask questions each time. Counseling should include a discussion of the risks related to seizures and AEDs during pregnancy. It should stress that most women with epilepsy have healthy pregnancies, but should also emphasize that early pre-partum planning can optimize fetal outcome.

References

1. Fairgrieve SD, Jackson M, Jonas P, et al. Population based, prospective study of the care of women with epilepsy in pregnancy. *BMJ (Clinical research ed)* 2000; 321 (7262):674–5.

2. Bell GS, Nashef L, Kendall S, et al. Information recalled by women taking anti-epileptic drugs for epilepsy: a questionnaire study. *Epilepsy Res* 2002; 52(2):139–46.

3. May TW, Pfafflin M, Coban I, et al. Fears, knowledge, and need of counseling for women with epilepsy. Results of an outpatient study. *Der Nervenarzt* 2009; 80 (2):174–83.

4. Vazquez B, Gibson P and Kustra R. Epilepsy and women's health issues: unmet needs–survey results from women with epilepsy. *Epilepsy Behav* 2007; 10(1): 163–9.

5. Winterbottom JB, Smyth RM, Jacoby A, et al. Preconception counselling for women with epilepsy to reduce adverse pregnancy outcome. *Cochrane Database Syst Revi* 2008; (3):CD006645.

6. Crawford P. Best practice guidelines for the management of women with epilepsy. *Epilepsia* 2005; 46(Suppl 9): 117–24.

7. Aguglia U, Barboni G, Battino D, et al. Italian consensus conference on epilepsy and pregnancy, labor and puerperium. *Epilepsia* 2009; 50(Suppl 1):7–23.

8. Davis AR, Pack AM, Kritzer J, et al. Reproductive history, sexual behavior and use of contraception in women with epilepsy. *Contraception* 2008; 77(6):405–9.

9. Crawford P and Hudson S. Understanding the information needs of women with epilepsy at different lifestages: results of the "Ideal World" survey. *Seizure* 2003; 12(7):502–7.

10. Helbig KL, Bernhardt BA, Conway LJ, et al. Genetic risk perception and reproductive decision making among people with epilepsy. *Epilepsia* 2010; 51(9):1874–7.

11. Winawer MR and Shinnar S. Genetic epidemiology of epilepsy or what do we tell families? *Epilepsia* 2005; 46(Suppl 10): 24–30.

12. Ottman R, Hirose S, Jain S, et al. Genetic testing in the epilepsies–report of the ILAE Genetics Commission. *Epilepsia* 2010; 51(4):655–70.

13. Kullman D. Genetics of Epilepsy. *J Neurol Neurosurg Psychiatry* 2002; 73(Suppl 2): ii32–ii5.

14. Holmes LB, Harvey EA, Coull BA, et al. The teratogenicity of anticonvulsant drugs. *New Engl J Med* 2001; 344(15): 1132–8.

15. Morrow J, Russell A, Guthrie E, et al. Malformation risks of antiepileptic drugs in pregnancy: a prospective study from the UK Epilepsy and Pregnancy Register. *J Neurol Neurosurg Psychiatry* 2006; 77(2): 193–8.

16. Artama M, Auvinen A, Raudaskoski T, et al. Antiepileptic drug use of women

with epilepsy and congenital malformations in offspring. *Neurology*. 2005; 64(11):1874–8.

17. Hernandez-Diaz S, Smith CR, Shen A, et al. Comparative safety of antiepileptic drugs during pregnancy. *Neurology* 2012; 78(21):1692–9.

18. Tomson T, Battino D, Bonizzoni E, et al. Dose-dependent risk of malformations with antiepileptic drugs: an analysis of data from the EURAP epilepsy and pregnancy registry. *Lancet Neurol* 2011; 10(7): 609–17.

19. Vajda FJ, Graham J, Roten A, et al. Teratogenicity of the newer antiepileptic drugs–the Australian experience. *J Clin Neurosci* 2012; 19(1):57–9.

20. Wide K, Winbladh B and Kallen B. Major malformations in infants exposed to antiepileptic drugs in utero, with emphasis on carbamazepine and valproic acid: a nation-wide, population-based register study. *Acta Paediatr* 2004; 93(2): 174–6.

21. Molgaard-Nielsen D and Hviid A. Newer-generation antiepileptic drugs and the risk of major birth defects. *JAMA* 2011; 305(19):1996–2002.

22. Cunnington MC, Weil JG, Messenheimer JA, et al. Final results from 18 years of the International Lamotrigine Pregnancy Registry. *Neurology* 2011; 76(21): 1817–23.

23. Tomson T and Battino D. Teratogenic effects of antiepileptic drugs. *Lancet Neurol* 2012; 11(9):803–13.

24. FDA Drug Safety Communication: risk of oral clefts in children born to mothers taking Topamax (topiramate). 2011. www. fda.gov/Drugs/DrugSafety/ucm245085. htm.

25. Vajda FJ, Hitchcock A, Graham J, et al. The Australian Register of Antiepileptic Drugs in Pregnancy: the first 1002 pregnancies. *Aust N Z J Obstet Gynaecol* 2007; 47(6): 468–74.

26. Harden CL, Meador KJ, Pennell PB, et al. Practice parameter update: management issues for women with epilepsy – focus on pregnancy (an evidence-based review): teratogenesis and perinatal outcomes: Report of the Quality Standards Subcommittee and Therapeutics and Technology Assessment Subcommittee of the American Academy of Neurology and American Epilepsy Society. *Neurology* 2009; 73(2): 133–41.

27. Shallcross R, Bromley RL, Irwin B, et al. Child development following in utero exposure: levetiracetam vs sodium valproate. *Neurology*. 2011; 76(4):383–9. PubMed PMID: 21263139.

28. Banach R, Boskovic R, Einarson T, et al. Long-term developmental outcome of children of women with epilepsy, unexposed or exposed prenatally to antiepileptic drugs: a meta-analysis of cohort studies. *Drug Saf* 2010; 33(1): 73–9.

29. Meador KJ, Baker GA, Browning N, et al. Effects of fetal antiepileptic drug exposure: outcomes at age 4.5 years. *Neurology* 2012; 78(16):1207–14.

30. Meador K, Reynolds MW, Crean S, et al. Pregnancy outcomes in women with epilepsy: a systematic review and meta-analysis of published pregnancy registries and cohorts. *Epilepsy Res* 2008; 81(1): 1–13.

31. Holmes LB, Mittendorf R, Shen A, et al. Fetal effects of anticonvulsant polytherapies: different risks from different drug combinations. *Arch Neurol* 2011; 68(10):1275–81.

32. Blencowe H, Cousens S, Modell B, et al. Folic acid to reduce neonatal mortality from neural tube disorders. *In J Epidemiol* 2010; 39(Suppl 1):i110–i21.

33. Prevention of neural tube defects: results of the Medical Research Council Vitamin Study. MRC Vitamin Study Research Group. *Lancet* 1991; 338 (8760):131–7.

34. Kaaja E, Kaaja R and Hiilesmaa V. Major malformations in offspring of women with epilepsy. *Neurology* 2003; 60(4): 575–9.

35. Kjaer D, Horvath-Puho E, Christensen J, et al. Antiepileptic drug use, folic acid supplementation, and congenital abnormalities: a population-based case-control study. *BJOG* 2008; 115(1): 98–103.

36. Pittschieler S, Brezinka C, Jahn B, et al. Spontaneous abortion and the prophylactic effect of folic acid supplementation in epileptic women undergoing antiepileptic therapy. *J Neurol* 2008; 255(12):1926–31.

37. Harden CL, Pennell PB, Koppel BS, et al. Practice parameter update: management issues for women with epilepsy – focus on pregnancy (an evidence-based review): vitamin K, folic acid, blood levels, and breastfeeding: Report of the Quality Standards Subcommittee and Therapeutics and Technology Assessment Subcommittee of the American Academy of Neurology and American Epilepsy Society. *Neurology* 2009; 73(2):142–9.

38. Meador KJ, Baker GA, Browning N, et al. Foetal antiepileptic drug exposure and verbal versus non-verbal abilities at three years of age. *Brain* 2011; 134(2): 396–404.

39. Wilson RD, Davies G, Desilets V, et al. The use of folic acid for the prevention of neural tube defects and other congenital anomalies. *J Obstet Gynaecol Can* 2003; 25(11):959–73.

40. Harden CL, Hopp J, Ting TY, et al. Practice parameter update: management issues for women with epilepsy–focus on pregnancy (an evidence-based review): obstetrical complications and change in seizure frequency: Report of the Quality Standards Subcommittee and Therapeutics and Technology Assessment Subcommittee of the American Academy of Neurology and American Epilepsy Society. *Neurology* 2009; 73(2):126–32.

41. Pennell PB, Peng L, Newport DJ, et al. Lamotrigine in pregnancy: clearance, therapeutic drug monitoring, and seizure frequency. *Neurology* 2008; 70(22 Pt 2):2130–6.

42. Sabers A and Petrenaite V. Seizure frequency in pregnant women treated with lamotrigine monotherapy. *Epilepsia* 2009; 50(9):2163–6.

43. Kaplan PW, Norwitz ER, Ben-Menachem E, et al. Obstetric risks for women with epilepsy during pregnancy. *Epilepsy Behav* 2007; 11(3):283–91.

44. Adab N, Kini U, Vinten J, et al. The longer term outcome of children born to mothers with epilepsy. *J Neurol Neurosurg Psychiatry* 2004; 75(11): 1575–83.

45. EURAP Study Group. Seizure control and treatment in pregnancy: observations from the EURAP epilepsy pregnancy registry. *Neurology* 2006; 66(3): 354–60.

46. Rauchenzauner M, Ehrensberger M, Prieschl M, et al. Generalized tonic-clonic seizures and antiepileptic drugs during pregnancy-a matter of importance for the baby? *J Neurol* 2013; 260(2): 484–8.

47. Chen YH, Chiou HY, Lin HC, et al. Affect of seizures during gestation on pregnancy outcomes in women with epilepsy. *Arch Neurol* 2009; 66(8): 979–84.

48. Klein A. The postpartum period in women with epilepsy. *Neurol Clin* 2012; 30(3):867–75.

49. Meador KJ, Baker GA, Browning N, et al. Effects of breastfeeding in children of women taking antiepileptic drugs. *Neurology* 2010; 75(22):1954–60.

50. Lossius MI, Hessen E, Mowinckel P, et al. Consequences of antiepileptic drug withdrawal: a randomized, double-blind study (Akershus Study). *Epilepsia* 2008; 49(3):455–63.

51. Hunt S. Russell A, Smithson WH, et al. Topiramate in pregnancy: preliminary

experience from the UK Epilepsy and Pregnancy Register. *Neurology* 2008; 71(4):272–6.

52. Mawhinney E. Craig J, Morrow J, et al. Levetiracetam in pregnancy: results from the UK and Ireland epilepsy and pregnancy registers. *Neurology* 2013; 80(4): 400–5.

<table><tr><td>Chapter</td><td rowspan="2">**12**</td></tr><tr><td></td></tr></table>

Teratogenicity and antiepileptic drugs

Georgia Montouris

Key points:

- Teratogenicity associated with antiepileptic drugs (AEDs) is likely multifactorial
- Epidemiological data on teratogenicity and AEDs are derived from international pregnancies, including the North American registry, UK registry, and EURAP
- Older AEDs are categorized as category D (evidence for human fetal risk but potential benefits may warrant use), whereas the newer agents are categorized as category C (animal studies showing adverse fetal effects), with the exception of topiramate
- Valproate has the highest risk of major congenital malformations, with the highest risk associated with polytherapy

Introduction

The first report that AEDs may have teratogenic effects dates back over 40 years. Since that time, evidence has been accumulated demonstrating that AEDs are associated with an increased risk of congenital malformations and may have long-term effects on intellectual development during childhood [1].

It is estimated that 0.3–0.5% of all children are born to mothers with epilepsy, corresponding to approximately 25,000 children each year in the USA alone. With the increasing use of antiepileptic drugs for other indications, such as psychiatric conditions, migraines, and pain disorders, the number of women using AEDs during pregnancy is likely to be considerably higher [2].

Since the mid-1990s, several new antiepileptic drugs have been introduced. For a number of reasons, these drugs appear to be more favorable than the older ones as treatments for epilepsy in women of childbearing age. They possess a good pharmacokinetic profile making them more stable during pregnancy, and they have a low potential for interaction with other drugs. They are less likely than the older drugs to be metabolized to compounds that are teratogenic [3].

Teratology

Teratology is the study of abnormal prenatal development that results from exposure to a "teratogen," which can produce structural or functional abnormalities in the conceptus [3].

Women with Epilepsy, ed. Esther Bui and Autumn Klein. Published by Cambridge University Press.
© Cambridge University Press 2014.

The teratogenicity of an agent is determined by a number of factors: (i) the physical and chemical nature of the agent; (ii) its administration at a specific dose and by a specific route; (iii) the gestational time at which it is administered; and (iv) the biological susceptibility of the mother and the conceptus [4].

Principles of teratogenesis

Five main principles of teratogenesis have been defined. First, susceptibility depends on the genotype of the conceptus and its interaction with the environment. Susceptibility is related to an inherited set of genes, that, when interacting with the teratogen, produce an alteration of normal morphogenetic and metabolic pathways, resulting in birth defects. The inter-action between a susceptible maternal and fetal genotype and the teratogen determines the degree of fetal sensitivity and the expression of different phenotypes [3, 4]. Second, susceptibility varies with the developmental stage at which the exposure occurs, resulting in different patterns of birth defects [4]. Organogenesis, which occurs between weeks 4 and 8, is the period most sensitive to teratogenic insults. In particular, the stage between weeks 3 and 5 is the most critical for central nervous system (CNS) development, whereas weeks 7 to 9 are crucial for urogenital system development; the embryo is most susceptible to cardiopathic events during days 20 through 42 [4, 5]. During the fetal period, beyond week 8 after conception, teratogenic exposure does not result in major malformations, but may cause growth retardation and functional disorders. These effects may continue after birth, particularly if they involve the CNS, as myelination, for example, continues for at least 2 years after delivery [3]. Third, teratogenic agents act through a number of specific mechanisms to initiate abnormal embryogenesis, such as mitotic inhibition, alteration of nucleic acid and its functions, reduction of precursors and substrates needed for biosynthesis, and alteration of enzymatic functions involved in differentiation and growth processes [3]. Fourth, access of a given agent to developing tissue depends on the nature of the agent. Drugs are subject to maternal metabolism and their teratogenic potential depends not only on placental transfer but also on maternal dose, route of administration, the physical properties of the drug, and the rate of absorption into the systemic circulation. Maternal metabolism has some detoxification enzyme systems that can reduce the amount of drug that reaches the fetus. However, as occurs for some established AEDs, the metabolites themselves may have a teratogenic potential [3]. Finally, embryotoxicity is a function of the dose of the exposure. The occurrence of abnormal development increases in degree as the dose rises beyond a threshold level [3].

Older antiepileptic drugs

Different mechanisms for the teratogenicity of AEDs have been postulated. Phenytoin, phenobarbital, and carbamazepine are metabolized via CYP-dependent oxidation. Oxidative intermediates are formed and further metabolized via hydroxylation by epoxide hydrolase, a hepatic cytosolic enzyme. Lower levels of this enzyme in fetuses as compared with adults may cause the accumulation of oxidative intermediates. The formation of oxidative intermediates is believed to be partly responsible for birth defects [6].

Valproic acid inhibits the metabolism of oxidative intermediates and of folic acid. Interference with folic acid metabolism has been widely accepted as a mechanism of teratogenesis. Folic acid is involved with the biosynthesis of DNA and RNA, and with the metabolism of certain amino acids. Valproic acid can cause neural tube defects and interfere with folate metabolism by inhibiting glutamate formyltranferase [6].

Newer antiepileptic drugs

Unlike the evidence of the older anticonvulsant drugs associated with teratogenicity, the limited data with newer AEDs does not allow conclusions to be drawn.

Even though animal reproductive studies are not sensitive and selective predictors of human teratogenicity, there is evidence to suggest that the newer AEDs may be less teratogenic. Intrauterine growth retardation and delayed skeletal ossification is found with both the older and newer AEDs and may be a consequence of maternal toxicity. The congenital malformations associated with the older AEDs, including neural tube, orofacial, cardiovascular, and urogenital defects, have not been found with some of the newer AEDs in the preclinical studies [6]. More recently Molgaard-Nielsen and Hviid reported the outcomes of 1,532 infants exposed to lamotrigine, oxcarbazepine, topiramate, gabapentin, or levetiracetam during the first trimester. A major birth defect was diagnosed in 38 out of 1,019 (3.7%) exposed to lamotrigine during the first trimester (APOR, 0.86; 95% Cl, 0.83–1.68), in 11 out of 393 infants (2.8%) exposed to oxcarbazepine (APOR, 0.86; 95% Cl, 0.46–1.59), and in 5 out of 108 infants (4.6%) exposed to topiramate (APOR, 1.44; 95% Cl, 0.58–3.58). Gabapentin (n=59) and levetiracetam (n=58) exposure during first trimester was uncommon, with only 1 (1.7%) and 0 infants diagnosed with birth defects. The authors concluded that the first trimester exposure of the five aforementioned AEDs compared to no exposure was not associated with an increased risk of major malformations [7].

Malformations

The Food and Drug Administration has assigned pregnancy categories to drugs defining potential risk to the fetus. Categories A, B, C, D, and X are as follows [8]:

Categories C and D pertain to anticonvulsant medications. Older AEDs are categorized as category D, whereas the newer agents are categorized as category C, with the exception

Category A: Adequate and well-controlled studies have failed to demonstrate a risk to the fetus in the first trimester of pregnancy (and there is no evidence of risk in later trimesters).

Category B: Animal reproduction studies have failed to demonstrate a risk to the fetus and there are no adequate and well-controlled studies in pregnant women.

Category C: Animal reproduction studies have shown an adverse effect on the fetus and there are no adequate and well-controlled studies in humans, but potential benefits may warrant use of the drug in pregnant women despite potential risks.

Category D: There is positive evidence of human fetal risk based on adverse reaction data from investigational or marketing experience or studies in humans, but potential benefits may warrant use of the drug in pregnant women despite potential risks.

Category X: Studies in animals or humans have demonstrated fetal abnormalities and/or there is positive evidence of human fetal risk based on adverse reaction data from investigational or marketing experience, and the risk involved in use of the drug in pregnant women clearly outweighs potential benefits.

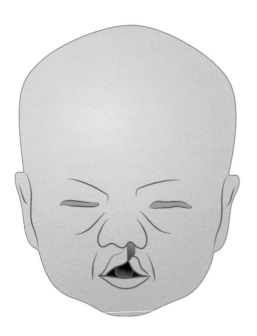

Figure 12.1: Oral facial clefts picture gallery. © 2009 Nucleus Medical Media, Inc.

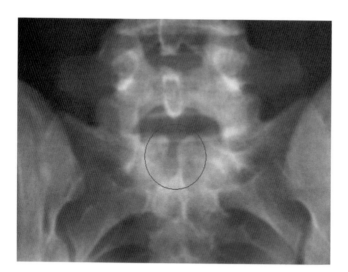

Figure 12.2: Spina bifida, Wikipedia.

of topiramate. As a result of an increased risk of oral clefts, the FDA changed the designation of topiramate from category C to category D in 2010.

The rates of malformations in the general population are 2–4%, which rises to 4–6% in women with epilepsy taking older AEDs. Newer agents appear to be associated with malformation risks similar to that of the general population [9].

Major congenital malformations (MCMs) are described above, involving oral facial (Figure 12.1), cardiac, urogenital, neural tube defects (Figure 12.2); however, minor malformations also exist. These, unlike the major, do not require surgical intervention, and include, but are not limited to, coarse hair, epicanthal folds, small nail beds, and skin tags [10].

Major malformation syndromes

In 1975, the fetal hydantoin syndrome was described and was the most commonly reported defect associated with a specific AED. It is characterized by craniofacial abnormalities, limb defects, deficient growth, and mental retardation. The craniofacial anomalies include a low and broad nasal bridge, epicanthal fold, short upturned nose, hypertelorism, ptosis, strabismus, prominent ears that are low-set and malformed, a wide mouth with prominent lips, and variations in the size and shape of the head, with sutural ridging or widening of the fontanels. The limb defects include hypolplasia of the distal phalanges and nails, which tend to assume a more normal appearance with time, finger-like thumbs, and variations in palmar creases and dermatoglyphics. There is intrauterine growth failure that results in small stature despite normal growth postnatally. The degree of mental retardation is mild to moderate [10].

From a historical point of view, a second fetal disorder was described associated with maternal AED, the trimethadione syndrome, first reported in 1970. Trimethadione, an oxazolidinedione, was first synthesized in 1944 in the course of a systematic search for drugs with analgesic properties. Shortly thereafter, its anticonvulsant properties in animals were described. Clinical trials soon followed and trimethadione's value in the treatment of petit mal epilepsy was established [11]. Trimethadione was marketed in 1946. It was noted that the casual relationship between fetal exposure and malformation was more established for trimethadione than for any other AED. These infants had developmental delay, speech disturbances, V-shaped eyebrows, epicanthal fold, and low-set ears with anteriorly folded helix, palatal anomalies, and irregular teeth. Additional features in some infants included intrauterine growth retardation, short stature, cardiac anomalies, ocular defects, simian creases, microcephaly, and hypospadias.

The fetal hydantoin syndrome later became known as the "fetal anticonvulsant syndrome" to include carbamazepine, phenobarbital, primidone, and sodium valproic acid [9].

Drug exposure and outcome

In addition to phenytoin as described above, outcome data from exposure to carbamazepine, phenobarbital, topiramate, and valproate have been extensively reported.

Carbamazepine (CBZ): In 1997 the relative risk for a major congenital malformation in children exposed to CBZ monotherapy was 4.9 (95% confidence interval (CI), 1.3–18.0). In the study by Holmes et al., in 2001 [12], the frequency of major malformations, microcephaly, and growth retardation, but not of facial or digit hypoplasia was higher in the 58 infants exposed to CBZ monotherapy. In a review by Matalon et al., in 2002 [13], the risk for major congenital malformations was higher when CBZ was used in polytherapy. For neural tube defects (NTDs), Rosa reported that 1% of CBZ-exposed infants had spina bifida [14]. Hernandez-Diaz, in 2007 [15], reported on findings in the NA AED Pregnancy Registry with CBZ monotherapy. The rate of major congenital malformations was 2.5 (95% CI, 1.6–3.7%) The Hungarian registry reported an increased risk of posterior cleft palate with CBZ, whereas the large UK pregnancy Register suggested no increase risk for major congenital malformations for CBZ [16].

Phenobarbital (PB): As for phenobarbital, early reports suggested it had less teratogenic risk than other AEDs; however after careful examination of the data, the risk appeared higher than in the general population (11%) and a possible dose-response relationship for dose greater than 60 mg per day. Subsequent studies have shown an increased risk and specific anomalies associated (cardiac) [16].

Topiramate (TPM): Full outcome data was reported on 203 pregnancies [17]. Of these, 178 resulted in live birth; 16 had major congenital malformations (9.0%, 95% CI, 5.6–14.1%). Three major congenital malformation (MCMs) were observed in 70 cases of monotherapy exposure (4.8%, 95% CI, 1.7–13.3%), and 13 in case exposed to topiramate as part of a polytherapy regimen (11.2%, 95% CI, 6.7–18.2%). Four of the MCMs were oral clefts (2.2%, 95% CI, 0.9–5.6%). Four cases of hypospadias were reported (5.1%, 95% CI, 0.2–10.1%) among 78 known live male births, of which two were classified as major malformations. Data from the North American Pregnancy Registry reported in 2011 that infants exposed to topiramate as a single therapy in the first trimester of pregnancy had a 1.4% prevalence of oral clefts compared with 0.38–0.55% for infants exposed to other antiepileptic drugs [18]. In information from the North American Pregnancy Registry in 2010 [19, 20], a total of 11 cases out of 289 (3.8%) demonstrated major congenital malformations. No unusual malformations were reported. Four of the eleven had oral clefts, two isolated, and two cleft lip and palate, and other anomalies [19].

Valproate (VPA): VPA has the highest rate of MCM among studied spina bifida aperta, and hypospadias have been associated with exposure to VPA and, to a lesser extent, CBZ. In pregnant women receiving VPA, the risk of spina bifida aperta in the fetus is approximately 1–2%, a 10-fold increase relative to the general population risk of 0.1–0.2%. In women taking CBZ, the risk is about 0.5–1%, whereas the risk is only 0.3–0.4% for those taking phenytoin and/or barbiturates [21–23]. In addition to the anatomical malformations associated with VPA, in utero VPA exposure has also been shown to impact on neurocognitive function. Meador et al. reported findings from The Neurodevelopmental Effects of Antiepileptic Drugs (NEAD) demonstrating 3-year-olds whose mothers took VPA during pregnancy had an average IQ 6–9 points lower than children exposed to other AEDs. The effects on the child's IQ appear to be dose-dependent. Additional reports on cognitive abilities and behavior of children exposed to antiepileptic drugs during pregnancy revealed an increase risk in children exposed to VPA over others [24]. Other studies support similar findings [25, 26]. Language impairment in children exposed to VPA was reported as well [27].

In 1997, a large multicenter prospective study of AED exposure reported that VPA appeared to have an increased risk of MCMs versus other AEDs. This study also demonstrated a relationship to VPA dose, with a significantly increased risk occurring for mothers taking more than 1000 mg per day. This finding has been replicated in subsequent publications from several large registries, including the North American Pregnancy Registry (10.7% vs. 2.9% other AED monotherapies), The Australian Pregnancy Registry (17.1% vs. 2.4% other AEDs), the Swedish Medical Birth Registry (9.7% vs. 4.0% carbamazepine), the Finnish National Medical Birth Registry (10.7% vs. 3.5% carbamazepine), the United Kingdom Pregnancy Register (6.2% vs. 2.2% carbamazepine), and the International Lamotrigine Pregnancy Registry (12.5% polytherapy with valproate vs. 2.7% polytherapy without valproate). Most recently, the Neurodevelopmental Effects of Antiepileptic Drugs (NEAD) Study Group confirmed both the increased risk of poor fetal outcome (MCM or death) and the dose-dependent effect of VPA in a prospective study (20.3% with VPA vs. 10.7% in phenytoin, 8.2% in carbamazepine, and 1% in lamotrigine) [39].

Furthermore, an association with VPA and childhood autism has been reported. In a report of a population-based study of 655,515 children born in Denmark from 1996 to

2006, 5,437 were identified as having autism spectrum disorder, including 2,067 with childhood autism. When examining the relationship of fetal valproate exposure to developmental outcome, increased risk of autism spectrum disorder (absolute risk, 4.42%; adjusted hazard ratio, 2.9 (95% CI, 1.7–4.9)) and childhood autism (absolute risk, 2.5%; adjusted hazard ratio, 5.2 (95% CI, 2.7–20.0)) were observed among the 508 children exposed to valproate [40].

Given the risks, both anatomical and cognitive, to the developing fetus from valproate exposure, alternative antiepileptic medications should be considered as first line therapy in women of childbearing potential.

Gabapentin: Results from the Gabapentin Pregnancy Registry, prospective and retrospective data concerning 51 fetuses, including 3 twin gestations, were collected from 39 women with epilepsy and other disorders (neuropathic pain) exposed to gabapentin during pregnancy. No increased risk of major congenital malformation was found. Two newborns had major congenital malformation with polytherapy exposure and one had minor malformation. Sample size is too small to make any conclusions [28].

Lamotrigine (LMT): Data form the International Observational Study revealed among 802 exposures, the frequency of MCMs was 2.7% (95% CI, 1.8–4.2%). A logistic regression analysis showed no difference in the risk of MCMs as a continuous function of dose. There was no effect of dose, up to 400 mg/d, on the frequency of MCMs [29]. Cunningham reported in 2005 that among 414 first trimester exposures to lamotrigine monotherapy, 12 outcomes with MCMs were reported (2.9%, 95% CI, 1.6–5.1%) [30]. The conclusion was that the risk of all major birth defects after first trimester exposure to lamotrigine monotherapy (2.9%) was similar to that in the general population. The North American Pregnancy Registry reported lamotrigine compared favorably to other AEDs, with a 1% risk of major congenital malformations, and appeared to have no increased risk compared with mothers not taking AEDs [1]. Holmes et al. reported in 2008 that a total of 16 (2.3%) of 684 infants exposed to lamotrigine had major malformations that were identified at birth. Five infants (0.73%) had oral clefts: isolated cleft palate [3], isolated left lip [1], and cleft lip and palate [1]. The rate among the lamotrigine-exposed infants showed a 10.4-fold increase (95% CI, 4.3–24.9) [19]. These findings were not reported in any other worldwide registries. The UK Pregnancy Register reported the major congenital malformation rate for pregnancies exposed to LTG was 3.2% (95% CI, 2.1–4.9%) [16].

Levetiracetam (LEV): In an early report in 2005, 11 cases of LEV-exposed pregnancies were registered in the European Registry of Antiepileptic Drugs and Pregnancy in the Netherlands. LEV was prescribed in monotherapy in two women and in combination with other AEDs in eight. No fetal malformations were detected [31]. Data from EURAP, an international registry of antiepileptic drugs and pregnancy, with 126 exposed pregnancies, reported two major congenital malformation cases yielding a major congenital malformation rate of 1.6% [32]. The North American Antiepileptic Drug Pregnancy Registry (NAAPR) reports a 2.1% major congenital malformation rate with 11 major congenital malformation cases among 450 exposed pregnancies [33], and among 133 exposed pregnancies reported by the UK Register, there were no major congenital malformation cases, yielding a rate of 0% [34]. Current reports of major congenital malformation among levetiracetam monotherapy exposures were 7.7% (UCB Registry) among 297 exposed pregnancies and 26 cases of major congenital malformation [34]. All of the other registries have reported lower rates of major congenital malformation in

LEV-exposed infants. Differences in methodology include data collection time points. The definition of major congenital malformations also varies from registry to registry. NAAPR exclude minor abnormalities, genetic and chromosomal abnormalities, ventricular septal defect (VSD) unless of large size, and symptomatic. UK and EURAP registries include VSD and exclude minor abnormalities. In addition, in the UCB registry, minor abnormality is considered as a major congenital malformation if more than one minor abnormality exists. Differences in methodology among the registries (see below) along with different comparators may account for the discrepancy seen in the results of the UCB registry and the others. When an internal comparator was available (in UCB registry, no internal comparator was used, only external), the rates of major congenital malformation and VSD were no greater in levetiracetam-exposed patients than in those treated with other AEDs [35].

Oxcarbazepine (OXC): In a review of studies of over 300 pregnancies exposed to oxcarbazepine, it was found that there was no evidence of increased risk of major congenital malformations with monotherapy (2.4%) [9]. A case series in Argentina included 35 women on OXC monotherapy and all infants were healthy; 1 of the 20 infants exposed to polytherapy with OXC had a cardiac malformation [16].

Zonisamide: Kondo et al. reported on a series of 26 pregnancies with zonisamide. Of the 26, 2 (7.7%) had major congenital malformation, although one was exposed to phenytoin (PHT) and the other to PHT and VPA [16].

Benzodiazepines: Information on risk of major malformation in this class of drugs is limited. The use of this class of drugs extends well beyond the use in epilepsy therapy. Benzodiazepines have been shown to have a mildly increased risk of major malformation as reported by Kluger in 2009 [1]. Enato et al. concluded in an update meta-analysis of the safety of benzodiazepines that while benzodiazepines do not appear to increase teratogenic risk in general, case-controls suggest a 2-fold increased risk in oral clefts [36]. In 2007, Wilker et al. reported maternal use of benzodiazepines and/or hypnotic benzodiazepine receptor agonists may increase the risk for pre-term birth and low birth weight, and cause neonatal symptoms, but does not appear to have a strong teratogenic potential. The tentative association with pyloric stenosis and alimentary tract atresia was seen in a higher than expected number of infants and needs confirmation [37]. Bellantuono et al. noted that data published in the last 10 years did not indicate an absolute contraindication in prescribing benzodiazepines during the first gestational trimester. However, studies analyzed in this article suffered from a number of methodological limitations, such as lack of careful report of benzodiazepine patterns of use in pregnancy, possible influences of recall bias, lack of controlling for confounding factors, and lack of data concerning possible major malformations in aborted fetuses. They report that even data from more recent studies suggest some caution in prescribing clonazepam and lorazepam in the first trimester of pregnancy due to reports of higher risk of MCMs.

History of prior major congenital malformations

In a large cohort drawn from the United Kingdom Epilepsy and Pregnancy Register, data was extracted for women who prospectively registered more than one pregnancy, calculating the recurrence risk for fetal malformations. Outcome data were available for 1,534 pregnancies born to 719 mothers. For those whose first child had a congenital malformation, there was a 16.8% risk of having another child with a congenital malformation, compared with 9.8% for women whose first child did not have a malformation (relative risk 1.73, 95% CI, 1.01–2.96). The risk was 50% for women who had two previous children with a congenital malformation. There was a trend toward a higher risk of recurrent malformations in pregnancies exposed to valproate (21.9%, relative risk 1.47, 95% CI, 0.68–3.20) and topiramate (50%, relative risk 4.50, 95% CI, 0.97–20.82), but not for other drugs such as carbamazepine and lamotrigine. Recurrence risks were also higher for pregnancies exposed to polypharmacy and for those where the dose of antiepileptic drug treatment had been increased after the first pregnancy [41].

Comparison of worldwide pregnancy registries

Three key pregnancy registries are discussed in this chapter, including: (1) EURAP, an International Registry of Antiepileptic Drugs and Pregnancy with over 18,000 enrolled pregnancies from many European, Asian, South American, and Middle Eastern countries, in addition to Australia; (2) the North American Antiepileptic Drug Pregnancy Registry (NAAPR) with over 8,500 enrolled pregnancies; and (3) the UK Epilepsy and Pregnancy Registry with over 5,000 enrolled pregnancies. As the majority of information on teratogenicity associated with AEDs stem from these three registries, highlighting key differences in these registries puts this data in appropriate context. In addition, a pharmaceutical-sponsored registry (UCB AED pregnancy registry) is also briefly discussed.

Definitions of congenital malformations between the different registries

Genetic disorders and chromosomal abnormalities:
- Included as a major congenital malformation in the UCB AED pregnancy registry
- Not included as a major congenital malformation in the NAAPR, UK Epilepsy and Pregnancy Register, and EURAP

Ventral septal defects:
- Included as birth defects in the UCB AED pregnancy registry, UK Registry and EURAP
- Only included in NAAPR if large and symptomatic

Minor abnormalities:
- Included as a major congenital malformation in the UCB AED registry if infant has more than one minor congenital abnormality
- Not included as a major congenital malformation in NAAPR, UK Epilepsy and Pregnancy Register, and EURAP

Comparators

Most pregnancy registries have internal comparators, typically other AEDs. EURAP and the UK Register have other AEDs as internal comparators. NAAPR has internal comparators of different AEDs and health family/friend controls; the external comparator is the Active Malformation Surveillance Program at Brigham and Women's Hospital (Boston). The UCB Registry has no internal comparator and the external comparator is MACDP (Metropolitan Atlanta Congenital Defects Program) (UCB abstract).

Table 12.1: Referral source, data collection points, and exposure data among the different registries

	EURAP	UK	NAAPR
Referral source			
Health care professional	X	X	
Self-referral		X	X
Data collection points			
At time of enrollment	X	X	X
Each trimester	X		
7th month of pregnancy			X
At birth	X	X	X
3 months postpartum		X	X
12 months postpartum	X		
Source of exposure data			
Health care professional	X	X	X
Patient			X

Table 12.2: Prevalence of major congenital malformations of AEDs taken as monotherapy in the first trimester of pregnancy by 50 or more enrolled participants

Compound name	Brand name	Total malformations	Enrolled pregnancies	Prevalence of malformations	95% CI
Lamotrigine	Lamictal®	31	1,562	2.0%	1.4 to 2.8%
Carbamazepine	Tegretol®	31	1,033	3.0%	2.1 to 4.2%
Phenytoin	Dilantin®	12	416	2.9%	1.5 to 5.0%
Levetiracetam	Keppra®	11	450	2.4%	1.2 to 4.3%
Topiramate	Topamax®	15	359	4.2%	2.4 to 6.8%
Valproate	Depakote®	30	323	9.3%	6.4 to 13.0%
Phenobarbital	phenobarbital	11	199	5.5%	2.8 to 9.7%
Oxcarbazepine	Trileptal®	4	182	2.2%	0.6 to 5.5%
Gabapentin	Neurontin®	1	145	0.7%	0.02 to 3.8%
Zonisamide	Zonegran®	0	90	0%	0.0 to 3.3%
Clonazepam	Klonipin®	2	64	3.1%	0.37 to 2.6%

Summary of prevalence of major congenital malformations, North American data

Between 1997 and 2011, the North American Pregnancy Registry enrolled a total of 7,370 pregnant women who were taking AEDs for any reason. Of these enrolled participants,

4,899 were taking an AED as monotherapy in the first trimester of pregnancy and were eligible for analysis. In 2011, participants in the Registry most commonly reported using the newer generation AEDs. Table 12.2 demonstrates the prevalence of major congenital malformation with AEDs taken as monotherapy in the first trimester of pregnancy by 50 or more enrolled participants. An internal control group, comprising pregnant women *not* taking any AEDs, was used as the unexposed comparison group for this analysis. The total number of malformations was 5 out of 442 enrolled pregnancies, with a prevalence of 1.1% and 95% CI, 0.37 to 2.6 [38].

In order to evaluate the safety of these drugs, as well as those most recently marketed agents (rufinamide, lacosamide, vigabatrin, ezogabine, clobazam), more observational data is required using standardized methodology.

References

1. Kluger S and Meador K. Teratogenicity of antiepileptic drugs. *Semin Neurol* 2008; 28(3): 328–35.

2. Tomson T and Batinno D. Teratogenic effects of antiepileptic medications. *Neurol Clin* 2009; 27:993–1002.

3. Palmieri C and Canger R. Teratogenic potential of the newer antiepileptic drugs. *CNS Drugs* 2002: 16(11):755–64.

4. Finnel RH. Teratology: general considerations and principles. *J Allergy Clin Immunol* 1999; 103:S337–42.

5. Polifka J and Friedman J. Clinical teratology: identifying teratogenic risks in humans. *Clin Genet* 1999; 56: 409–20.

6. McAuley JW and Anderson GC. Treatment of epilepsy in women of reproductive age. *Clin Pharmacokinet* 2002; 41(6):559–79.

7. Molgaard-Nielson D and Hvidd A. Newer-generation antiepileptic drugs and the risk of major birth defects. *JAMA* 2011; 305(19):1996–2002.

8. Drugs/FDA Categories, available at http://depts.washington.edu/druginfo/Formulary/Pregnancy.pdf.

9. Montouris G. Pregnancy and epilepsy management and outcome: an update. *Future Neurol* 2010; 5(3):449–59.

10. Montouris G, Fenichel GM and McLain LW Jr. The pregnant epileptic. *Arch Neurol* 1979; 36:601–3.

11. Booker HE. Trimethadione and other oxazolidinediones, chemistry and methods for determination, antiepileptic drugs. In: Woodbury DM, Penry JK and Schmidt RP, eds. *Epilepsy: a comprehensive textbook*, Vol 3. New York, NY: Raven Press, 1972.

12. Holmes LB, Harvey EA, Coull BA, et al. The teratogenicity of anticonvulsant drugs. *N Eng J Med* 2001; 344:1132–8.

13. Matalon S, Schechtman S, Goldzweig G, et al. The teratogenic effect of carbamazepine: a meta analysis of 1255 exposures. *Reprod Toxicol* 2002; 16:9–17.

14. Rosa F. Spina bifida in infants of women treated with carbamazepine. *N Engl J Med* 1991; 324:674–7.

15. Hernandez-Diaz S, Smith CR, Wyzszynski DF, et al. Risk of major malformations among infants exposed to carbamazepine during pregnancy. *Birth Defects Res A Clin Mol Teratol* 2007; 17:357.

16. Pennell P. Antiepileptic drugs during pregnancy: what is known and which AED seems to be the safest. *Epilepsia* 2008; 49 (Suppl 9):43–55.

17. Hunt S, Russell A, Smithson WH, et al. Topiramate in pregnancy. *Neurology* 2008; 71(4):272–6.

18. Lowes R. Topiramate linked to birth defects. *Medscape Medical News*. www.medscape.com/viewarticle/738432.

19. Holmes LB, Smith CR, Hernandez-Diaz S. Pregnancy registries: larger sample sizes essential. *Birth Defects Res A Clin Mol Teratol* 2008; 82:307 (abstract).

20. Hernandez-Diaz S, Mittendorf R and Holmes LB. Comparative safety of

topiramate during pregnancy. *Birth Defects Res A Clin Mol Teratol* 2010; 88:408 (abstract).

21. Lindhout D and Omtzigt JGC. Teratogenic effects of antiepileptic drugs: implications for the management of epilepsy in women of childbearing age. *Epilepsia* 1994; 35 (Suppl 4):S19–S28.

22. Wide K, Winbladh B and Källén B. Major malformations in infants exposed to antiepileptic drugs in utero, with emphasis on carbamazepine and valproic acid. A nation-wide population-based register study. *Acta Pediatr* 2004; 93:174–6.

23. Wyszynski D, Nambisan M and Surve T. Increased rate of major malformations in offspring exposed to valproate during pregnancy. *Neurology* 2005; 64:961–5.

24. Bromley RL, Baker GA and Meador KJ. Cognitive abilities and behavior of children exposed to antiepileptic drugs in utero. *Curr Opin Neurol* 2009; 22(2):162–6.

25. Viinikainen K, Eriksson K and Mönkkönen A. The effects of valproate exposure in utero on behavior and the need for educational support in school-aged children. *Epilepsy Behav* 2006; 9:636–40.

26. Erikkson K, Viinikainen K, Mönkkönen A, et al. Children exposed to valproate in utero – population-based evaluation of risks and confounding factors for long-term neurocognitive development. *Epilepsy Res* 2005; 65:189–200.

27. Nadebaum C, Anderson VA, Vajda F, et al. Language skills of school-aged children prenatally exposed to antiepileptic drugs. *Neurology* 2011; 76(8):719–26.

28. Montouris G. Gabapentin exposure in human pregnancy: results form the gabapentin pregnancy registry. *Epilepsy Behav* 2003; 4:310–7.

29. Cunnington M, Ferber S, Quartey G, et al. Effect of dose on the frequency of major birth defects following fetal exposure to lamotrigine monotherapy in an international observational study. *Epilepsia* 2007; 48(6):1207–10.

30. Cunningham TP and International Lamictal Pregnancy Registry Scientific Advisory Committee. Lamictal and risk of malformation in pregnancy. *Neurology* 2005; 64:955–96.

31. ten Berg K, Samren EB, van Oppen AC, et al. Levetiracetam use and pregnancy outcome. *Reprod Toxicol* 2005; 20(1):175–8.

32. Tomson T, Battino D, Bonizzoni E, et al. Dose dependent risk of malformations with antipepileptic drugs: an analysis of data from EURAP Epilepsy and Pregnancy Registry. *Lancet Neurol* 2011; 10(7):609–17.

33. UCB AED Pregnancy Registry. Interim Report, January 2012.

34. Kennedy F, Morrow J, Hunt S, et al. Malformation risk of AEDs in pregnancy: an update from the UK Epilepsy and Pregnancy Register. *Epilepsia* 2010; 51:S4–10.

35. Montouris G, Harden C, Albano J, et al. Incidence of congenital malformations in infants born to patients with epilepsy, a comparison of levetiracetam malformation rates from the UCB AED Pregnancy Registry to other Pregnancy Registries. American Academy of Neurology Annual Meeting, platform presentation, 2012.

36. Enato E, Moretti M and Koren G. The fetal safety of benzodiazepines: an updated meta-analysis. *J Obstet Gynaecol Can* 2011; 33(1):46–8.

37. Wikner BN, Stiller CO, Bergman U, et al. Use of benzodiazepines and benzodiazepine receptor agonists during pregnancy: neonatal outcome and congenital malformations. *Pharmacoepidemiol Drug Saf* 2007; 16:1203–10.

38. NAAPR. Annual Report, January 3, 2012.

39. Kluger BM and Meador KJ. Teratogenicity of antiepileptic medications. *Semin Neurol* 2008; 28(3):326–35.

40. Meador KJ and Loring DW. Risks of in utero exposure to valproate. *JAMA* 2013; 309(16):1730–31.

41. Campbell E, Devenney E, Morrow J, Russell A, et al. Recurrence risk of congenital malformations in infants exposed to antiepileptic drugs in utero. *Epilepsia* 2013; 54(1): 165–71.

Seizure management in pregnancy

A. Gabriela Lizama and Pamela Crawford

Key points:

- Majority of women with epilepsy (WWE) have a normal pregnancy and delivery; most WWE experience either an unchanged or improved seizure frequency
- Labor and delivery in addition to the 24-hour postpartum period is associated with a heightened risk of seizures, seen in 2–4% of WWE
- Antiepileptic drugs (AEDs) should be titrated based on monthly serum levels
- Intrapartum or peripartum seizures can be managed with optimization of AEDs, add-on clobazam, or intravenous AED depending on severity of seizures
- Lamotrigine serum levels significantly fluctuate during pregnancy and in the postpartum period

Most women with epilepsy have a normal pregnancy and delivery, without a change in seizure frequency. Despite such reassuring statistics, pregnancies in women with epilepsy warrant special attention by both medical and obstetric teams, given the increased risk of complications which include seizures during pregnancy and delivery.

Occurrence of seizures during pregnancy and the effect of pregnancy on epilepsy

The effect of pregnancy on seizure control has been discussed since the nineteenth century, and recent reports have varied in their estimate of this effect. A frequently cited meta-analysis by Schmidt, in which 2,065 pregnancies published in articles up to 1980 were analyzed, concluded that seizure frequency increased in 24% of cases, decreased in 23% of cases, and was unchanged in 53% of cases [1]. Studies published in the 1990s estimated that between 8% and 46% of pregnant women with epilepsy will experience an increase in seizure frequency [2].

The EURAP International Antiepileptic Drug and Pregnancy Registry has the primary objective of comparing the teratogenic potential of different antiepileptic drugs. Data from this registry has also permitted analysis of seizure control and occurrence of status epilepticus during pregnancy. At each trimester, the occurrence of seizures and status epilepticus during pregnancy is collected prospectively, and this has allowed for the analysis of seizure control and treatment changes during pregnancies of WWE. In 2006, the EURAP Study Group published their findings regarding seizure control and treatment in pregnant women

Women with Epilepsy, ed. Esther Bui and Autumn Klein. Published by Cambridge University Press.
© Cambridge University Press 2014.

with epilepsy in a large analysis that involved 1,956 pregnancies of 1,882 women with epilepsy. Women taking AEDs for any indication at the time of conception were eligible for inclusion in the registry, and only pregnancies registered within week 16 of gestation and before fetal outcome was known contributed to the prospective study. Pregnancies lost to follow-up or involving women taking AEDs for indications other than epilepsy were excluded from the study. Of the 1,956 pregnancies, 220 ended prematurely: 57 cases due to induced abortions, 133 cases due to spontaneous abortion, and 30 cases due to stillbirth. This left 1,736 complete pregnancies from which information about seizure control throughout the entire pregnancy was available. This data showed that 58.3% of all cases were seizure-free throughout pregnancy. This is close to the seizure freedom rate reported in people with epilepsy in general practice. Of the 41.6% cases with seizures, 23.4% of cases involved nonconvulsive seizure and 18.3% were convulsive [3].

A more recent study from Taiwan reported that 49.5% of untreated women recently diagnosed with epilepsy experienced a seizure during pregnancy [4]. Similarly, another very recent study from India of 1,297 pregnancies of women with epilepsy, followed under the Kerala Registry of Epilepsy and Pregnancy, found that 47.8% were seizure-free during pregnancy [5]. Unfortunately, the EURAP study is limited in that seizure frequency before pregnancy was not collected, therefore assessment of the effect of pregnancy on seizure control could not be fully assessed, but only changes in seizure frequency during pregnancy and across trimesters could be described. Nevertheless, the high proportion of seizure-free patients throughout pregnancy is in line with previous population-based studies from the 1980s [3], as well as other recent large population-based studies [3, 4, 5].

In the EURAP study, out of the 736 pregnancies in women with generalized epilepsies, 503 (68.3%) were seizure-free, again similar to the seizure freedom rate in the community. Of the 913 cases with localization-related epilepsy, 451 cases (49.4%) remained seizure-free [3]. The group also found that there was a higher risk of any type of seizures during pregnancy in women with localization-related epilepsy with an odds ratio (OR) 2.5 (confidence interval (CI) 1.7 to 3.9) [3]. In the Thomas study based in India, women with partial seizures had higher risk of relapse (OR 1.6, 95% CI, 1.2–2.0) compared to women with generalized epilepsies [5]. The EURAP group also described that use of polytherapy was associated with an increased risk of occurrence for any seizure type with OR 9 (CI, 5.6 to 14.8), and also was specifically associated with tonic-clonic convulsive seizures (OR 4.2, CI, 2.5 to 7.0) [3]. Oxcarbazepine monotherapy was also associated with a greater risk of convulsive seizures (OR 5.4, CI, 1.6 to 17.1) [3]. The recent study based in India also described an increased risk of seizures on polytherapy (OR 2.98, 95% CI, 2.3–3.9) compared to monotherapy [5]. This is likely to reflect that polytherapy is used in women with more refractory seizure disorders who are less likely to be seizure-free entering pregnancy.

The EURAP group also attempted to identify changes in seizure frequency throughout pregnancy. Using the first trimester as a reference, they found that seizure control remained unchanged in 63.6% of 1,718 completed pregnancy cases. In the cohort of completed pregnancies, 92.7% of women who were seizure-free entering pregnancy remained seizure-free during the entire pregnancy [3]. For those women who had a change in seizure frequency across trimesters, 17.3% experienced an increase in seizure frequency, while 15.9% experienced a decrease in seizure frequency [3]. Seizures during delivery occurred in only 3.5% of cases (60 cases) and were more common in women who had experienced seizures earlier in the pregnancy (OR 4.8, CI, 2.3 to 10) [3]. The risk of increase in seizure frequency was higher in localization-related epilepsies (OR 1.9, CI, 1.1 to 3.5), in pregnancies with polytherapy (OR 3.9, CI, 2.2 to 7.1), and oxcarbazepine monotherapy (OR 4.6, CI, 1.3 to 15.4) [3]. Data from the Kerala Registry of Epilepsy and Pregnancy in India suggests that women who had seizures in the preconception month had higher risk (OR 15, 95% CI, 9.0–25.1) of seizures during pregnancy when compared to those who were seizure-free during that period. Preconception seizures were the most important predictor of seizures during pregnancy [5].

There are many reasons why seizure control may change during pregnancy. Factors include deliberate or poor antiepileptic drug adherence, inappropriate reductions in anti-epileptic drug dosage, pregnancy-related falls in drug concentrations (known to occur with phenytoin, carbamazepine, phenobarbitone, and lamotrigine), hormonal changes, and vomiting of medication due to hyperemesis gravidarum. Additional stressors, such as emotional stress and sleep deprivation, may also contribute.

Sudden epileptic death in epilepsy (SUDEP)

In the latest review of maternal deaths from 2006 to 2008, 14 women died either while pregnant or within the year after pregnancy as a result of epilepsy. In 11 of these 14 cases, this was due to sudden epileptic death (a rate of 0.61 per 100,000 maternities). The quoted risk of SUDEP is 1:1000 patient-years for the general population. In the majority of cases the mother was not referred for review by a neurologist despite a known history of epilepsy. Only six women were referred for neurology review and in one case the neurologist's advice was not acted on. Nine of these women were treated with lamotrigine, and in seven of these nine cases, lamotrigine was used as monotherapy. One of the specific areas of advice was that most women with epilepsy would require an increased lamotrigine dose in pregnancy to maintain good seizure control and that management protocols should be altered accordingly. The other comment was that women with epilepsy or undiagnosed loss of consciousness are still unaware of the very rare but real risk of drowning while bathing unattended. In the women who died, nine died during the pregnancy, one died four weeks after a miscarriage, and four women died in the postpartum period. Of the eleven women who had sought antenatal care, only six had been seen by a health care provider with an interest in epilepsy. It was commented that in some cases the obstetrics and midwifery team did not appear to have perceived maternal epilepsy as a high-risk condition, and only six of the fourteen women with epilepsy had received pre-pregnancy counselling. However, it had been noted that a third of the women with epilepsy had difficult social circumstances that were likely to cause them to be excluded from mainstream health care [6].

Status epilepticus during pregnancy

The risk for status epilepticus in the general population during pregnancy remains a concern for both patient and clinician, as older data has suggested that convulsive status epilepticus in pregnancy is associated with high mortality. Previous studies have reported a less than 1% incidence of status during pregnancy. In the European study of 1,882 women with epilepsy, there were 36 cases (1.8%) of status epilepticus reported from the 1,956 pregnancies [3]. The risk of status epilepticus in the rest of the population with epilepsy is unknown. Only 12 cases were convulsive status. Of the status epilepticus cases, 13 (3 of which were convulsive) occurred in the first trimester, 11 (4 of which were convulsive) in the second, and 13 (5 of which were convulsive) in the third trimester (including one patient who had convulsive status at delivery and also in the second trimester). No cases of miscarriage or maternal death were attributed to status epilepticus [3]. No risk factors for status epilepticus could be identified; 19 patients had been seizure-free during pregnancy until the onset of status. Additionally, 34 out of 36 cases resulted in delivery of live-born offspring [3]. One patient with nonconvulsive status during the first trimester had a spontaneous abortion, which was reportedly not in close proximity to the status episode, and there was one report of a stillbirth attributed to status [3]. Possibly, the higher rate of status reported in the European study is due to missed cases of nonconvulsive status in earlier reports from the 1980s and 1990s.

Seizures surrounding labor and delivery

Most studies agree that the time around labor and delivery is associated with a higher risk of seizures. Estimates are that 1–2% of women with active epilepsy will have a tonic-clonic seizure during labor and another 1–2% will have a seizure in the following 24 hours [7]. The EURAP study reported that seizures occurred during delivery in 3.5% of patients (60 cases), with one case of convulsive status epilepticus during delivery. Of 60 patients with seizures during delivery, 14 had been seizure-free throughout the entire pregnancy, and 5 of the 29 patients with tonic-clonic seizures at delivery had only nonconvulsive seizures during pregnancy. The only factor significantly associated with the risk of seizures during delivery was the occurrence of seizures earlier during the pregnancy (OR 4.8, CI, 2.3 to 10) [3]. Data from the Kerala Registry of Epilepsy and Pregnancy in India shows that seizure relapse is highest during the three peripartum days [5].

Another recent study of women with epilepsy in the USA sought to characterize seizures during labor and delivery. Katz et al. retrospectively analyzed 89 consecutive pregnancies of women with epilepsy on antiepileptic drugs treated at their center. A total of 99 pregnancies between August 1990 and April 2000 were reviewed, and 10 pregnancies were excluded because the women took no AEDs during pregnancy (none were complicated by seizures during labor or delivery) [8]. The women were categorized as having primary generalized or partial epilepsies. The data was analyzed according to seizure type, duration of labor, complications at delivery, delivery type, and antiepileptic blood level closest to date of delivery. The study sample consisted of 32 pregnancies in women with primary generalized epilepsy and 57 pregnancies in women with partial epilepsy; 78% of the women were on monotherapy during the pregnancy, 20% on two antiepileptic drugs, and 3% took three antiepileptic drugs [8]. Seizures during labor and delivery occurred in 12.5% (4/32) of patients with primary generalized epilepsy, but did not occur in any of the 57 women with partial epilepsy (p<0.05) [8]. Katz suggested that insufficient AED may have contributed to three cases, while sleep deprivation may have contributed to one case. Of the four patients with seizures, three had a generalized tonic-clonic seizure and one had myoclonic status epilepticus. Of the 75 pregnancies with serum AED levels available for review, 49.3% (37 cases) had subtherapeutic levels at time of delivery. Of the women with subtherapeutic levels, 8.1% (3 cases) had a seizure during labor and delivery; there were no reported seizures in the 38 patients with therapeutic AED levels (p>0.05). Although the Katz study was limited by a small sample size and random sampling bias, the study supports the importance of maintaining therapeutic AED levels during the last trimester of pregnancy in order to try to prevent seizures during labor and delivery, and maintenance of therapeutic levels appears to be especially important for women with generalized epilepsies [8].

Effect on the fetus of having seizures during pregnancy

Unless associated with trauma, there is no evidence that a nonconvulsive seizure will adversely affect the developing fetus. Tonic-clonic seizures during the last trimester have been reported to cause fetal bradycardia and miscarriage [9]. A generalized tonic-clonic seizure during labor can cause transient fetal bradycardia, reduced beat-to-beat variability and decelerations for approximately 30 minutes after a seizure [10]; however, fetal bradycardia probably does not develop unless the mother also develops acidosis [11]. Tonic-clonic status epilepticus in pregnancy has been thought to carry a high mortality rate for both mother and fetus [12], but this data was assembled from case reports that were likely flawed by publication bias favoring reporting of adverse outcomes.

In the EURAP study, 74.1% of pregnancies ending in spontaneous abortion had occurred in patients who were completely seizure-free during their pregnancy. In cases ending in stillbirth, 50% had been seizure-free. Only one stillbirth and none of the spontaneous abortions ended in close proximity to a seizure or status epilepticus [3]. There was one miscarriage that seemed associated with a case of status epilepticus, but no single seizure was linked to miscarriage or stillbirth.

A recent retrospective cross-sectional study of women with epilepsy in Taiwan suggested that seizures during pregnancy are associated with certain adverse outcomes [4]. By using Taiwan's National Health Insurance Research Data (NHIRD), a large database consisting of monthly summaries of inpatient and ambulatory care claims, as well as a registry of contracted beds, medical facilities, board-certified specialists, and beneficiaries for over 98% over Taiwan's population, Chen et al. studied 1,016 women with epilepsy. The participants were 477,006 women who had a single birth in Taiwan between January 1, 2001 and December 31, 2003. The study cohort consisted of women who were diagnosed with epilepsy or convulsions within 2 years prior to their delivery. Women with a diagnosis of another chronic disease, which could increase the risk of adverse outcomes in pregnancy, such as hypertension, diabetes, psychiatric disorder, systemic lupus erythematosus, rheumatoid arthritis, gout, sarcoidosis, or ankylosing spondylitis, were excluded from the study. Importantly, women who were receiving antiepileptic drugs were also excluded from the study, thereby eliminating the confounding effect of antiepileptic drug use on adverse outcomes. The remaining 1,016 women with epilepsy were then stratified into two groups: women who did and did not have seizures during pregnancy. The comparison cohort was derived from the remaining women, again excluding women with chronic diseases that could affect outcomes. Compared to women without epilepsy and after adjusting for confounders (such as family income, infant sex and parity, mother's age, educational level and marital status, father's age and educational level), Chen found that epileptic seizures during pregnancy were independently associated with a 1.36-fold (95% CI, 1.01–1.88) increased risk of low birth weight infants, a 1.63-fold (95% CI, 1.21–2.19) increase in pre-term delivery, and a 1.37-fold (95% CI, 1.09–1.70) increase in small gestational age. Also, the risk for small gestational age increased 1.34-fold (95% CI, 1.01–1.84) for women with epilepsy and seizures during pregnancy compared to women with epilepsy without seizures during pregnancy. There was no significant difference in the risk of low birth weight or small gestational age infants between women with epilepsy and no seizures during pregnancy and women without epilepsy, but the risks of pre-term delivery increased to some extent, with OR 1.39 (95% CI, 1.03–1.93). Based on this data, it appears that a woman with epilepsy may be reassured that if seizure control is achieved throughout the pregnancy, the risk for small gestational age or low birth weight is no different to a women without epilepsy; however, there remains an associated risk of pre-term delivery associated with the diagnosis of epilepsy itself. Although the diagnosis of epilepsy itself cannot be said to have no risk, the evidence supports the importance of maintaining good seizure control throughout pregnancy in order to prevent adverse outcomes. The authors admit that the data likely underestimates adverse pregnancy outcomes, as the women with epilepsy who had seizures during pregnancy must have presented with seizures severe enough to seek care in an emergency department. Also, the study excluded women with epilepsy on antiepileptics, possibly limiting our ability to extrapolate the findings to women with epilepsy on antiepileptics, as this group is very different from the study cohort. Although concerns about the risks of antiepileptic drug use to the fetus are often the focus of prospective mothers and contribute to medication nonadherence, evidence supports optimizing seizure control during pregnancy. A multiple regression analysis of a retrospective study of 249 children aged 6 and over suggested that both valproate exposure and frequent tonic-clonic seizures in pregnancy may be significantly associated with a lower verbal IQ, despite adjusting for other confounding factors [13].

Preconception antiepileptic management

Current practice holds that women should enter pregnancy having complete seizure control or as few seizures as possible. Although the teratogenic potential of antiepileptic drugs concerns most expectant mothers, the need to achieve seizure control is supported by substantial evidence. It is important to review the need for continuing antiepileptic drug therapy in women with epilepsy. Women who have only had simple partial seizures or short-lived complex partial seizures and do not wish to drive may be willing to reduce or stop antiepileptic drug therapy. If a woman has juvenile myoclonic epilepsy or another primary generalized epilepsy with tonic-clonic seizures, even if seizure-free, they are at high risk of recurrence of the tonic-clonic seizures with the risk of injury and, although rare, sudden epileptic death. It is also essential that the known teratogenic risks of certain antiepileptic drugs are discussed and these risks put into perspective. Older studies have reported that the risk of significant fetal malformation is approximately 3% when one antiepileptic is taken, and up to 17% if more than two antiepileptics are taken [14]. Most major malformations develop in the earlier stages in pregnancy, often before a woman knows about the pregnancy.

AED management during pregnancy

Plasma concentrations of certain antiepileptic drugs have been reported to decrease during pregnancy. Ideally, drug levels should be measured at least twice before pregnancy and therapeutic serum levels should be maintained by increasing dosages as appropriate throughout the pregnancy. Drug dosage should be reduced to the pre-pregnancy dosage within 10 days after delivery [15]. The EURAP group reported that antiepileptic drug treatment was unchanged in 62.7% of 1,956 pregnancies of the 1,882 women with epilepsy participating in their registry. As would be expected, the number or dose of antiepileptic drug was increased or decreased in pregnancies complicated by seizure (OR 3.6, CI, 2.8–4.7, and 2.1, CI, 1.5–3.0) [2]. Monotherapy with lamotrigine (OR 3.8, CI, 2.1–6.9) or oxcarbazepine (OR 3.7, CI, 1.1–12.9) was also associated with an increase in AED load [3].

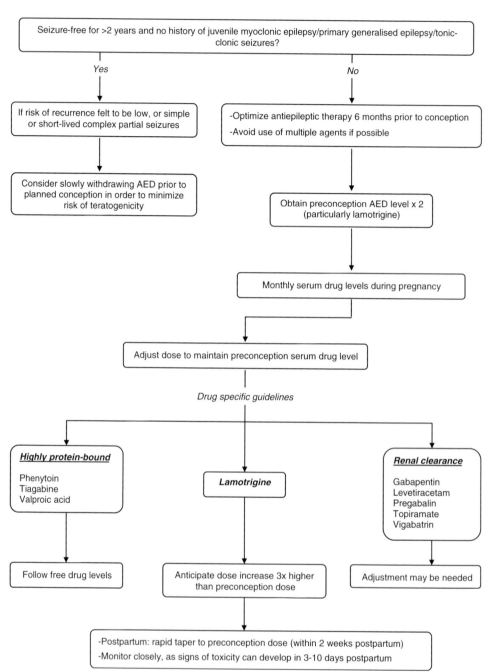

Seizure-free for >2 years and no history of juvenile myoclonic epilepsy/primary generalised epilepsy/tonic-clonic seizures?

Yes

No

If risk of recurrence felt to be low, or simple or short-lived complex partial seizures

-Optimize antiepileptic therapy 6 months prior to conception
-Avoid use of multiple agents if possible

Consider slowly withdrawing AED prior to planned conception in order to minimize risk of teratogenicity

Obtain preconception AED level x 2 (particularly lamotrigine)

Monthly serum drug levels during pregnancy

Adjust dose to maintain preconception serum drug level

Drug specific guidelines

Highly protein-bound

Phenytoin
Tiagabine
Valproic acid

Lamotrigine

Renal clearance

Gabapentin
Levetiracetam
Pregabalin
Topiramate
Vigabatrin

Follow free drug levels

Anticipate dose increase 3x higher than preconception dose

Adjustment may be needed

-Postpartum: rapid taper to preconception dose (within 2 weeks postpartum)
-Monitor closely, as signs of toxicity can develop in 3-10 days postpartum

Figure 13.1

Recommendation for seizure management

Hyperventilation, sleep deprivation, pain, and emotional stress can increase the risk of seizures during labor. In a study by Katz analyzing seizures in women with epilepsy during labor and delivery, the mean duration of labor for the four patients who had seizures during labor and delivery was 14.0 +/-6.0 hours, compared to 10.1 +/-11.0 hours for women without seizures during labor and delivery (p>0.05) [6]. In the Katz study, the patient who had myoclonic status required cesarean section for fetal heart rate decelerations [8]. One woman required cesarean section for fetal malposition, and the other two patients delivered vaginally, with one requiring induction [8]. Again, possible precipitants included insufficient AED doses in three of four cases, and sleep deprivation in one of four cases [8].

During labor, it is important to continue antiepileptic drug therapy. Use of oral clobazam 5 mg to 10 mg may also be beneficial to decrease anxiety as well as the risk of seizures around delivery [14]. It would be appropriate to offer epidural anesthesia early during labor in order help alleviate some degree of pain and emotional stress. Of note, magnesium sulfate is not an adequate medication for the management of epileptic seizures during labor and delivery. Convulsive seizures should be treated with intravenous benzodiazepines, such as lorazepam. If needed, intravenous phenytoin may be used and can additionally provide a longer duration of action. It is important to be aware that medications such as benzodiazepines, primidone, and phenobarbital can cause neonatal sedation and even a neonatal withdrawal syndrome. Other available intravenous anticonvulsants include iv levetiracetam, iv valproate, and iv lacosamide. However there is limited data available on the use of these drugs in the acute management of seizures in pregnancy.

Status epilepticus in pregnancy should be managed similar to status epilepticus in the general population; however, the differential diagnosis should include eclampsia, central venous thrombosis, and stroke in addition to exacerbation of underlying seizure disorder. Neuroimaging should be considered.

An epidural is often suggested, as it means that a woman is less likely to get exhausted and sleep-deprived and, if necessary, can be converted to spinal anesthesia if an emergency cesarian section is indicated.

AEDs and pharmacokinetics during pregnancy

If a woman is seizure-free before pregnancy, seizures usually remain well controlled throughout the pregnancy. Deliberate medication nonadherence, stress, and sleep deprivation may contribute to an increase in seizure frequency during pregnancy. Even with good adherence, breakthrough seizures may occur due to the effect of pregnancy on antiepileptic drug levels. Alteration of AED levels can be due to altered plasma protein-binding and albumin concentration, and increased drug clearance that occurs during pregnancy. Such changes in pharmacokinetics make it even more important for a clinician to monitor serum AED levels in AEDs such as lamotrigine or oxcarbazepine.

Certain antiepileptics are well documented to have altered metabolism during pregnancy. Studies have shown that during pregnancy, total concentrations decline by an average of 50% for phenobarbital, an average of 50–60% for phenytoin, and up to 25% for carbamazepine [16]. Phenytoin, valproate, and tiagabine are highly protein-bound. It is important for the physician to be aware that decreased binding to plasma proteins during pregnancy may cause measurements of lower total drug levels, while the unbound plasma concentration changes only slightly and the pharmacologically active concentration of the

Table 13.1

Drug	Metabolism	Expected change in pregnancy	Protein-binding	Additional comments
Carbamazepine	Hepatic	Decline up to 25%	CB: 75% Epoxide metabolite: 50%	
Ethosuximide	Hepatic	Data lacking	Negligible	
Lamotrigine	Hepatic	Decline by 60–90%	55%	Postpartum: requires rapid return to preconception dose to avoid toxicity
Levetiracetam	Renal	Decline >50%	Negligible	May require renal adjustment
Gabapentin	Renal	Data lacking	0	
Oxcarbamazepine	Hepatic	Decline >50%	40% for 10-monohydroxy metabolite	
Phenobarbital	Hepatic	Decline by 25–50%	45% protein-bound	
Phenytoin	Hepatic	Decline by 25–50%	Highly protein-bound, 90%	
Pregabalin	Renal	Data lacking	0	
Tiagabine	Hepatic	Data lacking	Highly protein-bound, >90%	
Topiramate	Renal predominance	Data lacking	15%	
Valproic acid	Hepatic	Decline by 25–50%	Highly protein-bound, 90%	Unbound concentration is often unchanged. Follow free level to avoid inappropriate drug increase
Vigabatrin	Renal	Data lacking	0	
Zonisamide	Hepatic	Decline by 25–50%	40–50%	

drug may be unchanged. Thus, for antiepileptics with known high protein-binding, it is recommended that free drug levels be measured during pregnancy rather than total drug levels, in order to avoid unnecessary drug dose increases. Studies of valproic acid have described up to a 50% decrease in total plasma concentrations by the end of the third trimester; however, the unbound plasma concentrations changes only slightly [16]. This information is particularly relevant for valproic acid, as a failure to obtain free drug levels may lead to inappropriate increases in dosage.

Less information is available about the effects of pregnancy on the newer AEDs. Studies have shown that the active metabolite of oxcarbazepine, the monohydroxy derivative (MHD), which is metabolized by glucuronide conjugation, declines by 36–50% in the last trimester [16]. Pregabalin and vigabatrin are both eliminated unchanged renally, and have insignificant amount of protein-binding; therefore, changes in serum concentrations of these drugs are expected to change as GFR changes. Levetiracetam, which is also predominantly eliminated renally, still requires enzymatic hydrolysis for 25% of its clearance, and plasma levels are reported to be reduced to 50% in the third trimester [16]. Two case reports showed a slightly lower maternal plasma concentration of zonisamide at delivery compared to the first 2 weeks postpartum [16]. Data regarding the pharmacokinetics of topiramate and gabapentin is limited, but case reports have shown no significantly different levels 2–4 weeks postpartum [16]. In a recent study of 12 women with epilepsy and 15 pregnancies using topiramate (TPM) as monotherapy or polytherapy, Westin et al. described a gradual decline in dose-corrected serum concentration of TPM. The authors proposed that increased GFR may play a major role in this decline, but reported pronounced inter-individual variability, and the data could not show a correlation with increased seizure frequency and decline in the TPM concentration to dose ratio [17].

Many studies have looked at lamotrigine metabolism in pregnancy. Reports have shown that lamotrigine metabolism is altered during pregnancy, with marked decreased serum concentration. The effect has been attributed to multiple factors, including altered drug metabolism, increased renal clearance, impaired absorption from the GI tract, and reduced plasma protein-binding resulting in redistribution of the drug. Lamotrigine is metabolized almost exclusively by hepatic glucuronic acid conjugation. Its major metabolite is lamotrigine-2-N-glucuronide (2-N-GLUC). Studies have shown that the 2-N-glucuronide pathway is enzymatically induced during pregnancy [18]. Levels have been shown to decrease by 60–90% through the induction of UDP-glucuronosyltransferase (UGT) enzymes, lamotrigine's main metabolic enzymes. In a recent study following nine women on lamotrigine (LTG) monotherapy during pregnancy, delivery, and approximately 3 weeks postpartum, it was found that lamotrigine clearance rates differed in each trimester, with an average increase in lamotrigine clearance of 197% above baseline in the first trimester, an increase of 236% above baseline in the second trimester, a 248% increase in the third trimester, and a 264% increase above baseline at delivery [19]. These findings are similar to previous reports showing the degree of change in clearance of lamotrigine during pregnancy, and suggests that an almost 3-fold dosage increase in LTG may be necessary to avoid subtherapeutic levels and breakthrough seizures [19].

Therefore, it is expected that lamotrigine dosages may need to be increased early in the pregnancy, and large increases in drug dosage may be required to maintain therapeutic drug levels. The clinician should also expect a quick normalization of lamotrigine metabolism and clearance in the next 2–3 weeks postpartum [19, 20]. After delivery, drug dosage should return back to preconception dose to avoid postpartum toxicity, even though this may appear to be a very rapid decrease over 1–2 weeks.

In a study of 12 pregnancies in women on lamotrigine monotherapy, 3 of 7 women whose LTG dose was adjusted during pregnancy developed signs of LTG toxicity, including dizziness, ataxia, and diplopia, between 3 to 10 days after delivery [20]. Of note, the effects of pregnancy on LTG plasma levels are minor in women who are also taking valproic acid, which is known to inhibit glucuronidation [16].

Conclusion

It is important that women with epilepsy receive pre-pregnancy counseling so that they end the pregnancy on optimal drug therapy, both for seizure control and fetal wellbeing. Antiepileptic drug concentrations need to be measured before pregnancy and the level maintained through drug dosage alteration, particularly for lamotrigine and oxcarbazepine. The need for medication adherence should be stressed, and women, especially those who are approaching delivery, need therapeutic blood levels in order to decrease the risk of seizures during delivery. After delivery, antiepileptic drug dosages need to be reduced back to pre-pregnancy levels. Women need to be counseled about factors that can precipitate seizures during pregnancy, but advised that only rarely will the seizure affect the developing fetus, and the majority of women with epilepsy remain free of seizures through both pregnancy and delivery.

References

1. Schmidt D. The effect of pregnancy on the natural history of epilepsy: a review of the literature. In: Janz D, Dam M, Bossi L, et al., eds. *Epilepsy, pregnancy, and the child*. New York, NY: Raven Press, 1982; 3–14.

2. Tomson T. Seizure control during pregnancy and delivery. In: Tomson T, Gram L, Sillanpaa M, et al., eds. *Epilepsy and pregnancy*. Petersfield: Wrightson Biomedical Publishing Ltd, 1997; 113–23.

3. EURAP Study Group. Seizure control and treatment in pregnancy: observations from the EURAP epilepsy pregnancy registry. *Neurology* 2006; 66:354–60.

4. Chen YH, Chiou HY and Lin HL. Affect of seizures during gestation on pregnancy outcomes in women with epilepsy. *Arch Neurol* 2009; 66(8): 979–84.

5. Thomas SV, Syam U and Devi JS. Predictors of seizures during pregnancy in women with epilepsy. *Epilepsia* 2012; 53(5):e85–e8.

6. Lewis G, Cantwell R, Clutton-Brock T, et al. Confidential Enquiries for Maternal and Child Deaths. The Centre for Maternal and Child Enquiries. *Br J Obstet Gynaecol* 2011; 118(Suppl 1):1–30.

7. Bardy A. *Epilepsy and pregnancy. A prospective study of 154 patients in epileptic women*. Helsinki: University of Helsinki, 1982.

8. Katz JM and Devinsky O. Primary generalized epilepsy: a risk factor for seizures in labor and delivery. *Seizure* 2003; 12(4):217–19.

9. Betts T and Crawford P. *Women in epilepsy*. London: Martin Dunitz, 1998.

10. Hiilesmaa VK, Bardy A and Terramo K. Obstetric outcome in women with epilepsy. *Am J Obstet Gynecol* 1985; 152:499–504.

11. Goetting MG and Davidson BN. Status epilepticus during labour. A case report. *J Reprod Med* 1987; 32:313–14.

12. Licht EA and Sankar R. Status epilepticus during pregnancy: a case report. *J Reprod Med* 1999; 44:370–72.

13. Adab N, Kini U, Vinten JA, et al. The longer term outcome of children born to mothers with epilepsy. *J Neurol Neurosurg Psychiatry* 2004; 75(11):1575–83.

14. Crawford P. Management of epilepsy in pregnancy. *Future Neurol* 2006; 1(3): 303–10.

15. Ohman I, Vitols S and Thomson T. Lamotrigine in pregnancy: pharmacokinetics during delivery, in the neonate during lactation. *Epilepsia* 2000; 41:709–13.

16. Sabers A and Tomson T. Managing antiepileptic drugs during pregnancy and lactation. *Curr Opin Neurol* 2009; 22: 157–61.

17 Westin AA, Nakken KO, Johannessen SI, et al. Serum concentration/dose ratio of topiramate during pregnancy. *Epilepsia* 2009; 50(3):480–5.

18. Öhman I, Beck O, Vitols S, et al. Plasma concentrations of lamotrigine and its 2-N-glucuronide metabolite during pregnancy in women with epilepsy. *Epilepsia* 2008; 49(6): 1075–80.

19. Fotopoulou C, Kretz R, Bauer S, et al. Prospectively assessed changes in lamotrigine-concentration in women with epilepsy during pregnancy, lactation and the neonatal period. *Epilepsy Res* 2009; 85:60–4.

20. de Haan GJ, Edelbroek P, Segers J, et al. Gestation-induced changes in lamotrigine pharmacokinetics: a monotherapy study. *Neurology* 2004; 63:571–3.

Obstetric and fetal monitoring in women with epilepsy

Dini Hui and Ori Nevo

Key points:

- The majority of women with epilepsy (WWE) have either no change in seizure frequency or decrease in seizure frequency. The risk of seizure during delivery remains small but significant (~3.5%)
- Neonates of WWE taking antiepileptic drugs (AEDs) are likely to be at an increased risk of being small for gestational age (SGA). However, there is no substantially increased risk of perinatal death in neonates born to WWE
- Routine antenatal fetal tests should be performed to rule out congenital malformations, such as the maternal serum biochemical screen, fetal anatomy ultrasound, and possibly fetal echocardiography
- Delivery should take place in an obstetric unit where resources for, and expertise in, maternal and fetal resuscitation are readily available
- WWE do not have a substantially increased risk of cesarean delivery. Cesarean section should be reserved for the usual obstetrical indications, or in the setting of recurrent uncontrolled generalized seizures in late pregnancy or labour

Effect of pregnancy on maternal epilepsy

The majority of patients with epilepsy maintain seizure control during pregnancy with the risk of increase in seizure frequency generally thought to be small. Potential reasons for seizure exacerbation may include poor compliance because of maternal concerns regarding teratogenicity, decreased drug levels related to nausea and vomiting in early pregnancy, physiological increase in metabolism during pregnancy, decreased free drug levels, lack of adjusting drug levels, sleep deprivation towards term and during labour, and lack of absorption of AEDs from the GI tract during labour. Several studies in the past have attempted to examine the change in seizure frequency, though no studies compared the change in seizure frequency in pregnant WWE to non-pregnant WWE [2–5]. Three studies in particular used each patient's pre-pregnancy seizure frequency as the control. Bardy et al. [2] prospectively evaluated 154 pregnancies in Finland over a 4-year period, and found that seizure frequency was unchanged in 54% (95% confidence interval (CI), 0.46–0.62), decreased in 14% (95% CI, 0.10–0.21), and increased in 32% (95% CI, 0.25–0.40) compared to pre-pregnancy seizure frequency. In a second study, 78 pregnancies in Norway were prospectively evaluated, and seizure frequency was unchanged in 72% (95% CI, 0.61–0.81)

Women with Epilepsy, ed. Esther Bui and Autumn Klein. Published by Cambridge University Press.
© Cambridge University Press 2014.

decreased in 14% (95% CI, 0.08–0.24), and increased in 14% (95% CI, 0.08–0.24) compared to pre-pregnancy baseline [3]. Finally a third study in Sweden prospectively evaluated 93 pregnancies in 70 patients over a 6-year period and found that seizure frequency as a whole was not different in pregnancy compared to baseline (p = 0.42). The percent change was reported as unchanged in 61%, decreased in 24%, and increased in 15% [4]. Combined, the studies available report that most women (54–72%) with epilepsy in pregnancy experience no significant change in seizure frequency. The rate of seizure decrease ranged from 14–24% whereas the rate of seizure increase ranged from 14–32%. Reassuringly, if women are seizure-free for at least 9–12 months prior to pregnancy, the majority of women (84–92%) will remain seizure-free during pregnancy [1]. A more recent large prospective study, again addressing the question of seizure control and treatment during pregnancy, recorded data from 1,956 pregnancies in 1,882 WWE participating in EURAP, an International Registry of Antiepileptic Drugs and Pregnancy [5]. Of all cases, 58.3% were seizure-free throughout pregnancy, similar to findings of prior studies discussed above. For those exhibiting a change in seizure frequency, 17.3% had an increase and 15.9% had a decrease. This prospective study also examined risk of seizures during delivery and found that seizures occurred in 60 pregnancies (3.5%), and was more common in those with seizures during pregnancy. There were 36 cases of status epilepticus (1.8% of pregnancies), resulting in one case of stillbirth, but no cases of miscarriage or maternal mortality. The authors concluded that pregnancy did not increase the risk of status epilepticus in WWE [5].

In summary, most WWE during pregnancy will not experience a change in seizure frequency (54–72%). For those experiencing a change in seizure frequency, the rate of seizure decrease ranged from 14–24% and that of seizure increase ranged from 14–32%. The risk of seizure during delivery remains small but significant (3.5%).

Effect of maternal epilepsy and anticonvulsant use on pregnancy

One of the foremost concerns regarding the effect of epilepsy on pregnancy is derived from the increased risk of congenital abnormalities associated with AEDs. This is discussed in Chapter 12 and will not be discussed here. Additionally, when a maternal medical disorder exists, parents become concerned regarding the chance that their offspring will develop the same problem. Epilepsy is a heterogeneous disorder resulting from multiple genetic and non-genetic factors. The maternal effect has been well described, though its mechanism is not fully understood. Mothers with epilepsy have higher rates of affected offspring (approximately 3–9%) compared to fathers with epilepsy (1–3%) [6]. The risk of epilepsy in siblings of individuals with epilepsy rises from approximately 3% to 8% if the parent is also affected [6]. If both parents have epilepsy, the risk may further increase [7].

Several other pregnancy outcomes have been investigated in WWE. This includes risk of perinatal death, in addition to other fetal morbidities such as small for gestational age infants, Apgar scores at birth, respiratory distress syndrome, and neonatal intensive care unit admission. Neonates of WWE taking AEDs are likely to be at an increased risk of being SGA. Though the definition of SGA varies widely, studies examining risk of SGA in WWE generally define this to be birth weight less than the 10th percentile for children of the same sex, born at the same gestational week. The increase in risk is approximately twice the expected rate. Three studies have examined this association [8–10]. In 2000, Hvas et al. found that pregnancies among WWE taking antiepileptic drugs had more than twice the risk of SGA (n = 87, OR 2.3, CI 1.3–4.0) [8]. Pregnant WWE not taking AEDs did not show a significantly increased risk of SGA. A second study in 2006 found similar outcomes, with OR 2.16 (CI, 1.34–3.47) for SGA in pregnant WWE taking AEDs [9]. In 2009 Veiby et al. examined pregnancy, delivery, and fetal outcome in maternal epilepsy from the Medical Birth Registry of Norway between 1999 and 2005 and found SGA infants occurred more frequently in both AED-exposed and unexposed pregnancies of WWE, with OR 1.2 (CI, 1.0–1.4) [10]. There is no substantially increased risk of perinatal death in neonates born to WWE. Hiilesmaa et al. and Richmond et al. examined the risk of perinatal death in those born to WWE and observed no increased risk (OR 0.57, CI 0.18–1.77) [11, 12]. Neonates of WWE taking AEDs possibly have an increased risk of 1-minute Apgar scores of <7, about twice the expected rate as examined by Viinikainen et al. (n = 127; OR 2.29, CI 1.29–4.05). For other perinatal outcomes such as respiratory distress, intra-uterine growth restriction, and neonatal ICU admission, insufficient data did not allow meaningful conclusions [13].

In terms of other pregnancy-related complications, a recent evidence-based review by the American Academy of Neurology examined whether WWE are at increased risk for cesarean delivery, pre-eclampsia, threatened pre-term labor or pre-term labor and delivery, bleeding complication, and spontaneous abortion [1]. Based on evidence available at the time of this review and guideline (2009), WWE are thought not to have a substantially increased risk of cesarean delivery. Evidence is insufficient to support or refute an increased risk of pre-eclampsia or pregnancy-induced hypertension in WWE taking AED amongst the studies included. There is also no strong evidence that WWE have an increased risk of pre-term labor and delivery, late pregnancy-related bleeding, or an increased risk of spontaneous abortion [1]. More recent studies have re-evaluated the risk of these pregnancy-related complications with conflicting results. Borthen et al. undertook a retro-spective hospital-based study of 205 women with a past or present history of epilepsy delivering in Norway between 1999 and 2005 and a matched control group of women without epilepsy. The findings from this study revealed that WWE using antiepileptic drugs had an increased risk of severe pre-eclampsia (OR 5.0, CI 1.3–19.9), and cesarean section (OR 2.5, CI 1.4–4.7) [14]. The group also conducted a population-based cohort study examining delivery outcome of WWE from the Medical Birth Registry of Norway and compared 2,805 pregnancies in women with a past or current history of epilepsy and to 362,302 pregnancies in women without a history of epilepsy. This study found only a slight increased risk of cesarean section (OR 1.4, CI 1.3–1.6). It is thus possible that there may be a slight increased risk of cesarean section, though the reasons for this remain unclear [15].

Antenatal management

Prior to conception, women should be counseled and educated regarding the effects of epilepsy on pregnancy and vice versa. The lowest effective dose of the most appropriate AED should be continued and ideally, monotherapy is preferred where possible. It is suggested to avoid valproate (VPA) during pregnancy if possible, since the use of VPA is associated with the highest risk for in utero exposure [11]. If the change from VPA to another AED is planned, this should be done well in advance of pregnancy where possible, to make sure the new treatment adequately prevents seizures. Canadian recommendations suggest that all women receiving AEDs should also be advised to take folic acid 5 mg daily prior to conception [13, 17]. Though no formal recommendations from the USA exist,

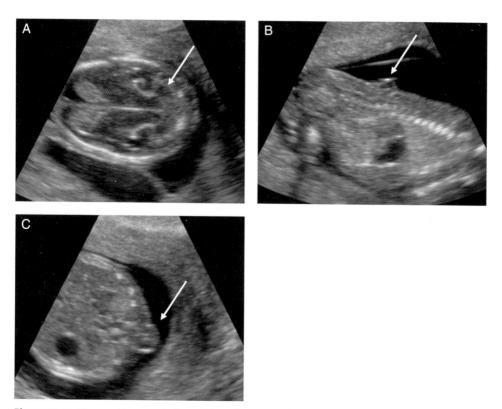

Figure 14.1: Ultrasound images of a fetus with myelomeningocele at 13 weeks gestation. (A) Deformation of the cerebellum known as banana sign (arrow). (B) and (C) Myelomeningocele at the level of the lumbar spine (arrow).

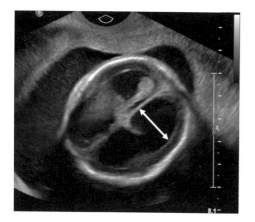

Figure 14.2: Ultrasound image of fetal head at 18 weeks showing ventriculomegaly. The lateral ventricles are dilated to 14 mm (arrow).

many epileptologists recommend a prenatal vitamin with an additional 4 mg of folic acid daily (for a total of 5 mg folic acid daily). More detailed discussion on preconception counseling and prenatal epilepsy management can be found in Chapters 11 and 12.

Non-invasive prenatal diagnosis via ultrasound and maternal serum screening for congenital abnormalities should be offered at 15–20 weeks gestation. Ultrasound imaging of the cranium (see Figure 14.1 and Figure 14.2) and identification of cranial scalloping

Table 14.1: Suggested maternal and fetal monitoring for women with epilepsy

Time period	Suggested management and monitoring
Pre-pregnancy	• Optimize AED(s) and start 5 mg folic acid daily • Preconception antiepileptic drug levels • Preconception counseling (Chapter 11)
First trimester	• Routine screening for Down syndrome
Second and third trimester	• Early anatomy scan at 14–15 weeks with special attention to neural tube defects, cardiac and facial anatomy • Maternal serum alpha-fetoprotein if not already assessed • Anatomy scan at 19–20 weeks. Monitor fetal growth every 4 weeks
Intrapartum	• Ensure proper hydration, pain control, and close monitoring for maternal seizures • Plan for normal vaginal delivery +/- epidural, with cesarean section reserved for obstetrical indications
Postpartum	• Ensure adequate pain control and adequate sleep • Postpartum antiepileptic drug levels • Postpartum safety and counseling (Chapter 19)

(lemon sign) and cerebellar crowding (banana sign) in association with mild ventriculo-megaly is diagnostic of an open myelomeningocele, even if the spinal defect is not easily identifiable due to fetal position, or maternal body habitus [17–20]. Fetal ultrasonography should also include detailed assessment of the heart (fetal echocardiogram if cardiac structures are not otherwise well visualized). Ongoing assessment for adequate fetal growth can be monitored either by the standard symphysis-fundal height measurements, or preferably by serial assessment of fetal growth via ultrasound. A list of suggested antenatal fetal testing can be found in Table 14.1.

Intrapartum and postnatal management

Labor management should be based on routine standards of obstetrical care. All health care providers should be informed of a woman's history of epilepsy. Women should continue their regular AEDs during labor. Though the risk of seizures during delivery remains small, with up to 3.5% of WWE experiencing a seizure during labor and 1–2% in the first 24 hours postpartum, women with major convulsive seizures should deliver in the hospital [21]. Several factors such as hyperventilation, sleep deprivation, pain, and emotional stress increase the chance of seizures during labour. It is thus reasonable to consider epidural analgesia at an early stage [16]. In patients with frequent seizures or who are anxious about seizures during delivery, oral clobazam (5 or 10 mg) can be useful in preventing seizures [16]. Alternatively, lorazepam 1–2 mg may be used as well. Generalized tonic-clonic seizures are likely to result in hypoxia, and this may have deleterious effects on the fetus [16, 22]. Delivery should take place in an obstetric unit where resources for, and expertise in, maternal and fetal resuscitation are readily available. Cesarean section should be reserved for the usual obstetrical indications, or if there are recurrent uncontrolled generalized seizures in late pregnancy or labor.

All neonates should receive vitamin K intramuscularly at birth. Recommendations by the American Academy of Neurology regarding vitamin K supplementation in women taking antiepileptic drugs in pregnancy were updated in 2009 [23–24]. Harden et al. evaluated evidence from relevant articles published between 1985 and 2007 [24]. According to these guidelines, there is inadequate evidence to determine if newborns of WWE taking AEDs have a substantially increased risk of hemorrhagic complications. Additionally, there is no convincing evidence that oral prenatal vitamin K supplementation in WWE diminishes neonatal bleeding complications. Thus, although some have recommended maternal oral vitamin K supplementation in the latter part of pregnancy, there is no good evidence to support its use. Vitamin K is routinely given to all neonates as an intramuscular injection.

References

1. Harden CL, Hopp J, Ting TY, et al. Management issues for women with epilepsy – focus on pregnancy (an evidence-based review): obstetrical complications and change in seizure frequency. *Epilepsia* 2009; 50(5): 1229–362.

2. Bardy AH. Incidence of seizures during pregnancy, labour and puerperium in epileptic women: a prospective study. *Acta Neurol Scand* 1987; 75:356–60.

3. Gjerde IO, Strandjord RE and Ulstein M. The course of epilepsy during pregnancy: a study of 78 cases. *Acta Neurol Scand* 1988; 78:198–205.

4. Tomson T, Lindbom U, Ekqvist B, et al. Epilepsy and pregnancy: a prospective study of seizure control in relation to free and total plasma concentration of carbmazepine and phenytoin. *Epilepsia* 1994; 35:122–30.

5. EURAP Study Group. Seizure control and treatment in pregnancy: observations from the EURAP epilepsy pregnancy registry. *Neurology* 2006; 66:354–60.

6. Winawer MR and Shinnar S. Genetic epidemiology of epilepsy or what do we tell families. *Epilepsia* 2005; 46(Suppl 10): 24–30.

7. Nelson-Piercy C. Epilepsy. In: *Handbook of Obstetric Medicine*, 4th edn. London: Informa UK Limited, 2010: 153–4.

8. Hvas CL, Henriksen TB, Ostergaard JR, et al. Epilepsy and pregnancy: effects of antiepileptic drug use and lifestyle on birthweight. *Br J Obstet Gynaecol* 2000; 107:896–902.

9. Viinikainen K, Heinonen S, Eriksson K, et al. Community-based prospective controlled study of obstetrical and neonatal oucome of 179 pregnancies in women with epilepsy. *Epilepsia* 2006; 47(1): 186–92.

10. Veiby G, Daltveit AK, Engelsen BA, et al. Pregnancy, delivery and outcome for the child in maternal epilepsy. *Epilepsia* 2009; 50(9):2130–39.

11. Hiilesmaa VK, Bardy AH and Teramo K. Obstetric outcome in women with epilepsy. *Am J Obstet Gynecol* 1985; 152(5): 499–504.

12. Richmond JR, Krishnamoorthy PK, Andermann E, et al. Epilepsy and pregnancy: an obstetric perspective. *Am J Obstet Gynecol* 2004; 190:371–9.

13. Harden CL, Meador KJ, Pennell PB, et al. Management issues for women with epilepsy – focus on pregnancy (an evidence-based review): II. Teratogenesis and perinatal outcomes. *Epilepsia* 2009; 50(5):1237–46.

14. Borthen I, Eide MG, Daltveit AK, et al. Obstetric outcome in women with epilepsy: a hospital-based retrospective study. *BJOG* 2011; 118:956–65.

15. Borthen I, Eide MG, Daltveit AK, et al. Delivery outcome of women with epilepsy: population-based cohort study. *BJOG* 2010; 117:1537–43.

16. Crawford PM. Managing epilepsy in women of childbearing age. *Drug Saf* 2009; 32(4):293–307.

17. Wilson RD. The use of folic acid for the prevention of neural tube defects and other congenital anomalies. *J Obstet Gynaecol Can* 2003; 25(11):959–65.

18. Chodirker BN, Cadrin C, Davies GAL, et al. Canadian guidelines for prenatal diagnosis. Techniques of prenatal diagnosis. SOGC Clinical Practice Guidelines, No.105, July 2001. *J Obstet Gynaecol Can* 2001; 23 (7):616–24.

19. Monteagudo A and Timor-Tritsch IE. Fetal face and central nervous system. In: Jaffe R, Bue TH, eds. *Textbook of fetal ultrasound*. New York, NY: Parthenon, 1999; 109–11.

20. Pilu G and Hobbins JC. Sonography of fetal cerebrospinal anomalies. *Prenat Diagn* 2002; 22:321–30.

21. Sabers A. Complications during pregnancy and delivery. In: Tomson T, Gram L, Sillanpaa M, et al., eds. *Epilepsy and pregnancy*. Chichester: Wrightson Biomedical Publishing Ltd, 1997; 105–11.

22. Teramo K, Hiilesmaa V, Bardy A, et al. Heart rate during a maternal grand mal epileptic seizure. *J Perinat Med* 1979; 7 (1):3–6.

23. Kazmin A, Wong RC, Sermer M, et al. AED in pregnancy and hemorrhagic disease of the newborn: an update. *Can Fam Physician* 2010; 56:1291–2.

24. Harden CL, Pennell PB, Koppel BS, et al. Practice parameter update: management issues for women with epilepsy-focus on pregnancy (an evidence based review): vitamin K, folic acid, blood levels, and breastfeeding: Report of the Quality Standards Subcommittee and Therapeutics and Technology Assessment Subcommittee of the American Academy of Neurology and American Epilepsy Society. *Neurology* 2009; 73(2):142–9.

Pregnancy and epilepsy: neuroimaging

Kalliopi A. Petropoulou

Key points:

- Multidisciplinary decision in triaging imaging modality is recommended, as protocols can be optimized or deferred to minimize potential harm to fetus
- Computed tomography (CT) of the head does expose the fetus to scattered radiation, though radiation dose is relatively low
- Iodinated contrast for CT may be associated with neonatal hypothyroidism; rated a class B category drug
- Gadolinium contrast for MR has associated fetal developmental anomalies in animal studies; rated as a class C category drug
- Imaging helps differentiate causes of seizures in pregnancy including eclampsia, cerebral venous thrombosis, postpartum angiopathy, and tumors

Pregnant women who present with seizure may or may not have a prior history of seizure or epilepsy. The imaging approach would vary depending on the medical history and presentation. The imaging protocols should be tailored to address the clinical question and for that, adequate and accurate history should be provided. For example, a pregnant woman with eclampsia should be approached from an imaging standpoint differently from a patient with known epilepsy prior to her pregnancy. The main focus of this chapter is discussion of pregnancy-related conditions, which are associated with epilepsy and seizure among other neurologic symptoms, along with their appropriate imaging.

Neuroimaging in pregnancy

Computed tomography (CT) and magnetic resonance imaging (MRI) are the two main modalities available for evaluation of the brain. Patients with epilepsy are evaluated almost exclusively with MRI. However CT may be the only modality available in a case of acute onset of seizure or when the patient's condition does not allow the lengthy imaging often required for MRI.

CT can accurately show acute intracranial hemorrhage, brain edema, mass effect, hydrocephalus and many times, dural sinus thrombosis. Modern scanners allow the completion of imaging within seconds, which may be quite desirable for a patient with altered level of consciousness and otherwise limited available history. The multiplanar capability and superior soft tissue resolution renders MRI as the modality of choice for evaluation of the brain parenchyma.

Women with Epilepsy, ed. Esther Bui and Autumn Klein. Published by Cambridge University Press.
© Cambridge University Press 2014.

Pregnancy represents a challenge when it comes to choosing the appropriate imaging modality since potential risks to the fetus have to be taken into consideration. Pregnancy as well as breastfeeding may raise questions as to the appropriateness of the intravenous, iodinated or gadolinium-based, contrast administration. It is imperative that existing guidelines are followed any time a pregnant woman undergoes either CT or MR imaging.

Safety considerations for the unborn child
CT imaging and radiation exposure

It has long been recognized that ionizing radiation can induce detrimental biological effects in organs and tissues by producing free radicals and damaging important molecules such as DNA. The amount of biological damage depends on the total energy deposited (dose) and the type of radiation. X-rays produce less biological damage than alpha particles for the same amount of energy (dose) deposited in the tissue. Data on the detrimental effects of radiation comes from studies on atomic bomb survivors, radiation workers, and radiation therapy. The effects are categorized as deterministic and stochastic (random).

Determinist effects occur at high doses of radiation (dose >0.5Gy), generally result in cell death, and are characterized by a threshold dose. Typical manifestations include skin erythema, cataract, hair loss, and induction of sterility. Exposure of the fetus to radiation dose >0.5Gy may result in malformations, growth or mental retardation.

Stochastic effects occur at low doses (doses <0.5Gy) of radiation, reflect damage to one cell, and may result in carcinogenesis and genetic damage. The severity of the radiation-induced stochastic effects is independent of the radiation dose and there is no associated dose threshold. The radiation dose only affects the probability of the stochastic effects. The important goal of radiation protection is to prevent the occurrence of deterministic effects and minimize the radiation dose, and thus the potentially associated stochastic effects.

The International Commission on Radiological Protection in its 2007 recommendations stated that no deterministic effects of practical significance are likely to occur on the fetus or embryo when exposed to a cumulative dose below 100mGy [1]. In contrast there is no dose threshold for stochastic effects of radiation exposure. Stochastic effects reflect damage to one cell, which can lead to carcinogenesis. Exposure of the fetus to radiation up to 1mGy is acceptable given the very low likelihood for carcinogenesis (less than 1/10,000).

CT studies above the diaphragm and below the knee fall into this category. In addition, during the head CT study, the fetus is exposed mainly to attenuated scattered rather than direct radiation exposure. The estimated fetal exposure from a head CT is 1.0–10mGy [1, 2]. Although the use of lead on the pregnant woman's abdomen does not protect from the scattered radiation, most radiology departments recommend its use. In the case of unintended exposure to radiation solely for imaging purposes, the American College of Obstetricians and Gynecologists has stated that abortion is not recommended [3].

Iodinated contrast medium and the effect on the fetus and newborn

Iodinated contrast agents can cross the placenta. They have not been proven to have either mutagenic or teratogenic effect in animal studies and are rated as class B category drugs by the FDA. However, there is the potential of a deleterious effect on the development and function of the fetal thyroid gland resulting in neonatal hypothyroidism. Untreated neonatal hypothyroidism impacts the development, especially the mental development, of the fetus [1]. It is standard pediatric practice to screen newborns for hypothyroidism during the first week of life in cases of iodinated contrast medium administration during pregnancy. In general, administration of iodinated contrast medium during pregnancy should be avoided. If no alternative test is available and the contrast-enhanced CT is absolutely necessary for the diagnosis of the pregnant woman's condition, it could be administered after the risks and benefits have been explained to the patient and written informed consent has been obtained. The risk of neonatal hypothyroidism is practically negligible, especially in the past 30 years when water-soluble iodinated contrast agents are in use instead of lipid-soluble ones used in the past [1].

Iodinated contrast media are excreted into the breast milk however, as high molecular weight, non-ionized, and water-soluble drugs have little affinity in binding to milk. Their use in breastfeeding women is considered safe, with exception placed on women nursing pre-term infants, as their immature auto regulatory thyroid axis puts them at increased risk for transient hypothyroidism. Nursing mothers should be informed, and if concerned, may be instructed to discard milk for 24 hours. The administration of contrast agents takes into consideration the mother's safety as well. In our institution, the renal function is checked routinely prior to administration of contrast agents.

MR imaging and high magnetic field exposure

When a pregnant woman undergoes MR imaging, the fetus is exposed too strong magnetic field (10,000 times higher than the Earth), energy deposition that has the potential of minimal increase in body temperature, and high acoustic noise level. Although there has been no documented harm to the fetus so far [4, 5] and the use of MR imaging is considered safe, caution in the use of this imaging modality during pregnancy has been suggested. The American College of Radiology has eliminated restrictions related to gestational age in the 2007 update and suggested that the benefits for the mother and fetus must always outweigh the risks and, if necessary, to defer MR imaging until after the delivery [3].

Gadolinium-based contrast medium and the effect on the fetus and newborn

So far there have been no controlled studies in pregnant women regarding the adverse effects of gadolinium-based contrast on the human fetus. Animal studies use higher doses of gadolinium than usually used in imaging of humans, but they have shown that it may result in aborted fetuses or cause developmental anomalies. The gadolinium-based contrast agents are rated as class C drugs by the FDA, based on the fact that animal studies have shown adverse effects on the fetus at much higher doses than routinely administered and no controlled studies on women exist. According to the current American College of Radiology recommendation (2010), such agents should be used with extreme caution and only if the administration is essential in making the diagnosis [1]. In general, gadolinium-based contrast agents should be avoided during pregnancy. As with the iodine contrast medium, informed written consent should be obtained prior to using a gadolinium-based medium [4], if the use is deemed absolutely necessary and the benefits to the mother and fetus outweigh the risks.

Gadolinium-based contrast agents are excreted into the breast milk. They share similar properties with iodinated contrast media, resulting in minimal binding to milk and plasma proteins and thus minimal delivery to the infant. It is considered safe to continue breast-feeding following gadolinium administration. Again, if the nursing mother is concerned, she may be instructed to discard breast milk for 24 hours, which is the necessary time for the contrast agent to be cleared from the blood stream. All radiology departments have policies in place as how to appropriately image pregnant and nursing women and minimize the exposure to the fetus of any risk related to modality or contrast medium.

Epilepsy in pregnancy-related conditions: neuroimaging

Comorbid conditions in pregnancy, such as the ones discussed below, may affect women otherwise healthy as well as women with epilepsy.

Pre-eclampsia and eclampsia

Pre-eclampsia and eclampsia are the most severe stages of a complex, multisystem disorder that occurs in later stages of the pregnancy as well as in the first 6–8 weeks postpartum. Pre-eclampsia, which occurs in 2–8% of all pregnancies, is a disorder characterized by the onset of hypertension, peripheral edema, and proteinuria in pregnant women after the 20th week of gestation. Patients with pre-eclampsia may also experience headache, visual changes, confusion, and altered mentation. Eclampsia refers to complications of seizures or coma, unrelated to other causes superimposed on the pre-eclamptic status. In reality, women with eclampsia may have variable, if present, hypertension and proteinuria, and thus eclampsia may not represent just the next step of pre-eclamptic status [6, 7]. Delayed eclampsia, following delivery, may not be associated with hypertension or proteinuria [8].

Pre-eclampsia/eclampsia also known as toxemia of pregnancy is associated with Posterior Reversible Encephalopathy Syndrome (PRES) [9]. This is a distinct syndrome referring to specific imaging findings in the brain seen in a variety of toxicity settings, not just eclampsia. The pathophysiology is complex and remains unclear in many aspects. However, several observations have been established and are shared among the several toxicity settings (eclampsia, severe hypertension, transplantation, infection/sepsis, auto-immune disease, chemotherapy, and cancer). The explanations for brain edema, the hallmark finding in PRES, vary [10]. They are focused on the disruption of the blood-brain barrier and include the hypothesis of hypertension with failed auto regulation and hyperperfusion [6], with an alternative hypothesis of vascular endothelial damage, hypoperfusion, and vasoconstriction [11, 12]. Regardless, endothelial cell damage and abnormal activation have been proven and are accepted as on inciting factor in the development of eclampsia [13, 14]. T-cell activation and cytokine production (TNF-α, IL-1, INF, IL-6), and systemically increased VEGF levels are common findings and contribute to development of brain edema [6, 8, 12, 15]. The diffuse endothelial activation also affects the platelet function resulting in platelet adhesion, degranulation, hemolysis, protein/fluid leak, and edema. Magnesium, protein, and fluid loss are also encountered as result of glomerular endothelial malfunction [9]. Decreased levels of magnesium have been found in patients with abnormal brain MR findings [12]. Endothelial cell activation and associated "leakiness," along with vasoconstriction and hypertension are believed to affect the utero-placental unit, which becomes dysfunctional.

Neuroimaging can accurately contribute to the diagnosis of PRES. CT imaging performed in an emergency situation may exclude other etiologies for acute onset of seizures, such as an intracranial hemorrhage, but may also reveal hypodense areas in the parieto-occipital regions which are considered manifestations of eclampsia [16]. The imaging modality of choice is MR, which can be diagnostic for eclampsia and also rule out other potential causes. The pertinent findings on MR imaging are patchy areas of T2 hyperintensity involving the parietal occipital regions and distributed along the posterior as well as anterior watershed zones [17]. Other areas of the brain, such as cerebellum,

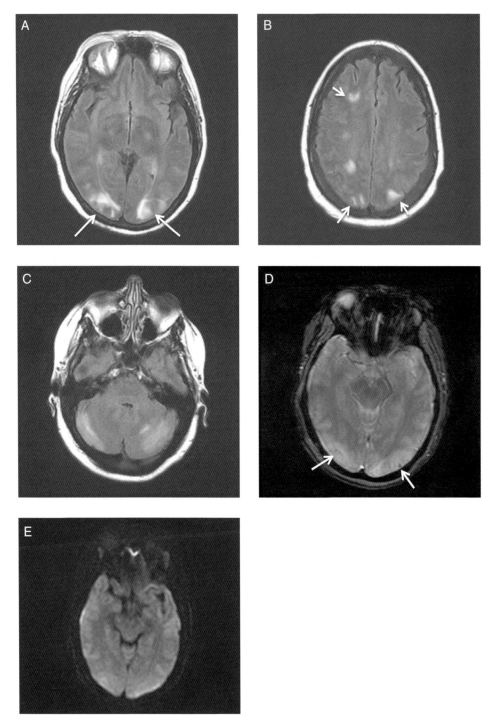

Figure 15.1: 34-year-old female with eclampsia and seizure. Axial FLAIR sequences demonstrate vasogenic edema in the occipital lobes (Figure A arrows), along the watershed zones in the frontoparietal vertex (Figure B arrows), as well as in the cerebellum (Figure C). Punctate areas of susceptibility artifact suggestive of micro hemorrhage are shown on GRE sequence (Figure D arrows). DWI showed no evidence of restricted diffusion (Figure E).

brainstem, and thalami, may also be involved [18]. The lesions are located at the subcortical white matter with some involvement of the overlying cortex (Figure 15.1). Occasionally they may be associated with micro hemorrhages [19].

The type and etiology of the brain edema in eclampsia has been extensively discussed in the literature. MR imaging findings and laboratory data suggest vasogenic-type edema [6, 8, 10, 20, 21] corresponding to the subcortical white matter signal abnormality on MR. Rarely, focal, cortical-based DWI abnormalities, surrounded by vasogenic subcortical white matter edema, and associated with either restricted diffusion or pseudo normalization of DWI, have been observed. Both findings are indicative of a severe form of PRES, with worst outcome linked to the presence of true restricted diffusion, indicative of acute infarct [18, 19, 20]. Therefore DWI contributes in the diagnosis and assessment of severity of PRES in addition to its well-known specificity in the diagnosis of territorial stroke. The PRES findings are often distributed along the watershed zones or in a random fashion, but do not follow the vascular territory distribution which is the typical presentation of the arterial ischemic stroke. MR of the brain obtained soon after seizure activity may demonstrate cortical swelling and T2-signal hyperintensity, perceived as edema along the involved cortex due to seizure activity. The finding is transient without any residual abnormality. The lesions in eclampsia rarely show any enhancement; therefore unenhanced MR imaging, which is generally all that can be used during pregnancy, suffices. The suggested MR protocol should include T1-weighted (T1W), fluid attenuated inversion recovery (FLAIR), fast spin echo T2-weighted (FSET2), diffusion-weighted imaging (DWI) and gradient echo (GRE) sequences, in order to delineate even the most subtle of the findings (FLAIR, FSET2) and assess for micro hemorrhages (T1W, GRE) [22, 23]. The use of DWI is recommended to exclude true ischemic event in more complicated situations (Figure 15.1, E). Catheter angiography as well as MR angiography have shown reversible findings in PRES, such as focal stenosis or diffuse lumen irregularity, pruning, or even a beaded appearance of intracranial vessels. Of course catheter angiography involves radiation exposure as well iodine contrast administration, which is not exactly advisable in pregnancy, but can be performed postpartum. MR angiography can be performed without gadolinium-based contrast medium and therefore can be part of the protocol. The appearance of PRES on routine unenhanced MR sequences is almost pathognomonic; therefore the MR angiography would be useful in exclusion of other entities rather than contributory to the diagnosis of PRES in a pregnant patient.

Thrombotic thrombocytopenic purpura (TTP), which also occurs in pregnancy, shares similar MR imaging findings with pre-eclampsia/eclampsia. Follow-up studies usually show resolution of the abnormalities when patients improve clinically, although TTP may be complicated with infarction or intracerebral hemorrhage. HELLP syndrome (Hemolysis, Elevated Liver Enzymes, Low Platelets) is another hypertensive disorder of pregnancy sharing much of the pathophysiology with pre-eclampsia/eclampsia [10, 24, 25].

Cerebral venus thrombosis

The association of pregnancy and the puerperium with cerebral venous thrombosis is well known, with the majority of the cases occurring during peripartum or postpartum [26, 27]. The estimated risk of cerebral venous thrombosis is 11.6 cases per 100,000 deliveries [28]. Risk factors include hypertension, cesarean delivery, infections, pre-eclampsia/eclampsia [28], and anemia [27]. Clinical symptoms vary and include headache, seizures, papilledema, focal neurologic deficits, and even coma [29].

The thrombosed venous structures on non-contrast-enhanced CT imaging appear hyperdense. Along the superior sagittal sinus, the clot has the shape of the Greek letter delta, the popularized "delta sign." The contrast-enhanced CT shows enhancement around the relatively hypodense clot (empty delta sign) [16]. MR is the preferred imaging modality when it comes to assessment of the intracranial venous structures. In addition to the multiplanar capability and higher soft tissue resolution, there is better delineation of the dural sinuses and deep central veins. Most importantly, there is no exposure to radiation when the patient is pregnant and, in most cases, there is no absolute need for administration of gadolinium-based contrast medium in order to confidently reach the diagnosis. Routine MR imaging of the brain provides clues regarding the patency of major intracranial vessels and dedicated MR venogram (MRV) confirms patency or not (Figure 15.2, A, B). Thrombosed vessels on routine imaging show lack of signal void, a finding quite reliable on sequences such as PD (Proton Density) and FLAIR (Figure 15.3, A, B), and a variable degree of hyperintensity on T1W sequences (Figure 15.2, A). The affected vessels show no detectable flow on MRV (Figure 15.2, B). Pitfalls on MR imaging do exist. Clots exhibiting very low signal on FSET2W sequences should not be misinterpreted as flow void. Developmentally small dural sinuses may appear as occluded, especially on maximum projection images (Figure 15.4). Partially thrombosed dural sinus may appear as completely occluded, since MR angiographic techniques overestimate vascular lumen stenosis [30]. Careful analysis, however, of routine brain imaging in conjunction with MRV findings allows accurate diagnosis on most occasions. Diagnosis, however, of cavernous sinus thrombosis, often a sign of ongoing infection, requires intravenous contrast administration [22]. CT venogram (CTV) is not subject to the MRV limitations, but the application includes radiation exposure as well as exposure to iodinated contrast agent. It is an excellent choice as a follow-up study after the delivery.

Although cerebral venous thrombosis in puerperium has a more benign course than in other patient categories [27], complications may occur and are evident on MR imaging. Ischemic infarcts, especially in non-arterial territory distribution as well as intraparenchymal hemorrhages, may occur (Figure 15.2, C, D, E, F). Alternatively, these findings may serve as clues to the interpreting radiologist to look for signs of intracranial venous thrombosis or recommend further imaging. The value of DWI in the diagnosis of ischemic stroke is well established. Venous stroke, however, is associated with more variable patterns of DWI and ADC [31]. Three types of lesions have been described [32]: (a) lesions with elevated diffusion suggestive of vasogenic edema, which resolved; (b) lesions with low diffusion suggestive of cytotoxic edema found in patients without seizure activity, that persisted; and (c) lesions with low diffusion seen in patients with seizure, that also resolved [27]. Reversibility of brain abnormalities in a setting of cerebral venous thrombosis has been documented [28, 33]. Following treatment, MR imaging can be used to assess the brain and recanalize large venous structures such as dural sinuses.

Catheter angiography dynamically assesses the central venous system; however, it is not the first choice of imaging, because of increased risks as an interventional procedure and the exposure to radiation in the case of pregnancy.

Postpartum cerebral angiopathy

Postpartum cerebral angiography is an idiopathic form of the reversible cerebral segmental vasoconstriction syndrome first described in 1988 [34, 35]. It can afflict postpartum women within 1–4 weeks following delivery and is characterized by thunderclap headache, seizure,

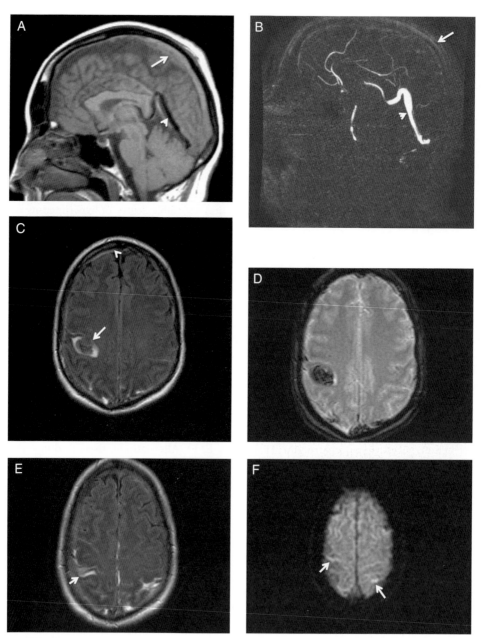

Figure 15.2: 28-year-old female with superior sagittal sinus thrombosis complicated with hemorrhage in the right posterior frontal lobe. Sagittal T1W image shows lack of flow void along the SSS (Figure A arrows), while the straight sinus remains patent (Figure A short arrow). Corresponding sagittal MIP image of the MRV shows no flow-related enhancement along the SSS (Figure B arrow), but is present along the straight sinus (Figure B short arrow). Parenchymal hemorrhage is noted in the right posterior frontal lobe on FLAIR (Figure C arrow) and GRE (Figure D) sequences. In addition, a thin subdural hematoma is noted (Figure C arrowhead). Further axial FLAIR sequences show cortical edema in the frontoparietal vertex (Figure E arrows). Subtle abnormalities in the same areas on the DWI are suggestive of infarct due to cortical vein thrombosis (Figure F arrows).

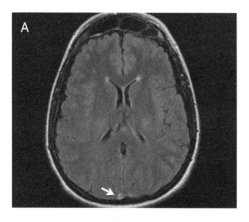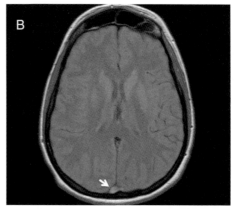

Figure 15.3: Uncomplicated superior sagittal sinus thrombosis. The presence of clot in the SSS is evident on axial FLAIR (Figure A arrow) as well as axial PD (Figure B arrow). This patient's examination did not include MRV; however the original diagnosis was made based on the routine MR imaging findings. Sagittal T1W sequences (not shown) also demonstrated lack of flow void.

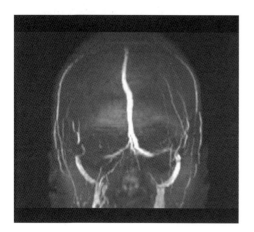

Figure 15.4: MIP images of MR venogram show narrowing of the transverse sinuses which was not confirmed on the source images. It is a pitfall that can be addressed by carefully evaluating the source images and not to rely on the MIP images only.

focal neurologic deficits, and segmental narrowing and dilatation of large and medium-sized cerebral arteries, which is very similar to angiographic findings seen with eclampsia [36]. MR imaging of the brain reveals T2 hyperintensities in the white as well as gray matter, often along watershed zones [2] (Figure 15.5, A, B, C). Complication with intracerebral hemorrhages can occur [37, 38]. Tests for cerebral vasculitis are negative; however, MR angiography, CT angiography, or catheter angiography demonstrate areas of stenosis or dilatation in intracranial arteries, which eventually resolve [29, 31] (Figure 15.5, D, E). Both CT and catheter angiography require intravenous administration of iodine contrast.

Brain tumors
Meningioma and choriocarcinoma are tumors that are either influenced or directly related to the pregnancy.

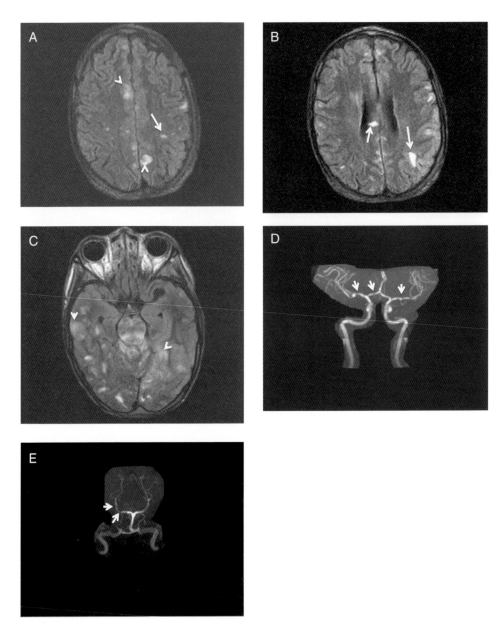

Figure 15.5: 28-year-old female presented with severe headache and seizure 2 weeks following delivery. Axial FLAIR multiple abnormalities involving white matter (Figure A, B arrows) as well as gray matter (Figure A, C arrowheads). Midbrain is also involved (Figure C). MR angiography shows multiple areas of focal constriction in the anterior (Figure D arrows) as well as posterior circulation (Figure E arrows).

Meningioma

The presence of hormonal receptors found in some meningiomas may promote their growth during pregnancy [39]. Depending on their location they may present with seizure, along with other symptoms. Meningiomas may calcify, which makes them more easily recognizable on non-contrast-enhanced CT, more often though they are isodense to the brain parenchyma. MRI is far more sensitive in detecting meningiomas, especially in a situation like pregnancy when intravenous contrast medium is not advocated. They share the same MR characteristics with meningiomas found in non-pregnant patients. They are isointense to gray matter on T1W and moderately hyperintense on T2W sequences, may show restricted diffusion, and enhance avidly.

Metastatic choriocarcinoma

Choriocarcinoma is a malignant trophoblastic tumor, specifically associated with pregnancy—normal, molar, or ectopic pregnancy—metastasizes to the brain in 10% of cases [20, 29]. As any other metastasis, choriocarcinoma may manifest itself with seizure, and as a highly vascular tumor, may bleed; this lends the variable signal characteristics of the brain metastasis on MR imaging. The variability of signal characteristics depends on the age of hemorrhage. The mass enhances and is usually surrounded by extensive vasogenic edema. The MR imaging should include GRE or other sequences sensitive to susceptibility artifact generated by blood byproducts [2] (Figure 15.6, A, B, C).

Other primary brain tumors

Glioblastoma multiforme may be diagnosed prior to, or during, pregnancy. Recent data also suggests that the glioblastoma multiforme can double in growth in pregnancy [45]. Management and treatment of the pregnant woman can represent a challenge, since treatment of the tumor includes radiation and chemotherapy.

Epilepsy in non pregnancy-related conditions: neuroimaging

Pregnant women may present with epilepsy for reasons unrelated to pregnancy [40]. It is likely that neuroimaging workup of a known epileptic woman has been completed prior to commencement of the pregnancy and appropriate consultation has taken place. However, even patients with congenital brain anomalies known to represent a substrate for epilepsy may experience first time seizures later in life. Detailed analysis of these conditions is beyond this chapter's scope; however, it is important for the neuroradiologist to approach the interpretation of neuroimaging studies from a broader perspective and recognize the imaging findings. Other conditions which evolve over time, such as cavernous hemangiomas are known to be associated with seizures which present any time during the course of life [41, 42].

Pregnant women may also be subject to central nervous system infection. Listeria meningitis, epidural abscesses, or brain infections with space occupying lesions, such as neurocysticercosis, may present with seizures [43, 46]. Imaging will be challenging, since contrast-enhanced MR may be necessary to fully disclose the extension of the disease.

Pregnancy sets certain limitations when it comes to imaging. Developmental anomalies in general can be worked up satisfactorily without intravenous contrast administration. Optimization of the protocol with the inclusion of high-resolution 3D images (SPGR, MPRAGE, etc.) is all that is needed for accurate diagnosis without exposing the pregnant woman and unborn child to any contrast medium [44]. Diagnosis of vascular malformations and tumors, however, usually require the administration of intravenous contrast

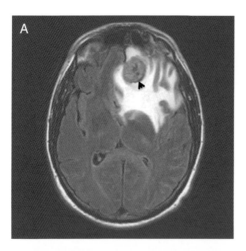
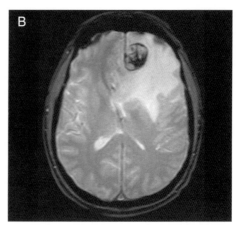
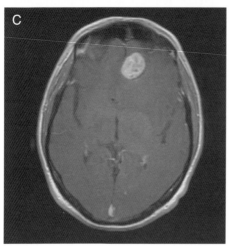

Figure 15.6: Metastatic choriocarcinoma. Axial FLAIR sequences demonstrates a mass in the left frontal lobe surrounded by extensive vasogenic edema (Figure A). There is hemorrhage in the mass as clearly shown on axial GRE sequence (Figure B). Just a subtle rim of hemosiderin can be seen on the FLAIR image (Figure A arrow). The mass enhances avidly on the axial post-contrast T1W sequence (Figure C).

medium, either iodinated, e.g., catheter angiography, or gadolinium-based contrast for MR imaging. Postponement of imaging after pregnancy may be entertained, especially if the treatment is postponed as well. The final, often multidisciplinary, decision as how to handle these pregnant women will be based on the principle that benefits should outweigh potential risks.

Neuroimaging of pregnant women: protocol suggestions

The above review of the imaging findings of the most frequent medical conditions related to pregnancy which present with epilepsy, in conjunction with the existing safety recommendations, set the framework for the imaging protocols. Every radiology department is required to establish policies on how to handle pregnant or nursing women in terms of safety. Pregnant or nursing women should be informed of potential consequences and be allowed to make the final decision. Written informed consent should be obtained.

Non-contrast-enhanced CT of the brain is accessible and accurately depicts acute intracranial hemorrhage, which may accompany many of the discussed conditions. Although often less available, MR imaging is the preferred imaging modality when it comes to evaluation of neurological conditions. Pregnant women can be imaged on 1.5T magnets, which are widely available.

The exact MRI sequences to be utilized will depend on the available software, which may differ from one MRI platform to another. However, the absolutely necessary T1W, FSET2W, FLAIR, GRE, DWI sequences are widely available. The addition of GRE or any other (e.g., SWAN) sequence sensitive to blood by products provides important information regarding the hemorrhagic nature of a lesion. DWI is important in detecting acute stroke that may complicate many of the pregnancy-related conditions presenting with seizures or epilepsy. Given the overlapping clinical and imaging findings of the main pregnancy-related conditions with seizure, the addition of MR venography may provide important information and thus be part of the routine protocol.

Contrast media, whether iodinated or gadolinium-based, should be avoided during pregnancy. The administration may be considered only if the use is absolutely necessary to reach a diagnosis which would be beneficial to the pregnant woman as well as the unborn child. The American College of Radiology (ACR), in the updated Manual on Contrast Media in 2010, stated that existing data suggest that it is safe for both mother and infant to continue breastfeeding after contrast agent administration. That includes both iodinated and gadolinium-based contrast.

The instructions for pregnant women and lactating mothers undergoing MR imaging and potentially receiving contrast medium, as well as the consent form for MR imaging of pregnant women, which are in place in our institution, are summarized in Tables 15.2 and 15.3, respectively.

Table 15.1: Recommendations on using head magnetic resonance imaging and computed tomography in pregnant patients

1. Discuss and document indications, risks and benefits, and alternatives with patient.
2. Involve and inform the radiologists and obstetrician when deciding on CT and MRI in the pregnant patient. Some CT and MRI examinations can be modified to provide diagnostically critical information while exposing the embryo or fetus to as little risk as possible.
3. MRI is thought to be preferable to CT, although conclusive data to this effect is not available.
4. During head CT examination of the mother, the fetus is exposed only to radiation that is scattered through the body; therefore, shielding of the abdomen does not significantly reduce the minimal fetal radiation dose, but may help to alleviate maternal anxiety.
5. Delay elective MRI until after pregnancy.
6. Avoid MRI in the first trimester unless no alternative exists.
7. Iodinated contrast is rated by the FDA as a category B drug.
8. Avoid gadolinium in pregnancy unless no alternative exists—gadolinium is rated by the FDA as a category C drug.

FDA, U.S. Food and Drug Administration

Table 15.2: Instructions for lactating mothers and pregnant women receiving contrast

POLICY
It is the policy of the Imaging Services, Department of Radiology to provide instructions to lactating mothers who receive contrast agents during radiology examinations.

PROCEDURE
The use of iodinated or gadolinium-based contrast media in pregnant or lactating women often raises concerns owing to the desire to avoid exposure to drugs in the fetus or neonate. The following policy and procedure is based on a review of the literature and recommendations by the Contrast Media Safety Committee of the European Society of Urogenital Radiology. As always, the risk and potential benefits of the imaging procedures must be considered.

Pregnant women:
1) Free iodine in radiographic contrast medium given to the mother has the potential to depress fetal/neonatal thyroid function.
   - Recommendation: Check neonatal thyroid function within the 1st week of life if iodinated contrast medium was given to the mother during pregnancy. (Standard practice for most neonates).
2) Gadolinium:
   - No teratogenic or other effects on the fetus or neonate have been detected. Nevertheless, pregnancy is considered a relative contraindication to the use of gadolinium-based MRI contrast agents.

Lactating mother:
Iodinated contrast medium & gadolinium-based contrast medium:
   - Only tiny amounts of contrast medium given to the mother reach breast milk, and only a minute proportion is absorbed through the baby's intestine.
   - Recommendation: There is no scientific basis for stopping breastfeeding for a lactating mother who has received iodinated or gadolinium-based contrast medium.

Table 15.3: Consent for magnetic resonance imaging during pregnancy

Patient name:	Date:

Magnetic Resonance Imaging, (MRI), is an imaging method that uses magnetic fields to create images of human anatomy and pathology. Because of the strength of the magnetic field used in the study, you will be screened prior to your exam. All metalic items must be removed before you may enter the MRI scan room.

There are no known serious risks to a properly performed MRI procedure. Although there are no known safety issues related to MRI and pregnancy, the safety of this examination for the pregnant patient and her unborn fetus may not be completely known. Your doctor has recommended that this exam is necessary for you. There may be other types of tests that may help diagnose your condition, but a review of your case has determined that your undergoing an MRI examination is indicated and would be among the least risky of all available diagnostic options.

By signing below you are attesting to your having the opportunity to ask any questions you may have had.

I request that the Radiologists, Technologists, and others proceed with performing and acquiring this examination on you.

Patient's signature:

M.D. signature:

Witness:

References

1. Tremblay E, Therasse E, Thomassin-Naggara I, et al. Quality initiatives: guidelines for use of medical imaging during pregnancy and lactation. *Radiographics* 2012; 32(3):897–911.

2. Klein JP and Hsu L. Neuroimaging during pregnancy. *Semin Neurol* 2011; 31(4):361–73.

3. ACOG Committee on Obstetric Practice. Opinion No. 299. *Obstet Gynecol* 2004; 104(3):1–5.

4. Kanal E, Barkovich AJ, Bell C, et al. ACR guidance document for safe MR practices: 2007. *AJR Am J Roentgenol* 2007; 188(6):1447–74.

5. De Wilde JP, Rivers AW and Price DL. A review of the current use of magnetic resonance imaging in pregnancy and safety implications for the fetus. *Prog Biophys Mol Biol* 2005; 87(2–3):335–53.

6. Cipolla MJ and Kraig RP. Seizures in women with pre-eclampsia: mechanisms and management. *Fetal Matern Med Rev* 2011; 22(2):91–108.

7. Ay H, Buonanno FS, Schaefer PW, et al. Posterior leukoencephalopathy without severe hypertension: utility of diffusion-weighted MRI. *Neurology* 1998; 51(5):1369–76.

8. Bartynski WS and Sanghvi A. Neuroimaging of delayed eclampsia. Report of 3 cases and review of the literature. *J Comput Assist Tomogr* 2003; 27(5):699–713.

9. van Loenen NT, Hintzen RQ and de Groot CJ. New onset seizures in pregnancy caused by an unexpected neurologic disorder. *Eur J Obstet Gynecol Reprod Biol* 2004; 117(1):109–11.

10. Bartynski WS. Posterior reversible encephalopathy syndrome, part 2: controversies surrounding pathophysiology of vasogenic edema. *AJNR Am J Neuroradiol* 2008; 29(6):1043–9.

11. Trommer BL, Homer D and Mikhael MA. Cerebral vasospasm and eclampsia. *Stroke* 1988; 19(3):326–9.

12. Bartynski WS. Posterior reversible encephalopathy syndrome, part 1: fundamental imaging and clinical features. *AJNR Am J Neuroradiol* 2008; 29(6):1036–42.

13. Dekker GA and Sibai BM. Etiology and pathogenesis of pre-eclampsia: current concepts. *Am J Obstet Gynecol* 1998; 179(5):1359–75.

14. Schwartz RB, Feske SK, Polak JF, et al. Pre-eclampsia-eclampsia: clinical and neuroradiographic correlates and insights into the pathogenesis of hypertensive encephalopathy. *Radiology* 2000; 217(2):371–6.

15. Paarlberg KM, de Jong CL, van Geijn HP, et al. Vasoactive mediators in pregnancy-induced hypertensive disorders: a longitudinal study. *Am J Obstet Gynecol* 1998; 179(6 Pt 1):1559–64.

16. Brass SD and Copen WA. Neurological disorders in pregnancy from a neuroimaging perspective. *Semin Neurol* 2007; 27(5):411–24.

17. Bartynski WS and Boardman JF. Distinct imaging patterns and lesion distribution in posterior reversible encephalopathy syndrome. *AJNR Am J Neuroradiol* 2007; 28(7):1320–7.

18. McKinney AM, Short J, Truwit CL, et al. Posterior reversible encephalopathy syndrome: incidence of atypical regions of involvement and imaging findings. *AJR Am J Roentgenol* 2007; 189(4):904–12.

19. Hefzy HM, Bartynski WS, Boardman JF, et al. Hemorrhage in posterior reversible encephalopathy syndrome: imaging and clinical features. *AJNR Am J Neuroradiol* 2009; 30(7):1371–9.

20. Schaefer PW, Buonanno FS, Gonzalez RG, et al. Diffusion-weighted imaging discriminates between cytotoxic and vasogenic edema in a patient with eclampsia. *Stroke* 1997; 28(5):1082–5.

21. Schwartz RB, Mulkern RV, Gudbjartsson H, et al. Diffusion-weighted MR imaging in hypertensive encephalopathy: clues to pathogenesis. *AJNR Am J Neuroradiol* 1998; 19(5):859–62.

22. Alvis JS and Hicks RJ. Pregnancy-induced acute neurologic emergencies and neurologic conditions encountered in pregnancy. *Semin Ultrasound CT MR* 2012; 33(1):46–54.

23. Acheson J and Malik A. Cerebral venous sinus thrombosis presenting in the puerperium. *Emerg Med J* 2006; 23(7):e44.

24. Knopp U, Kehler U, Rickmann H, et al. Cerebral haemodynamic pathologies in HELLP syndrome. *Clin Neurol Neurosurg* 2003; 105(4):256–61.

25. Stone JH. HELLP Syndrome: Hemolysis, Elevated Liver Enzymes, and Low Platelets, *JAMA* 1998; 280(6):559–62. doi:10.1001/jama.280.6.559.

26. Srinivasan K. Puerperal cerebral venous and arterial thrombosis. *Semin Neurol* 1988; 8(3):222–5.

27. Cantu C and Barinagarrementeria F. Cerebral venous thrombosis associated with pregnancy and puerperium. review of 67 cases. *Stroke* 1993; 24(12):1880–4.

28. Lanska DJ and Kryscio RJ. Risk factors for peripartum and postpartum stroke and intracranial venous thrombosis. *Stroke* 2000; 31(6):1274–82.

29. Angelov A. Intracranial venous thrombosis in relation to pregnancy and delivery. *Pathol Res Prac* 1989; 185(6):843–7.

30. Provenzale JM, Joseph GJ and Barboriak DP. Dural sinus thrombosis: findings on CT and MR imaging and diagnostic pitfalls. *AJR Am J Roentgenol* 1998; 170:777–83.

31. Ducreux D, Oppenheim C, Vandamme X, et al. Diffusion-weighted imaging of patterns of brain damage associated with cerebral venus thrombosis. *AJNR Am J Neuroradiol* 2001; 22:261–8.

32. Mullins M, Grant E, Wang B, et al. Parenchymal abnormalities associated with cerebral venous thrombosis: assessment with diffusion-weighted MR imaging. *AJNR Am J Neuroradiol* 2004; 25:1666–75.

33. Röttger C, Trittmacher S, Gerriets T, et al. Reversible MR imaging abnormalities following cerebral venous thrombosis. *AJNR Am J Neuroradiol* 2005; 26:607–13.

34. Call GK, Fleming MC, Sealfon S, et al. Reversible cerebral segmental vasoconstriction. *Stroke* 1988; 19(9):1159–70.

35. Neudecker S, Stock K and Krasnianski M. Call-Fleming postpartum angiopathy in the puerperium: a reversible cerebral vasoconstriction syndrome. *Obstet Gynecol* 2006; 107(2 Pt 2):446–9.

36. Shinghal AB. Postpartum angiopathy with reversible posterior leukoencephalopathy. *Arch Neurol* 2004; 61:411–16.

37. Ursell MR, Marras CL, Farb R, et al. Recurrent intracranial hemorrhage due to postpartum cerebral angiopathy: implications for management. *Stroke* 1998; 29(9):1995–8.

38. Zak IT, Dulai HS and Kish KK. Imaging of neurologic disorders associated with pregnancy and the postpartum period. *Radiographics* 2007; 27(1):95–108.

39. Smith JS, Quiñones-Hinojosa A, Farmon-Smith M, et al. Sex steroid and growth factor profile of a meningioma associated with pregnancy. *Can J Neurol Sci* 2005; 32(1):122–7.

40. Larner AJ, Smith SJ, Duncan JS, et al. Late-onset Rasmussen's syndrome with first seizure during pregnancy. *Eur Neurol* 1995; 35(3):172.

41. Hoeldtke NJ, Floyd D, Werschkul JD, et al. Intracranial cavernous angioma initially presenting in pregnancy with new-onset seizures. *Am J Obstet Gynecol* 1998; 178(3):612–3.

42. Aladdin Y and Gross DW. Refractory status epilepticus during pregnancy secondary to cavernous angioma. *Epilepsia* 2008; 49(9):1627–9.

43. Gowri V, Jacob PC, Jain R, et al. Neurocysticercosis in pregnancy. *Neurosciences (Riyadh)* 2005; 10(2):183–5.

44. Vezina LG. MRI-negative epilepsy: protocols to optimize lesion detection. *Epilepsia* 2011; 52(Suppl 4):25–7.

45. Pallud J, Mandonnet E, Deroulers C, et al. Pregnancy increases the growth rates of World Health Organization grade II gliomas. *Ann Neurol* 2010; 67(3):398–404.

46. Mylonakis E, Paliou M, Hohmann EL, et al. Listeriosis during pregnancy: a case series and review of 222 cases. *Medicine (Baltimore)* 2002; 81(4): 260–9.

Obstetrical anesthesia and the pregnant epileptic patient

Fatima Zahir and Jonathan H. Waters

Key points:

- Epilepsy is one of the most common neurological complications that will be encountered in pregnancy, and the majority of parturients will have an uneventful pregnancy with an excellent outcome
- The risk of intubation failure is 5-fold higher than in the non-pregnant patient. Mortality is secondary to hypoxia, secondary to difficult or failed intubation, or to pulmonary aspiration of gastric contents
- There is no contraindication to the use of regional anesthesia, including spinal, epidural, and combined spinal-epidural techniques, in the pregnant epileptic patient who presents in labor
- Local anesthetic toxicity as a differential diagnosis should be considered when confronted with a newly seizing parturient who has had recent neuraxial anesthesia
- Close cooperation and communication between the anesthesiologist and obstetric team is required in order to optimize the outcome and minimize perinatal and obstetrical risks

Introduction

The prevalence of epilepsy is 0.4–0.8% in the general population, with the incidence of epilepsy for childbearing women having been reported as 50 per 100,000 [1]. Consequently, epilepsy is one of the most common neurological complications that will be encountered in pregnancy. The majority of women with seizure disorders will have an uneventful pregnancy with an excellent outcome. However, pregnant women with epilepsy face a number of challenges during the course of their pregnancy. For example, there is conflicting evidence to suggest a higher risk of intrauterine growth retardation; however, the data at this time is limited. Approximately one-third of women with epilepsy will experience an increase in seizure frequency during pregnancy, and approximately one-half will experience no change [2]. The most important predictive factor is pre-pregnancy severity; women who remained seizure-free for at least 9 months prior to pregnancy had an 84–92% likelihood of remaining seizure-free during pregnancy [3].

Women with Epilepsy, ed. Esther Bui and Autumn Klein. Published by Cambridge University Press.
© Cambridge University Press 2014.

Obstetric anesthesia

Airway management

The first inclination of the anesthesiologist or intensivist when confronted with a seizing patient is to induce a general anesthetic and intubate the patient. This can be particularly hazardous in the obstetrical patient, in that the risk of intubation failure is 5-fold higher than in the non-pregnant patient. It has consistently been shown that maternal mortality is greater with general anesthesia than regional anesthesia. Most of the deaths are due to hypoxia from difficult or failed intubation, or to pulmonary aspiration of gastric contents [24, 25]. Failed endotracheal intubation and ventilation are still a major cause of anesthesia-related maternal mortality occurring during cesarean deliveries.

Intubation difficulty results from pregnancy associated-edema. One of the hallmarks in the diagnosis of pre-eclampsia/eclampsia is generalized edema. This edema includes the airway and trachea, making this type of patient notoriously difficult to intubate. Generalized edema of the eclamptic patient is compounded by the normal anatomic changes of the airway that occur during pregnancy. Capillary engorgement leads to increased edema and friability of the mucosal vasculature of the respiratory tract and swelling of the lining of the oropharynx, larynx, and trachea. Therefore, a smaller endotracheal tube is needed in order to avoid trauma, and subsequent swelling, to the airway. Additionally, large breasts can fall against the neck in the supine position, making insertion and manipulation of the laryngoscope blade difficult during direct laryngoscopy.

While there is no single method that will reliably predict a difficult airway, the Mallampatti classification is traditionally used to assess the airway. This classification assesses the visualization of the uvula and soft palate. More visualization of these structures reflects more room within the oropharynx with which to place a laryngoscope and endotracheal tube. Mallampatti classification should be evaluated just prior to anesthetic induction, as progesterone-induced water shifts during the course of labor itself can lead to progression of the score even in this brief time period.

Pregnancy-induced weight gain leads to an overall increase in body mass index (BMI). The average patient gains 17% of her body weight during pregnancy. Increased BMI has previously been shown to increase the risk of difficult intubation [9]. Failure to manage the airway appropriately in a gravid patient potentially threatens not one life, but two, as maternal complications are the leading cause of fetal insult and death [10].

Compounding the difficulty of placing an endotracheal tube, pregnant patients are more likely to desaturate while the airway is being secured, due to a combination of the parturient's increased oxygen demands in pregnancy and a 20–30% reduction in functional residual capacity (FRC) as a result of upward displacement of the diaphragm by the gravid uterus. The reduction in FRC is attributed to a reduction in expiratory reserve volume by 25% and residual volume by 15%. Therefore, maternal pre-oxygenation is of the utmost importance prior to securing the airway.

In addition, the pregnant patient has increases in gastric pressure from a gravid uterus pressing up against it, decreases in esophageal sphincter tone from hormonal influences, and decreased gastric emptying times. All of these changes make the pregnant patient more prone to aspirate upon anesthesia induction. In fact, the first description of aspiration pneumonitis was described in the gravid patient.

The supine position in the parturient can lead to aortocaval compression, decreased venous return to the heart, and an associated decrease in cardiac output, which in turn reduces uterine perfusion pressure. It should be avoided by left uterine displacement. This requires a wedge made of blankets or towels placed under the right hip to displace the uterus laterally and facilitate venous return to the heart.

Anesthesia and antiseizure medications

There is no contraindication to the use of regional anesthesia, including spinal, epidural, and combined spinal-epidural techniques, in the pregnant epileptic patient who presents in labor. Neuraxial anesthesia actually prevents the hyperventilation that accompanies pain of labor and its subsequent alkalosis, which could precipitate a seizure.

Other factors that may precipitate an episode include hypocarbia and hypoxia, which lower the seizure threshold and result in spontaneous, asynchronous firing of the neurons. Reduced brain oxygenation itself can trigger a seizure, as the neurons are exquisitely sensitive to depletion in their oxygen supply and respond to hypoxia by firing erratically. The seizure threshold may be further lowered by the associated acidity as a result of anaerobic cellular metabolism and lactic acid production. Hypocarbia-associated cerebral vasoconstriction can decrease the blood supply to the brain and aggravate the initial insult.

Hypercarbia most commonly associated with respiratory failure can lower the seizure threshold, and its concomitant cerebral vasodilation can increase the amount of local anesthetic delivery to the brain. The acidosis caused by hypercarbia can lead to ion-trapping and decreased protein-binding, which leads to an increase in the amount of free local anesthetic in the brain and potentiates their central nervous system toxicity. Chronic hyperventilation has been noted to increase the incidence of reactive hypoglycemia, reducing the glucose supply to the brain, which does not have its own stores and as such, is highly dependent on normoglycemic conditions. Hypoglycemia has been shown to lower the seizure threshold, and trigger "hypoglycemic seizures."

Acute and/or severe electrolyte imbalances frequently cause seizures, and these seizures may be the sole presenting symptom. Seizures are especially common in patients with sodium disorders, hypocalcemia, and hypomagnesemia. Successful management of patient seizures begins with the establishment of an accurate diagnosis of the underlying electrolyte disturbance, because rapid identification and correction of the disturbance is necessary to control seizures and prevent permanent brain damage.

While managing the patient with a seizure disorder, the potential influence of these anticonvulsant agents on the response to anesthesia must be kept in mind. Several anticonvulsants, notably phenobarbital, are known hepatic enzyme inducers. Phenobarbital acts on the hepatic microsomal enzymes, specifically on the cytochrome P450 enzymatic system, to accelerate the rate of biotransformation of anesthetic drugs. Increased biotransformation of volatile halogenated agents such as enflurane may increase the risk of organ toxicity. Drugs that compete with phenytoin for a common metabolic pathway, such as diazepam or sulfonamides, will increase phenytoin serum levels. The principal metabolic pathway of phenytoin in humans is aromatic hydroxylation, catalyzed by the cytochrome P450 isozymes (CYP2C9 and CYP2C19). Resistance to neuromuscular blocking agents is observed in patients chronically treated with anticonvulsants. This results from an increased hepatic metabolism consequent to enzymatic induction with an increased bio-elimination of these drugs.

It may be preferable to dose the anticonvulsants parenterally, when possible, given that oral absorption is erratic during the course of labor, due to pain and other physiologic changes of pregnancy. Pain frequently elicits nausea and vomiting which can also contribute to poor control of anticonvulsant drug levels.

Local anesthetics

Local anesthetics can be anticonvulsant in low doses, but when given in high doses, can be proconvulsant. The proconvulsant properties of all local anesthetics are exhibited with toxic blood levels following inadvertent intravascular injection, or from accumulation following repeated injections. Depending on the route of administration, seizures may present immediately, or with a delayed onset. In the laboring obstetrical patient, overdoses generally occur when an epidural catheter is inadvertently placed into a vein. In order to ensure that this does not happen, a small dose of local anesthetic is given to test the epidural placement. This "test dose" is typically 1.5% lidocaine with 1:200,000 epinephrine. From this test dose, the patient would exhibit signs of local anesthetic neurotoxicity, or sizeable changes in heart rate would result from the epinephrine, if the catheter were in a vein. With a negative test dose, a larger dose of local anesthetic is given. These larger doses of local anesthetic are necessary to achieve labor analgesia. If the test dose is not given, or is misinterpreted, the large dose of local anesthetic necessary to achieve labor analgesia can trigger a seizure. While not proven in humans, there appears to be animal data to suggest that a lipid emulsion is effective in treating local anesthetic overdoses.

While local anesthetic agents are proconvulsant in high doses, in lower doses, local anesthetics have been shown to have anticonvulsant properties in humans. Their anticonvulsant activity is exhibited at subtoxic plasma levels, for example, 1–2 mg/kg intravenously of lidocaine has been shown to terminate status epilepticus, as well as reduce the duration of electrically induced seizures in electroconvulsive therapy [4]. With this in mind, regional anesthesia is not contraindicated during pregnancy; however, local anesthetic toxicity as a differential diagnosis should be considered when confronted with a newly seizing parturient who has had recent neuraxial anesthesia.

Anesthetic induction agents (barbiturates, benzodiazepines, ketamine, etomidate)

Benzodiazepines are widely used in the emergency therapy of generalized tonic-clonic seizures because of their potent anticonvulsant properties. Overall, they are effective in controlling status epilepticus in more than 90% of patients with a generalized seizure disorder [11]. Midazolam is as effective in suppressing EEG seizure activity as diazepam, which is often the first line treatment in the emergency treatment of seizure disorders. If it is not possible to establish intravenous access, intramuscular midazolam and rectal diazepam are acceptable alternative routes of administration. The duration of antiseizure activity with lorazepam is longer than that achieved with intravenous diazepam, reducing the need for frequent redosing. Benzodiazepines, especially when taken during the third trimester, can cause a severe benzodiazepine withdrawal syndrome in the neonate, with symptoms including hypotonia, apneic spells, cyanosis, and impaired metabolic responses to cold stress and seizures. The neonatal benzodiazepine withdrawal syndrome has been reported to persist from hours to months after birth [26].

The ultra short-acting barbiturates are predominantly potent anticonvulsant agents. Thiopental specifically has well-known anticonvulsant properties and may be used to terminate seizure activity. It has also been used as an infusion to control intubated and ventilated patients with status epilepticus that are refractory to more conventional anticonvulsant agents [12]. The tendency of methohexital to provoke convulsions during intravenous use in epileptic patients is well known and, consequently, it should be avoided during induction.

Induction with etomidate in patients with epilepsy is associated with involuntary myoclonic movements that resemble generalized convulsive seizures and positive EEG findings [13]. Because of their proconvulsant properties, etomidate should be avoided while inducing the pregnant epileptic. Higher doses of etomidate suppress the low-dose-induced myoclonus therefore; dose and rate of administration will determine whether etomidate will exhibit pro- or anticonvulsant properties. It has been used in several instances to control refractory status epilepticus [16].

It seems prudent to avoid use of ketamine in the pregnant epileptic, since its ability to activate epileptogenic foci in patients with a known seizure disorder is well established [14]. As ketamine is a racemic mixture, the variability of the EEG pattern produced is attributed to the difference in anesthetic potency of the two isomers. The more potent S isomer causes a greater decrease in EEG amplitude, and subsequent burst suppression, than the less potent R isomer.

Propofol appears to possess anticonvulsant properties clinically, although it has been reported to cause excitatory activity, including myoclonus, hiccoughs, and muscle tremors, during induction of anesthesia. The findings have not been corroborated with positive EEG findings. Unlike etomidate, prolonged infusions of propofol have not been associated with persistent myoclonic movements, during or after termination of the infusion [15].

Volatile anesthetics (halothane, enflurane, isoflurane, sevoflurane, desflurane)

General anesthesia is typically initiated with the induction drugs previously described. Following induction and intubation, maintenance of anesthesia takes place typically with a volatile anesthetic. These volatile anesthetics are halogenated hydrocarbons. Of the volatile agents, enflurane has been associated with the development of tonic-clonic activity in normal subjects, as well as those with epilepsy [17]. The ability of enflurane to provoke seizure activity is dependent on its concentration, as well as the $PaCO_2$ level [18]. Hypocarbia with an end-tidal enflurane concentration between 2.5% and 3% causes an increase in the frequency and magnitude of positive EEG findings in monitored epileptics [19]. Sevoflurane has been associated with seizure-like activities during cesarean delivery [23]. The other volatile agents have not been found to cause seizures in patients with a pre-existing seizure disorder; in fact, they have been recommended for treatment of continuous seizures refractory to intravenous therapy. There have been reports of seizure-like activity following concurrent use of nitrous oxide with either halothane or isoflurane [21].

Neromuscular blocking agents (curare, pancuronium, rocuronium, atracurium, vecuronium)

Neuromuscular blockers, or what are more commonly referred to as muscle relaxants, are pervasive in the anesthetic management of patients. These drugs are used to relax the skeletal muscles to enhance surgical exposure. None of the muscle relaxants used in clinical practice have demonstrated seizure activity. However, atracurium is metabolized to lauda-nosine, which is known to cause neurotoxicity. Special consideration must be given to patients with hepatic failure in whom the half-life of the metabolite is prolonged [22]. As was discussed earlier, anticonvulsant medications will enhance liver metabolism so that muscle relaxants are more rapidly metabolized in the patient taking these drugs. As such, the neuromuscular blocker needs to be redosed more frequently.

Anticholinesterases are routinely used to reverse the effect of neuromuscular blockers. The anticholinesterases have not been reported to cause central nervous system excitation. Physostigmine is known to cross the blood-brain barrier to reverse the sedative effects of atropine and scopolamine. Rarely, the central nervous system (CNS) depressant effects of the centrally acting anticholinergics have been reversed and manifested as excitation and delirium [23].

Opiod analgesics (morphine, hydromorphone, fentanyl, alfentanyl, sufentanyl, remifentanil)

Pain control for the pregnant epileptic involves the use of opioid analgesics. Meperidine neurotoxicity is well known, manifesting clinically as tremors, myoclonus, and seizures. Its CNS manifestations are thought to be secondary to its biodegradation to its metabolite normeperidine. The chances of neurotoxicity are increased by repeated administration of meperidine, because normeperidine has a significantly longer half-life and will accumulate in the body, leading to toxic levels. The risk is greater with oral administration due to extensive first pass metabolism of meperidine. The seizures resolve over several days with discontinuation of the agent, as the body excretes the active metabolite. Patients with renal failure are more susceptible to developing neurotoxicity due to decreased metabolism and excretion of normeperidine. There is an increased rate of conversion to normeperidine with use of anticonvulsants [20].

Morphine alone has never been demonstrated to produce seizure activity in humans after intravenous administration. Although animal studies have shown proconvulsant proper-ties, the doses used in clinical practice do not appear to have any effect on the seizure threshold. There have been reports of grand mal seizures after low-to-moderate doses of intravenous fentanyl, sufentanil, and alfentanil [7]. These movements have not been found to be consistent with epileptic activity and are more likely to be non-epileptic myoclonic movements or exaggerated narcotic-induced rigidity. Although morphine does not exhibit seizure activity when given intravenously, there have been case reports documenting tonic-clonic seizures in patients after administration of epidural and intrathecal morphine [5, 6]. Animal studies have demonstrated seizures after epidural morphine administration, which are naloxone-reversible, while intrathecal morphine-induced seizure activity was not. This suggests that morphine mediates its seizure activity through both opiate and non-opiate receptors.

Although episodes of generalized tonic-clonic seizure-like activity after intravenous administration of low-to-moderate doses of fentanyl and alfentanil have been reported [7], current evidence suggests these findings are more consistent with myoclonic move-ments or exaggerated narcotic-induced rigidity. Prolonged administration of large doses of fentanyl and sufentanil may precipitate seizures and should be used cautiously in the patient with a pre-existing seizure disorder [8]. There have been no reports of seizure activity following intrathecal or epidural administration of fentanyl and its analogues.

The neonate of parturients with chronic opioid abuse may also present with withdrawal symptoms at birth. The predominant manifestations include central nervous system hyperirritability and autonomic nervous system dysregulation, such as sneezing, yawning, sweating, tachycardia and mydriasis, gastrointestinal dysfunction (including diarrhea, nausea, and vomiting), respiratory distress, and abnormal motor movements (for example, tremors, hypertonia, hyperreflexivity, and repetitive movements). Benzodiazepine withdrawal differs from opioid withdrawal, in that it does not cause gastrointestinal dysfunction and abnormal motor movements may be more pronounced [27]. Studies suggest no increase in congenital abnormalities in pregnant patients who underwent surgery during the course of their pregnancy, but a greater risk of abortion, growth restriction, and low birth weight. These studies concluded that problems resulted from primary disease or the surgical procedure itself rather than exposure to anaesthesia [28]. The current consensus is that benzodiazepines are not teratogenic and a single dose appears safe. Because of concerns about increased risk of cleft palate, regular use, particularly in the first trimester when the fetus is most vulnerable to drug use, should probably be avoided.

The majority of women with idiopathic epilepsy will have an uncomplicated pregnancy course with excellent maternal and fetal outcomes. In order to minimize perinatal and

Table 16.1: Anesthetic effects on seizure threshold

AGENT	EFFECT
Inhalational agents	
• Nitrous Oxide	Possible proconvulsant with enflurane or halothane
• Halothane	Terminates status epilepticus
• Enflurane	Proconvulsant
• Isoflurane	Terminates status epilepticus
• Sevoflurane	Possible proconvulsant role
• Desflurane	Terminates status epilepticus
Local anesthetics	Proconvulsant at toxic doses
Benzodiazepines	Anticonvulsant
Barbiturates	
• Thiopental	Anticonvulsant
• Methohexital	Proconvulsant
Etomidate	Proconvulsant; possible anticonvulsant at higher doses
Propofol	Anticonvulsant
Ketamine	Proconvulsant
Opioids	
• Morphine	Possible proconvulsant after neuraxial administration
• Meperidine	Proconvulsant due to normeperidine metabolite
• Fentanyl	Possible proconvulsant after prolonged IV administration
• Sufentanil	Similar to fentanyl
• Alfentanil	Similar to fentanyl
Neuromuscular agents	Atracurium degrades to laudanosine, which can produce seizure activity. None of the other agents are pro- or anticonvulsant

obstetrical risks, it is important for the patient to understand that prevention of seizures is the most important goal during her pregnancy. There are complex interactions among the mother, fetus, and epilepsy, as well as the changes associated with pregnancy. Consequently, close cooperation and communication between the anesthesiologist and obstetric team is required in order to optimize the outcome.

References

1. Brodie MJ and Dichter MA. Antiepileptic drugs. *N Engl J Med* 1996; 334:168–75.

2. Bader AM. Neurologic and neuromuscular disease. In: Chestnut DH, ed. *Obstetric anesthesia: principles and practice*, 9th edn. St Louis, MO: Mosby, 1999; 963–85.

3. Samuels P and Niebyl J. Neurological disorders: pregnancy and co-existing disease. In: Gabbe SG, Niebyl JR, Galan HL, et al., eds. *Obstetrics: normal and problem pregnancies*, 6th edn. Philadelphia, PA: Saunders, 2012.

4. Koppanyi T. The sedative, analgesic and anticonvulsant actions of local anesthetics. *Am J Med Sci* 1962; 244:646–54.

5. Borgeat A, Biollaz J, Depierraz B, et al. Grand mal seizure after extradural morphine analgesia. *Br J Anaesth* 1988; 60:733–5.

6. Jacobson L. Intrathecal and extradural narcotics. *Adv Pain Res Ther* 1984; 7: 199–236.

7. Bailey PL, Wilbrink J, Zwanikken P, et al. Anesthetic induction with fentanyl. *Anesth Analg* 1985; 64:48–53.

8. Young ML, Smith DS, Greenberg J, et al. Effects of sufentanil on regional glucose utilization in rats. *Anesthesiology* 1984; 61:564.

9. Reisner LS, Benumof JL and Cooper SD. The difficult airway: risk, prophylaxis and management. In Chestnut DH, ed. *Obstetric anesthesia: principles and practice*. St. Louis, MO: Mosby, 1999: 590–620.

10. Kuczkowski KM, Fouhy SA, Greenberg M, et al. Trauma in pregnancy: anaesthetic management of the pregnancy trauma victim with unstable cervical spine. *Anaesthesia* 2003; 58:822.

11. Tassinari CA, Daniele O, Michelucci R, et al. Benzodiazepines: efficacy in status epilepticus. *Adv Neurol* 1983; 34:465–75.

12. Brown AS and Horton JM. Status epilepticus treated by intravenous infusions of thiopentate sodium. *Br Med J* 1967; 1:27–8

13. Kreiger W, Copperman J and Laxer KD. Seizures with etomidate anesthesia. *Anesth Analg* 1985; 64:1226–7.

14. Bennett DR, Madsen JA, Jordan WS, et al. Ketamine anesthesia in brain-damaged: electroencephalographic and clinical observations. *Neurology* 1973; 23:449–60.

15. White PF. Propofol: pharmacokinetics and pharmacodynamics. *Sem Anesth* 1988; 7 (Suppl 1):4–20.

16. Hoffman P and Schockenhoff B. Etomidate as an anticonvulsive agent. *Anaesthesist* 1984; 33:142–4.

17. Botty C, Brown B, Stanley V, et al. Clinical experiences with compound 347, a halogenated anesthetic agent. *Anesth Analg* 1968; 47:477–505.

18. Michenfelder JD and Cucchiara RF. Canine cerebral oxygen consumption during enflurane anesthesia and its modification during induced seizures. *Aaesthesiology* 1974; 40(6):575–80.

19. Lebowitz MH, Blitt CD and Dillon JB. Enflurane-induced central nervous system excitation and its relation to carbon dioxide tension. *Anesth Analg* 1972; 51:355–63.

20. Pond SM and Kretschzmar KM. Effect of phenytoin on meperidine clearance and normeperidine formation. *Clin Pharmacol Ther* 1981; 30:680–6.

21. Smith PA, McDonald TR and Jones CS. Convulsions associated with halothane anesthesia. *Anaesthesia* 1966; 21:229–33.

22. Ward S and Weatherly BC. Pharmacokinetics of atracurium and its metabolites. *Br J Anaesth* 1986; 58 (Suppl):6S–10S.

23. Duvosin R and Katz R. Reversal of central anticholinergic syndrome in man by physostigmine. *JAMA* 1968; 206:163–5.

24. Department of Health et al. *Why mothers die 1997–1999. The Confidential Enquiries into Maternal Deaths in the United Kingdom*. London: RCOG Press, 2001.

25. Hawkins JL, Koonin LM, Palmer SK, et al. Anesthesia related deaths during obstetric delivery in the United States, 1979–1990. *Anesthesiology* 1997; 86:277–84.

26. McElhatton PR. The effects of benzodiazepine use during pregnancy and lactation. *Reprod Toxicol* 8(6): 461–75.

27. Anand KJS and Ingraham J. Tolerance, dependence, and strategies for compassionate withdrawal of analgesics and anxiolytics in the pediatric ICU. *Crit Care Nurs* 1996; 16:87–93.

28. Mazze RI and Kallen B. Reproductive outcome after anaesthesia and operation during pregnancy: a registry study of 5405 cases. *Am J Obstet Gynecol* 1989; 161: 1178–85.

Seizure management in the postpartum period

Elinor Ben-Menachem

Key points:

- Serum levels (total and free levels) of antiepileptic drugs (AEDs) should be determined prior to conception and monthly during pregnancy
- Serum levels of most AEDs need to be monitored directly after birth of the baby and followed closely for the first few weeks
- Doses of certain AEDs, such as lamotrigine, need to be adjusted directly after birth
- Breastfeeding is recommended in most cases, but the infant needs to be monitored for side effects when the mother is taking AEDs that pass significantly through breast milk
- Physician and mother should be cautious about adding new therapies early on in the postpartum period and during breastfeeding. New therapies should only be undertaken in difficult cases where seizure control is lost

Introduction

Although most attention is focused on the baby, the mother with epilepsy is in a critical period immediately after giving birth. The operational definition of the period directly after birth starts at the time of birth of the placenta until the woman has reached amenorrhea. This period extends for about 6 weeks after birth [1]. Biologically, it is the time during which the mother's body, including hormone levels and uterus size, returns to pre-pregnancy conditions. When lactating, the hormonal changes are, of course, different than when the mother decides not to breastfeed. Most important is seizure control during this time, and therefore the levels of AEDs must be monitored and the doses adjusted routinely during pregnancy and especially directly after birth until the levels have returned to the pre-pregnant state.

The problem of seizure control

In the immediate postpartum period, there are many changes that can occur in the concentration of AEDs due to fluctuations in bioavailability and a sharp increase in clearance. Blood concentrations of many of the AEDs need to be adjusted promptly postpartum, since changes can occur very rapidly causing an increase in seizures or symptoms of toxicity.

Women with Epilepsy, ed. Esther Bui and Autumn Klein. Published by Cambridge University Press.
© Cambridge University Press 2014.

Treating breakthrough seizures

Women with epilepsy (WWE) have a higher risk of seizures in the postpartum state than in the non-pregnant state or during pregnancy. This probably depends on the changes in blood concentrations of the AEDs, as well as hormonal changes, lack of sleep, and stress, which almost always occur when caring for a new baby [2]. There is no consensus as to how to treat break through seizures, especially in otherwise seizure-free patients. Therapeutic drug monitoring (TDM) is essential in this circumstance, as doses of AEDs may need to be titrated. However, not all AEDs are amendable to TDM. Available AEDs for TDM are phenytoin, carbamazepine, lamotrigine, topiramate, clobazam, and levetiracetam. The newer AEDs, such as lacosamide, pregabalin, and perampanel, cannot or are difficult to monitor by TDM at this time, and therefore, an increase in the dosage would probably need to be done in a more empirical fashion.

Rescue medication for acute seizures can also be used. Since the postpartum period is limited to about 6 weeks, increases of the chronic AED may be less advantageous for the patient then giving rescue medication. However, the goal is seizure freedom and that may not always be achieved alone by medication given acutely after a seizure. Diazepam is a proven rescue medication with effects on the nursing baby being only transitory when used acutely. Benzodiazepines like midazolam given buccally or as a nasal spray, or lorazepam, especially as a dissolvable tablet, can be used, but the effects on the nursing infant are not as well studied, but probably have the same transitory effect as diazepam [3].

Behavior of individual AEDs

Each AED behaves differently during this period, and strategies on how to adjust dosages can vary. Below is a synopsis of the different major AEDs and how their kinetics change postpartum. The basic observation is that after birth, clearance of all AEDs decreases rapidly, requiring immediate and careful dose adjustments. The mother risks toxicity and seizures if the drug levels are not adjusted fast enough. AED doses may have been increased, particularly for lamotrigine, during pregnancy because of an increased volume of distribution and then decrease postpartum. TDM is needed because the doses may differ from what was used pre-pregnancy. There is no substitute for careful monitoring of adverse effects balanced with seizure control.

Carbamazepine

Carbamazepine levels decrease during pregnancy, especially the bound carbamazepine levels. In several studies the range in total carbamazepine decreased up to 42% [4]. Unbound levels decreased much less or not at all [5], and therefore, like phenytoin, it is important to follow unbound concentrations of carbamazepine during and after pregnancy to determine if adjustments need to be made or not. Recovery to baseline levels in the postpartum period takes about 1 month. During this time, toxicity can occur if adjustments have been made during pregnancy, but in most cases dose adjustments are not necessary. According to the recommendation from the American Epilepsy Society and the American Academy of Neurology concerning breastfeeding, based on two Class II studies, the guidelines maintain that carbamazepine is safe and only penetrates into breast milk in clinically insignificant amounts (6).

Gabapentin

Gabapentin concentrations have not been followed through pregnancy. Since gabapentin is not metabolized nor protein-bound, there is little reason to believe there would be major changes in plasma concentrations [4]. There is no evidence that plasma levels need to be followed though pregnancy and afterwards. While blood levels can be analyzed, many hospitals will not have the assay readily available, and therefore analyses can take time. Concerning breastfeeding, the recommendation from the American Epilepsy Society and the American Academy of Neurology based on one Class II study is that gabapentin significantly penetrates into breast milk [6].

Lamotrigine

Lamotrigine (LTG) is probably the most studied of any AED in pregnant and postpartum women. This is because it is thought to be a drug with low teratogenic properties, and is preferably used as a first line drug in young women. When LTG was first marketed, many women on LTG monotherapy began reporting breakthrough seizures [7]. This led to studies monitoring the blood concentrations of LTG before, during, and after pregnancy to determine what was occurring. More is written on this subject in Chapter 12. All case series and prospective follow-ups have shown the same thing. In one study, for example, Fotopoulou et al. [8] followed 15 women through pregnancy. As in other studies [5, 6], the plasma clearance of LTG was 250% higher than at baseline by the end of pregnancy. During the first postpartum week, the levels dropped down 218% from baseline and by week 3, the clearance levels had recovered to baseline levels.

What does this mean practically? During pregnancy, patients on LTG risk having breakthrough seizures if the dose of LTG is not at least doubled over the course of the pregnancy. In fact, blood levels should be drawn consistently throughout pregnancy in order to maintain constant LTG concentrations. Then, at birth, levels of lamotrigine will return rapidly to the pre-pregnancy state, and this may even occur in the child as well, since significant amounts of lamotrigine are found in breast milk [8, 9]. In anticipation of this, doses of lamotrigine should be initially cut by 25% immediately following birth and then per week, especially in the case when blood tests of lamotrigine cannot be taken, and adjusted thereafter [10]. Preferably, blood samples should be taken every week after birth for 1 month to best readjust the levels until baseline values have been established. By anticipating the increasing blood levels after birth, potential overdosing can be effectively counteracted. Therefore, seizures are probably not a problem in the postpartum period for women on lamotrigine, except for the slight risk of seizure exacerbation with excessively high doses of lamotrigine. The recommendation from the American Epilepsy Society and the American Academy of Neurology based on one Class II study is that lamotrigine possibly penetrates into breast milk in clinically significant amounts [6].

Levetiracetam

Levetiracetam is a drug with favorable pharmacokinetic properties. It is not metabolized in the liver; it has complete bioavailability, linear pharmacokinetics, renal excretion, and no drug-drug interactions or plasma protein-binding [11]. In one prospective study [12], five patients were evaluated first before week 16 of pregnancy, during the pregnancy, at birth (with blood also taken from the umbilical cord,) and up to 12 months postpartum.

The women were maintained on the same dose of levetiracetam unless they had break-through seizures, and then the dose was adjusted, which happened in one patient. The four patients where the dosage was not changed showed similar results: the concentration of levetiracetam decreased by 17.6% during the 1st to 3rd trimester but the seizure frequency remained unchanged. The mean 3rd trimester concentration was only 47% of the immediate postpartum concentration. In other words the concentration of levetiracetam directly after birth increased spontaneously by 47% without dose adjustment. However, at 12 months postpartum, the concentration of levetiracetam was 38% more than during the 3rd trimester. There was extensive transfer of levetiracetam to the umbilical cord and the ratio in this study was 1.21. The recommendation from the American Epilepsy Society and the American Academy of Neurology based on two Class II studies is that levetiracetam probably penetrates into breast milk in clinically significant amounts [6].

Oxcarbazepine

Oxcarbazepine is rapidly metabolized to the active metabolite (monohydroxy derivative, or MHD), which is in turn metabolized by glucuronidation, and is 40% protein-bound. Protein-binding in oxcarbazepine's case is not significant, but the metabolism by glucuronidation is. It has the same metabolism as lamotrigine and has been shown in several studies to cause a decrease in the MHD levels by 30–40%. After pregnancy, the levels return to normal by about 1 week [4, 13]. Monitoring of the MHD levels should be considered during pregnancy, and if and when a dose adjustment has been made, readjustment of the dose needs to be made again after a week postpartum. Concerning breastfeeding, oxcarbazepine was not discussed in the recommendation from the American Epilepsy Society and the American Academy of Neurology concerning whether it penetrates significantly into breast milk or not [6].

Phenobarbital

Although few women take phenobarbital in western European countries, Canada, and the USA, it is used extensively in other parts of the world. Due to sedation of the fetus, it is not encouraged during pregnancy. Some early studies have looked at the concentration of phenobarbital in the blood during and after pregnancy. In one study, steady-state plasma AED concentrations were measured at intervals throughout pregnancy and during the postnatal period in 105 women who underwent 134 pregnancies [1]. In this study, the dosage of phenobarbital had to be increased by 85% from the pre-pregnancy dose to maintain the same concentration during pregnancy. The return to pre-pregnancy levels took over 4 weeks postpartum, but this is probably due to its long half-life. Therefore, the risk of seizure breakthrough due to phenobarbital postpartum is not high, but sedation and toxicity can occur if the dose is not appropriately adjusted. One way is to not adjust the phenobarbital at all during pregnancy unless the patient has seizure symptoms, so at the end of pregnancy the concentration will have returned to normal. On popular websites, breastfeeding is not recommended because of the possible sedative effects [14], but the recommendation from the American Epilepsy Society and the American Academy of Neurology based on one Class I and one Class II studies, maintains that phenobarbital is safe and only penetrates into breast milk in clinically insignificant amounts [6].

Phenytoin

For phenytoin the situation is similar to phenobarbital, as described above [1]. However, while phenobarbital is 50% bound to serum proteins, phenytoin is 90% bound. The half-life of phenytoin is much shorter than phenobarbital and adjustments are therefore easier. During pregnancy, protein-binding decreases as well as metabolism, which is induced. Thus total phenytoin concentration can decrease by 55–61%, but free phenytoin is more stable and decreases by 16–31% [4]. After pregnancy, it takes about 4 weeks for the blood concentration to return to normal [1]. If only total phenytoin levels are evaluated at this time and not free phenytoin levels, then the dose could be mistakenly adjusted upward during pregnancy, risking phenytoin toxicity after the birth as the protein-binding and clearance return to the pre-pregnancy state. Even slight increases of phenytoin can cause unwanted symptoms of ataxia, diplopia, and dizziness, so it is important to monitor patients carefully, especially by controlling free phenytoin levels. Concerning breastfeeding, the recommendation from the American Epilepsy Society and the American Academy of Neurology based on two Class II studies, maintains that phenytoin is safe and only penetrates into breast milk in clinically insignificant amounts [6].

Topiramate

Topiramate is primarily a renally metabolized drug and is only bound to serum proteins by 15%. It is only significantly metabolized by the liver if given in a dose >200 mg/day. There is a decline of about 30–40% in the last trimester. This is another instance where blood levels should be followed through pregnancy (and possibly adjusted for) and then immediately after both [4]. Concerning breastfeeding, the recommendation from the American Epilepsy Society and the American Academy of Neurology based on one Class II study, maintains that topiramate penetrates into breast milk in clinically significant amounts [6].

Valproic acid

Valproic acid is a drug that is used extensively throughout the world, and many women of childbearing age are treated with this drug. Due to the potential increase of teratogenic effects, the number of women on valproate during pregnancy is hopefully declining. However, it remains one of the most common medications, especially for women with primary generalized epilepsies, in spite of the knowledge that this drug is one of the most teratogenic of the antiepileptic drugs [15]. As with most of the AEDs which have high protein-binding, due to increased clearance during pregnancy and decrease in the bound fraction of valproate (about 90% is bound to proteins in the non-pregnant state), the concentration of bound VPA decreases and then there will be an increase again postpartum. The unbound fraction, however, remains largely unchanged [4]. Again, as with most other AEDs, except when breakthrough seizures do occur changes, in doses are not necessary [2]. Following free levels of valproate is usually the best indication of whether the effective levels of VPA have changed or not [4]. Concerning breastfeeding, the recommendation from the American Epilepsy Society and the American Academy of Neurology based on one Class I and two Class II studies maintains that valproate is safe and only penetrates into breast milk in clinically insignificant amounts [6].

Gabapentin, topiramate, oxcarbazepine

There is limited information concerning the pharmacokinetics of these drugs postpartum, which might be due to the observation that breakthrough seizures occur rarely after birth and dose adjustments are rarely necessary. Blood levels of these drugs can be done, but many hospitals will not have the assay readily available, and therefore analyses can take time.

Recommendations for routine postpartum care

After birth and 1 month, 3 months, and 6 months afterwards, AED blood levels (both free and total at peak and trough) should be assessed, as well as electrolytes, hematology (patients should not be allowed to become anemic), and glucose. Free AED levels are particularly important in carbamazepine, oxcarbazepine (monohydroxy derivative), phenytoin, and valproate. Blood pressure is important to follow after birth because of the risk for occult postpartum eclampsia that can occur at this time. Seizure control is important, and the patients should be encouraged to call immediately if there is any change at all.

Treatment of the refractory patient

Some patients who have successful pregnancies do have difficulties with control of seizures and continue to have them postpartum. If the mother is lactating, then it is hard to change the drug regimen during that period to more active therapies. Decisions on possible epilepsy surgery or participation in clinical trials have to wait.

Changes in the drug regimen with the addition of a new drug or increase in one of the existing drugs can be done, but monitoring of the infant has to be continuous so as not to cause changes in behavior and wakefulness in the infant. If possible, drastic alterations should be postponed until the mother is no longer lactating. If seizures worsen, then the mother may have to consider stopping breastfeeding and go on to drug adjustment.

Implantation of a vagus nerve stimulator (VNS) is not contraindicated at this time, but is not very practical when dealing with the birth of a new baby and lactation. Since the device is implanted on the left side under the left clavicle it could be uncomfortable during breastfeeding, and the baby could hit the device repeatedly while the implantation site is trying to heal. Thus, if the idea of adding VNS to a therapy arises, it probably should be postponed until lactation is over.

Status epilepticus

Postpartum eclampsia: Status epilepticus (even in the absence of a pre-eclampsia prodrome) can occur even in women with epilepsy being treated with antiepileptic drugs. This condition can be a diagnostic challenge and needs to be ruled out first. Blood pressure must be assessed immediately and should not be forgotten. MRI studies can also help in the diagnosis, often demonstrating mostly reversible, white matter hyperintensities on T2-weighted images [16]. MRI and MRI venography are also important to exclude cerebral venous thrombosis [17].

Status epilepticus should be treated in the same way as other cases. In the process, the patient's usual AED concentrations should be immediately checked and adjusted promptly when indicated. Other important blood tests should include electrolytes, glucose, and toxicity screen. According to the American Epilepsy Society and the American Academy of Neurology there is insufficient evidence to support or refute an increased risk of pre-eclampsia or status epilepticus [18].

Conclusion

Clearance of the AEDs invariably increases during pregnancy and abruptly decreases after delivery. The general rule and best practice when dealing with patients on AEDs would be to systematically take the plasma levels of the AEDs as soon as it is known that the patient is pregnant, and follow the levels monthly until delivery, and then weekly until the pre-pregnancy state is re-achieved.

References

1. Lander CM and Eadie MJ. Plasma antiepileptic drug concentrations during pregnancy. *Epilepsia* 1991; 3:257–66.

2. Lander CM. Antiepileptic drugs in pregnancy and lactation. *Aust Prescr* 2008; 31:70–2.

3. Adab N. Therapeutic monitoring of antiepileptic drugs during pregnancy and in the postpartum period: is it useful? *CNS Drugs* 2006; 20:791–800.

4. Tomson T, Landmark C and Battino D. Antiepileptic drug treatment in pregnancy: changes in drug disposition and their clinical implication. *Epilepsia* 2013; 54: 405–14.

5. Tomson T, Lindblom U, Ekqvist B, et al. Disposition of carbamazepine and phenytoin in pregnancy. *Epilepsia* 1994; 35:131–5.

6. Harden CL, Pennell PB, Koppel BS, et al. American Academy of Neurology; American Epilepsy Society. Management issues for women with epilepsy–focus on pregnancy (an evidence-based review): III. Vitamin K, folic acid, blood levels, and breast-feeding: Report of the Quality Standards Subcommittee and Therapeutics and Technology Assessment Subcommittee of the American Academy of Neurology and the American Epilepsy Society. *Epilepsia* 2009; 50(5):1247–55.

7. Ohman L, Beck O, Luef G, et al. Plasma concentrations of lamotrigine and its 2-N-glucuronide metabolite during pregnancy in women with epilepsy. *Epilepsia* 2008; 49:1075–80.

8. Fotopoulou C, Kretz R, Bauer S, et al. Prospectively assessed changes in lamotrigine-concentration in women with epilepsy during pregnancy, lactation and the neonatal period. *Epilepsy Res* 2009; 85:60–4.

9. Penell PB, Peng L, Newport DJ, et al. Lamotrigine in pregnancy: clearance, therapeutic drug monitoring, and seizure frequency. *Neurology* 2008; 70:2130–36.

10. Sabers A. Algorithm for lamotrigine dose adjustment before, during and after pregnancy. *Acta Neurol Scand* 2012; 126(1):e1–e4. doi: 10.1111/j.1600-0404.2011.01627.x.

11. Pastalos PN. Clinical pahrmacokinetics of levetiracetam. *Clin Pharmacokinet* 2004; 43:707–24.

12. López-Fraile IP, Cid AO, Juste AO, et al. Levetiracetam plasma level monitoring during pregnancy, delivery, and postpartum: clinical and outcome implications. *Epilepsy Behav* 2009; 15: 372–5.

13. Mazzucchelli I, Onat FY, Ozkara C, et al. Changes in the disposition of oxcarbazepine and its metabolites during pregnancy and the puerperium. *Epilepsia* 2006; 47:504–9.

14. www.netdoctor.co.uk/brain-and-nervous-system/medicines/phenobarbital.html.

15. Tomson T and Battino D. Teratogenic effects of antiepileptic drugs. *Lancet Neurol* 2012; 11:803–13.

16. R Veltkamp, A Kupsch, J Polasek, et al. Late onset postpartum eclampsia without pre-eclamptic prodromi: clinical and neuroradiological presentation in two patients. *J Neurol Neurosurg Psychiatry* 2000; 69:824–7.

17. Harden CL, Hopp J, Ting TY, et al. Management issues for women with epilepsy-focus on pregnancy (an evidence-based review): I. Obstetrical complications and change in seizure

frequency: Report of the Quality Standards Subcommittee and Therapeutics and Technology Assessment Subcommittee of the American Academy of Neurology and the American Epilepsy Society. *Epilepsia* 2009; 50:1229–36.

18. Demir CF, Inci MF, Ozkan F, et al. Clinical and radiological management and outcome of pregnancies complicated by cerebral venous thrombosis: a review of 19 cases. *J Stroke Cerebrovasc Dis* 2013; 22(8):1252–7.

Breastfeeding and use of antiepileptics

Weerawadee Chandranipapongse and Shinya Ito

Key points:

- Maternal use of antiepileptics is not contraindicated in breastfeeding of healthy infants
- However, it is prudent to be vigilant for possible adverse effects
- Benefits of breastfeeding need to be clearly communicated to patients
- Infant drug clearance is the major determining factor for drug accumulation in the breastfed infants
- Milk-to-plasma drug-concentration ratio has little clinical meaning as an indicator for safety of the drug in breastfeeding, unless other factors such as infant drug clearance are also considered

Epilepsy in pregnancy is estimated to occur in 3–7 women in every 1,000 pregnancies [1]. These pregnancies are considered high risk and usually require treatment to control seizures. Antiepileptic drug therapies are generally maintained during pregnancy and continued through lactation in the majority of these patients. Carbamazepine, valproic acid, and lamotrigine are the most commonly prescribed antiepileptic drugs across the pregnancy registries [2]. Other antiepileptic drugs used during pregnancy include cloba-zam, clonazepam, ethosuximide, felbamate, gabapentin, levetiracetam, oxcarbazepine, phenobarbital, phenytoin, primidone, tiagabine, topiramate, vigabatrin, and zonisamide.

Antiepileptic therapy during pregnancy poses a risk of anomalies to the developing fetus. In order to minimize the teratogenic risk, it is recommended that a single anti-epileptic drug be used with the lowest effective dose [3]. Similarly, assessing the safety of antiepileptic drugs during lactation is challenging. Despite the fact that the majority of drugs are excreted into milk at concentrations low enough to pose little toxicity risk, the adverse effects of antiepileptic drugs on nursing infants are still of great concern. Unlike pregnancy, in which eliminating drug exposure of infants in utero is not a realistic medical option, breastfeeding mothers and their health care providers may decide to discontinue breastfeeding while on antiepileptic therapy. However, the decision not to breastfeed must be justified by the fact that the risk to the baby outweighs the benefits of breastfeeding, which are often ignored due to lack of understanding.

Benefits of breastfeeding

Breastfeeding benefits not only infants but also their mothers. Health benefits to breastfed infants include a reduction in the risk of infectious diseases, such as acute otitis media,

Women with Epilepsy, ed. Esther Bui and Autumn Klein. Published by Cambridge University Press.
© Cambridge University Press 2014.

gastroenteritis, lower respiratory tract infection, immunologically mediated disorders including atopic dermatitis, asthma, type 1 diabetes, and other disorders such as obesity, type 2 diabetes, and sudden infant death syndrome [4]. A randomized trial of intense breastfeeding promotion showed breastfed infants have higher cognitive function than formula-fed infants [5]. Similarly, breastfeeding mothers have a reduced risk of type 2 diabetes, breast cancer, and ovarian cancer [4]. Moreover, breastfeeding also enhances maternal-infant bonding, which psychologically benefits both the mother and infant [6]. No breastfeeding, or early cessation of breastfeeding, is known to be associated with an increased risk of postpartum depression [4].

Assessing infant exposure levels to drugs in breast milk

Factors influencing the excretion of drugs into milk

The amount of drugs excreted into breast milk is determined by physicochemical characteristics of the drug, such as molecular weight, plasma protein-binding, lipophilicity, ionization, and the drug's pharmacokinetics in the mother. In addition, the composition of the milk changes over time from colostrum, transitional, to mature milk, and also within a feeding period (e.g. foremilk and hindmilk). These differences and specific mechanisms of mammary drug transfer (e.g., carrier-mediated transport) all contribute to the variation of drug excretion into milk. In general, low molecular weight (<500 Dalton), low plasma protein-binding, and high lipophilicity of the drug tend to be factors for increased drug excretion into milk [7]. Cationic nature of the drug is another factor for increased milk concentration. Namely, ionized drug molecules cannot pass the biological membrane by passive diffusion. The pKa (pH at which 50% of drugs are ionized) of a drug and the pH of its surrounding biological fluid determine the ionization status of that drug. As average plasma and breast milk pH are 7.4 and 7.2, respectively, cationic or basic drugs tend to be trapped in milk due to further ionization in the milk [7].

The selected pharmacokinetic and physicochemical properties of antiepileptic drugs are shown in Table 18.1. As described later, some of these parameters determine infant exposure levels to the drugs in milk. The drug concentration in maternal plasma depends on maternal pharmacokinetic processes, which are significantly altered during pregnancy compared to non-pregnant status. The physiological changes of pharmacokinetics during pregnancy does not return to a pre-pregnancy level until approximately 3 months postpartum [10]. Hence, maternal pharmacokinetics during breastfeeding is in a dynamic transition state.

The magnitude of drug transfer into milk is often expressed as the milk-to-plasma drug-concentration ratio (MP ratio). This ratio can be obtained from an experiment or calculated from an equation that takes into consideration the physicochemical characteristics of the drug [11]. However, MP ratio by itself has no direct clinical meaning as a predictor of drug exposure and safety in breastfed infants unless other factors are also considered. For example, MP ratio of more than one indicates the drug is concentrated in the milk rather than maternal plasma. However, if the infant is not exclusively breastfeeding or if the infant drug clearance is sufficiently high, the amount of drug the infant ingests would be much lower than what would be needed for therapeutic purposes. In such a case, the infant's exposure to the drug may be considered low, regardless of the MP ratio [11].

Table 18.1: Selected pharmacokinetic parameters of antiepileptic drugs [8, 9]

Drugs	Adult		Child		Molecular weight (Dalton)	Plasma protein-binding (%)	Milk-to-plasma ratio[a]	pKa
	Half-life (h)	Clearance (ml/kg/min)	Half-life (h)	Clearance (ml/kg/min)				
Carbamazepine	18–54	0.8–1.8	8–44	0.8–1.8	236	70–80	0.17–0.69	7.0
Clobazam	17–31	0.48–0.88	17–31	0.48–0.88	301	90	0.13–0.36	–
Clonazepam	18–50	–	–	–	316	50–86	0.33	1.5, 10.5
Ethosuximide	30–60	–	32–38	–	141	0	0.94	9.3
Felbamate	10–23	0.37–0.66	5–15	0.51–0.92	238	22–35	–	–
Gabapentin	5–9	1.3–1.9	5–9, 14	1.3–1.9	171	<3	0.73	3.68
Lamotrigine	14–60	0.46–1.21	5.9–9.5[b]	1.46–2.34[b]	256	53–60	0.40–0.67	5.7
Levetiracetam	6–8	–	–	–	170	<10	1	–
Oxcarbazepine	1–2.5	–	–	–	252	40	0.50–0.65	–
Phenobarbital	48–144	0.049–0.075	45–500	0.049–0.137	232	48–54	0.36–0.79	7.2
Phenytoin	7–50	0.14–0.99	15–160	0.05–0.14	252	89	0.03–0.55	8.3
Primidone	10–21	–	–	–	218	<20	0.72–0.80	–
Tiagabine	5–14	1.07–3.46	3–6[c]	2.5–7.5	412	96	–	–
Topiramate	18–30	0.3–0.5	–	–	339	13–17	0.67–1.10	6.3
Valproic acid	6–18	0.09–0.13	10–70	0.09–0.13	144	84–94	0.01–0.27	4.8
Vigabatrin (S, R enantiomers)[d]	5–11	1.16–1.85	5–11	–	129	0	S-: 0.04–0.22 R-: 0.14–0.87	9.72 4.02
Zonisamide	63	–	61–109	–	212	40	0.93	10.2

[a] The ratio between drug concentrations in breast milk and that in maternal plasma
[b] Treated with an enzyme inducer
[c] Concomitant other antiepileptics
[d] S-vigabatrin: active moiety; R-vigabatrin: inactive moiety

Determinants of infant drug exposure levels

Drug exposure of breastfed infants may be evaluated through the amount of drugs they ingest via breast milk. One of the direct methods to assess infant drug exposure is to measure the infant's serum/plasma drug concentrations [12]. Unfortunately, this approach is difficult to implement as it faces numerous ethical issues, especially in infants without symptoms. Hence, various surrogate endpoints are often used.

Indices of infant drug exposure

"Infant dose" described below is clearly the most basic index, which can be compared to an infant therapeutic dose, if known, or to a maternal dose per body weight basis (maternal weight-adjusted infant dose: see 2 below).

1. **Infant dose** (per body weight) is an estimated dose of drugs in milk ingested by an infant over a unit of time. It can be calculated from drug concentration in milk multiplied by an estimated milk volume ingested per day.

    $$\text{Infant dose}(\text{mg/kg/day}) = \text{drug concentration in milk}(\text{mg/L}) \times$$
    $$\text{volume of milk ingested per kilogram body weight per day}(\text{L/kg/day})$$

    Since the volume of ingested milk is not usually known, the estimated volume of 0.15L/kg/day may be used as a reference value for a mature infant, although it is likely to overestimate the actual ingested milk volume and infant dose. This estimated volume is often used for exclusively breastfed infants, until 4–6 months of age. The volume of milk intake then gradually decreases afterwards as the infant starts solids. The infant dose is best utilized by direct comparisons to known therapeutic doses of the drug in a neonate or infant. One of the challenges in an approach based on a drug concentration in milk, such as "infant dose" and "maternal weight-adjusted infant dose" (below), is a difficulty in estimating the average drug concentration in milk over time. In order to circumvent this, a maximum concentration is often used to estimate the infant drug exposure. The derived parameter called "maximum infant dose" is obviously an overestimate of the infant dose, and therefore must be interpreted cautiously

2. **Maternal weight-adjusted infant dose** is a widely used index for assessing an infant's drug safety during breastfeeding, because the infant "therapeutic" dose is not always established [6]. This index is expressed as a percentage of the dose per kilogram body weight of an infant received via milk (infant dose: see above) to maternal daily dose standardized by the mother's weight.

    $$\text{Maternal weight} - \text{adjusted infant dose } (\%) = \frac{\text{Infant dose per kg/day} \times 100}{\text{Maternal dose per kg/day}}$$

    This index is interpreted based on maternal usual therapeutic dose. The value of less than 10% may be considered inconsequential for pharmacological effects [6]. Clearly, if the infant "therapeutic" dose is substantially different from the maternal therapeutic dose, then the maternal weight-adjusted infant dose would lead to under- or over-estimation of the true infant exposure levels.

Table 18.2: Main responsible enzymes for metabolism of antiepileptics [9, 13]

Drug-metabolizing enzyme	Antiepileptics as a substrate
CYP3A (CYP3A4, 3A5, and 3A7)	carbamazepine, clobazam, clonazepam, ethosuximide, felbamate, phenytoin, tiagabine, valproic acid, zonisamide
CYP2C9	phenobarbital, phenytoin, valproic acid
CYP2C19	clobazam, phenobarbital, phenytoin, primidone
UGT	lamotrigine, valproic acid, oxcarbazepine

Infant drug clearance

In addition to the infant dose, drug clearance in breastfed infants is an important factor in determining the extent of the drug exposure in the infant. Pharmacokinetics of drugs in newborns and infants are different from adults because of their development, especially during the first year of life [13]. Moreover, individuals vary in their maturation rate. The elimination of drugs occurs mainly by either hepatic biotransformation or renal excretion. The function of both the liver and kidneys is relatively immature in neonates, thus making them prone to drug accumulation [9].

Through metabolism mainly in the liver, which is commonly divided into two phases, drugs are converted to more hydrophilic compounds. Phase I drug metabolism involves reactions such as oxidation, reduction, and hydrolysis, producing metabolites ready to undergo Phase II reactions. Phase II reaction represents conjugation (the addition of a small molecule to the drug), which includes glucuronidation (the addition of glucuronide), acetylation (the addition of an acetyl group), and sulphation (the addition of a sulphate group). Conjugated metabolites are water-soluble, and amenable to renal excretion.

As shown in Table 18.2, the main metabolizing enzymes may be identified for each of the antiepileptic drugs. Cytochrome P450 (CYP) enzymes represent groups of the main drug-metabolizing enzymes involved in phase I reactions. Major members of the CYP3A subfamily (i.e., CYP3A4, 3A5, and 3A7) are responsible for the metabolism of carbamazepine, clobazam, clonazepam, ethosuximide, felbamate, tiagabine, and zonisamide [9]. CYP3A4 and 3A7 have overlapping substrate specificity, but there is a clear developmental stage-specific expression of CYP3A4 and CYP3A7. Namely, CYP3A7 activity is very high in fetus and neonates, then rapidly declines to undetectable levels in most children and adults [14]. CYP3A4, the predominant CYP3A enzyme in adults, has very low activity levels at birth and gradually increases in the newborn period. Furthermore, premature neonates have lower CYP3A4 activity levels than full-term neonates. The CYP3A7 content remains higher than CYP3A4 until at least 6 months of age [13].

CYP2C9 and CYP2C19 have a role in metabolizing both phenytoin and phenobarbital. The ontogeny of CYP2C9 is better established compared to CYP2C19 [13]. The level of CYP2C9 activity is very low during fetal development. After birth, its activity increases dramatically during the first year of life [13, 14]. Like CYP3A, the activity of CYP2C9 in premature neonates is lower than term neonates. This corresponds with prolonged phenytoin half-life in pre-term newborns (approximately 75 hours), as opposed to approximately 20 hours in term neonates. Moreover, the phenytoin half-life in term neonates further decreases to approximately 8 hours after the second week of life [14].

In phase II reaction, glucuronosyltransferases (UGT) are enzymes responsible for the glucuronidation of antiepileptics, including lamotrigine (UGT1A4), valproic acid (UGT2B1), and oxcarbazepine [9]. Glucuronidation activity is low in neonates as a result of a low level of UGT. Maturation of UGT appears to be relatively slow and reaches adult values by 3–4 years of age [15].

Renal function in neonates is as low as 25% of the adult level per body weight basis, and the maturation is highly dependent on gestational age. Consequently, renal maturation in the pre-term neonates tends to occur more slowly than term neonates [14]. During the first 2 weeks of life, the renal function develops significantly due to the increase in renal blood flow, which allows for the additional recruitment of functional nephrons. Nevertheless, the overall renal function in the newborn period is still reduced and glomerular filtration rate (GFR) per body weight basis is only 25–30% of adult in term neonates, and even lower in premature neonates. The renal function increases to 50–75% of the adult level by 6 months of age, reaching the adult level by 2–3 years of life [9]. Theoretically, antiepileptic drugs eliminated by kidneys, particularly gabapentin, levetiracetam, and vigabatrin, may have prolonged excretion in the early neonatal period [9]. However, the amount of these drugs in milk is usually too low to cause accumulation in the neonate, although one study showed very low serum levetiracetam concentrations in breastfed infants [16].

In summary, as a result of reduced clearance, neonates and infants are at an increased risk of drug accumulation and their adverse effects if the drug amount in milk is sufficiently high and the exposure is prolonged.

Exposure Index

The Exposure Index has been proposed [17] as a theoretical indicator of a steady-state exposure of suckling infants to drugs in breast milk. An Exposure Index of 100% indicates the infant dose of the drug through breast milk is the same as the therapeutic dose (if known) for the infant. This index combines two independent factors, which are drug clearance (i.e., a pharmacokinetic parameter) and the MP ratio (i.e., a physicochemical parameter) [17]. The Exposure Index is directly proportional to the MP ratio and inversely proportional to the rate of clearance of the drug by the infant, as follows:

$$\text{Exposure Index}(\%) = [(A \times MP \text{ ratio})/\text{infant drug clearance}] \times 100$$

Where A is estimated milk intake (150 ml/kg/day or 0.1 ml/kg/min) and clearance is expressed as ml/kg/min. In this chapter, we also derive a maximum Exposure Index to estimate a maximum level by using the highest reported MP ratio and the lowest reported infant clearance on the drug in question. Similarly, the minimum Exposure Index was estimated by using the lowest reported MP ratio and the highest reported infant clearance of the drug of interest (Table 18.3).

The above equation is visually shown in Figure 18.1. Since the relation of the Exposure Index to infant drug clearance can be described in a hyperbolic curve at a given MP ratio, it is readily apparent that the Exposure Index becomes very high at a low clearance. If the infant drug clearance is low (e.g., renal dysfunction, or extreme prematurity), the MP ratio may have substantial impact on the exposure level. Hence, both the amount of drug transfer into the milk and infant pharmacokinetics (namely drug clearance) are important determinants of the exposure levels [1, 7, 17].

Table 18.3: Indices of drug excretion into milk with summary of adverse drug reactions in nursing infants of mothers treated with antiepileptic drugs [8, 9, 16]

Drugs	Serum drug level in breastfed infant (mg/l)[a]	Recommended therapeutic range (mg/l)	Drug level in breast milk (mg/l)[a]	Estimated infant dose (mg/kg/day)[b]	Recommended therapeutic dose in children (mg/kg/day)[a]	Maternal weight-adjusted infant dose (%)	Exposure Index (%)[c]	Reported adverse drug reactions[e] n case/n total[d]	Comments
Carbamazepine	0–2.6	5–10	0–6.7	1	10–20	0.4–8	3–8.6	9/36	**Monotherapy:** Transient cholestatic jaundice (three infants); and poor suckling (two). **Polytherapy:** Withdrawal symptoms (one: also exposed to phenobarbital and primidone); transient seizure-like activity (one: also exposed to fluoxetine and buspirone); and drowsiness (two: also exposed to phenytoin and primidone in one infant and phenytoin and clemastine in the other).
Carbamazepine Epoxide[f]	0–0.6	0.4–4	0–3.7						
Clobazam	-	-	0.13–033[g]	0.02–0.05	0.1–1	3–7.5[f]	1.5–7.5	-	-
Clonazepam	0.001–0.02	-	0.001–0.013	0.0002–0.002	0.01–0.03	2.5	-	3/35	**Monotherapy:** Periodic breathing (one infant); sedation (one); and

Table 18.3: (cont.)

Drugs	Serum drug level in breastfed infant (mg/l)[a]	Recommended therapeutic range (mg/l)	Drug level in breast milk (mg/l)[a]	Estimated infant dose (mg/kg/day)[b]	Recommended therapeutic dose in children (mg/kg/day)[a]	Maternal weight-adjusted infant dose (%)	Exposure Index (%)[c]	Reported adverse drug reactions[e] n case/n total[d]	Comments
									poor weight gain at 4 weeks of age (one).
Ethosuximide	16.9–29.5	40–80	18–70	2.7–10.5	15–40	32–115	–	2/5	**Monotherapy:** Hyperexcitability (one infant). **Polytherapy:** Sedation (one: also exposed to primidone and valproic acid).
Felbamate	–	–	–	–	15–45	–	–	–	–
Gabapentin	UD–0.4	–	1.2–8.7	0.18–1.3	10–15	1.3–3.8	3.8–5.6	0/8	–
Lamotrigine	<0.1–12.7	3–14	0.5–11.8	0.08–1.8	2	3.1–32.5	1.7–74	9/94	**Monotherapy:** Apnea (one infant; withdrawal symptoms after abruptly discontinued breastfeeding (one); and isolated elevated platelet count without adverse clinical effects (seven).

Levetiracetam	-	0.7–13	4.8–35.7	0.7–5.4	10	7.9	-	2/20	**Polytherapy**: Poor suckling (one infant: also exposed to phenytoin and valproic acid); and suspected withdrawal seizure (one: also exposed to primidone).
Oxcarbazepine	-	<0.1–0.1	0.2–1	0.03–0.15	8–10	1.5–1.7[f]	-	0/6	–
10-hydroxy-oxcarbazepine[h]		<0.1–0.2	2.85–10.4	0.43–1.56					
Phenobarbital	15–40	1–54.7	0.5–33	3–5	0.08–4.95	23–156	26–161	6/6	**Monotherapy**: Drowsiness (one infant); withdrawal symptoms after abruptly discontinued breastfeeding (one). **Polytherapy**: Methemoglobinemia, drowsiness, and poor suckling (one: also exposed to phenytoin); drowsiness and poor weight gain (one: also exposed to carbamazepine and primidone); withdrawal symptoms (one: also exposed to carbamazepine and

Table 18.3: (cont.)

Drugs	Serum drug level in breastfed infant (mg/l)[a]	Recommended therapeutic range (mg/l)	Drug level in breast milk (mg/l)[a]	Estimated infant dose (mg/kg/day)[b]	Recommended therapeutic dose in children (mg/kg/day)[a]	Maternal weight-adjusted infant dose (%)	Exposure Index (%)[c]	Reported adverse drug reactions[e] n case/n total[d]	Comments
									primidone in the other); and death (one: also exposed to phenytoin and primidone).
Phenytoin	0.13–0.2	10–20	0.26–4.2	0.04–0.63	5–8	0.5–8.9	2.1–110	8/36	**Monotherapy:** Withdrawal symptoms (two infants). **Polytherapy:** Drowsiness (four: also exposed to carbamazepine and clemastine in one infant, carbamazepine and primidone in the second infant, phenobarbital, primidone, and sulthiame in the third infant, and primidone in the last infant); methemoglobinemia, drowsiness, and poor suckling (one: also exposed to

phenobarbital); and death (one: also exposed to phenobarbital and primidone).								**Polytherapy:** Drowsiness (four infants: also exposed to carbamazepine and phenytoin in one infant, ethosuximide and valproic acid in the second infant, phenobarbital, phenytoin, and sulthiame in the third infant, and valproic acid in the last infant); withdrawal seizure (two: also exposed to carbamazepine and phenobarbital and phenobarbital in one infant, levetiracetam in the other); and death (one: also exposed to phenobarbital and phenytoin).
Primidone	0.7–2.5	5–12	0.8–13.7	0.12–2	12–20	18.5	–	7/9

Table 18.3: (cont.)

Drugs	Serum drug level in breastfed infant (mg/l)[a]	Recommended therapeutic range (mg/l)	Drug level in breast milk (mg/l)[a]	Estimated infant dose (mg/kg/day)[b]	Recommended therapeutic dose in children (mg/kg/day)[a]	Maternal weight-adjusted infant dose (%)	Exposure Index (%)[c]	Reported adverse drug reactions[e] n case/n total[d]	Comments
Tiagabine	-	-	-	-	32–56[i]	-	-	0/1	-
Topiramate	0.5–0.8	5–20	0.61–5.50	0.1–0.8	3–5	3–23	-	1/10	**Monotherapy:** Diarrhea (one infant).
Valproic acid	<0.004–14	50–100	0.18–7.20	0.03–1.08	10–20	0.4–7	0.77–30	2/16	**Monotherapy:** Thrombocytopenic purpura and anemia (one infant). **Polytherapy:** Drowsiness (one: also exposed to primidone).
Vigabatrin (S-enantiomer)[j]	-	-	0.26–1.07	0.04–0.16	50–150	0.001–0.005	-	-	-
Zonisamide	3.6–3.9	-	4.6–19.2	0.69–2.88	5–8	23–28	-	0/1	-

[a] Range
[b] Range of drug concentration in breast milk x 0.15 L/kg/day of milk intake
[c] $\frac{\text{Range of milk-to-plasma drug-concentration ratio}}{\text{Range of drug clearance in children}}$ ×100, based on the best and the worst case calculation
Range of drug clearance in children
[d] Number of infants with reported adverse events over total number of reported infant effects
[e] All reported adverse reactions were complicated with in utero exposure
[f] Active metabolite of carbamazepine
[g] Parent drug and its active metabolite
[h] Active metabolite of oxcarbazepine
[i] Adult dose; no established dose in neonate and pediatric
[j] Active moiety of vigabatrin
UD = undetectable

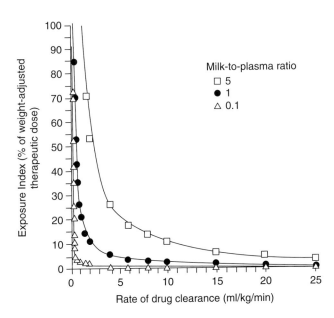

Figure 18.1: This graph shows the relation between the exposure levels and the infant clearance at 3 different milk to plasma ratios. Exposure index (EI) of 100% means that drug dose the infant would ingest through milk (per kg per day) is the same as the daily drug dose given to the infant for therapeutic purposes (per kg per day) [11].

As described above, the Exposure Index is conceptually equivalent to the infant dose that is expressed as a percentage of the infant therapeutic dose. Alternatively, it can be considered as a mean, steady-state serum drug concentration of breastfed infants, which is achieved after exposure to that drug in breast milk, and which is expressed as a percentage of the corresponding infant therapeutic serum level. An Exposure Index of less than 10% may be considered pharmacologically insignificant [7]. It is also important to note that many drugs have clearance values greater than 2–3 ml/kg/min in an adult. Even if the infant clearance is 25–50% of the adult level initially, it increases steadily during the infantile period. Given that most drugs have an MP ratio of one or less, infant exposure levels for most drugs in breast milk are predicted to be pharmacologically insignificant.

Maternal adherence during breastfeeding

As benefits of breastfeeding are evident, most mothers are willing to nurse their infants. This is reflected by high and increasing breastfeeding initiation rates in both developed and developing countries [18, 19]. However, when mothers need to take medication, they are often concerned about their drugs having adverse effects on their infants, which leads them to discontinue breastfeeding [20], even though most antiepileptic drugs are not contraindicated during breastfeeding and most of these infants born to epileptic mothers have already been exposed to antiepileptic drugs in utero. One study reported epileptic women tended to breastfeed at about half the rate of control subjects, and for a substantially shorter duration [21]. Moreover, less reassuring advice from physicians about the compatibility of drugs during breastfeeding is associated with a higher incidence of cessation of breastfeeding [21]. In contrast, reassuring advice is associated with a better chance of continuation of breastfeeding [20]. As described above, duration of breastfeeding in women on antiepileptics is shorter than control subjects. However, it is not known whether milk production is compromised in those women treated with antiepileptics.

Specific antiepileptic drugs in lactation

Carbamazepine

Carbamazepine is considered compatible with breastfeeding because the maximum estimated infant dose received via milk is far below the recommended initial therapeutic pediatric dosage (Table 18.3). Indeed, infant serum carbamazepine levels are usually below the therapeutic range [16]. Most infants have had no adverse reactions but sedation, poor suckling, and three cases of transient cholestatic jaundice have been reported [16]. These cases have all been complicated with intrauterine exposure and, in some cases, concurrent drug therapy. A study which assessed cognitive function at 3 years of age of infants whose mothers were exposed to antiepileptic drugs found no difference in the average intelligence quotient between breastfed (n = 26) and non-breastfed infants (n = 32) whose mothers were taking carbamazepine [22].

Clobazam

Data of clobazam use during lactation showed the maximum estimated infant dose received via milk is below the recommended therapeutic pediatric dosage (Table 18.3). Neither serum clobazam concentrations nor adverse effects in breastfed infants are published to date [16]. Breastfeeding during clobazam therapy is justified with monitoring of the infant for sedation and poor suckling [8].

Clonazepam

Only a few cases of breastfeeding with clonazepam have been reported, and all those cases have been complicated with its use during pregnancy. The maximum estimated infant dose through milk is below the recommended therapeutic pediatric dosage (Table 18.3). The highest maternal weight-adjusted infant dose is reportedly 2.5%. The Exposure Index cannot be calculated due to lack of pediatric clonazepam clearance. A study of the infants breastfed by the mother on benzodiazepines found a low rate of sedation (2/124; 1.6%), which was not correlated with the maternal doses or the length of breastfeeding hours [16]. Although most infants in these published reports have not experienced any adverse effects (Table 18.3), it is recommended to monitor breastfed infants for central nervous system depression or apnea [16].

Withdrawal symptoms in the neonates from intrauterine drug exposure are well known for some drugs, such as opioids and benzodiazepines. There are reports of alleviation of methadone withdrawal in the infants when they are breastfed by the mothers receiving methadone. However, no report has been published which clearly associates maternal benzodiazepine use during breastfeeding with improvement of the infant withdrawal symptoms. One study showed that breast milk intake had beneficial effects on the severity and outcome of neonatal withdrawal symptoms among the infants of the mothers who were abusing drugs, including benzodiazepines and opioids, although benzodiazepine-specific data were not shown in that study [23]. The existing data on benzodiazepine excretion into human milk suggest that the amount of the drugs in milk is insufficient for such effects.

Ethosuximide

Ethosuximide results in a high estimated infant dose through milk, which ranges from 18% to 70% of a recommended therapeutic dose of an infant (Table 18.3). The maternal weight-adjusted infant dose and the Exposure Index are similarly high. Adverse effects in breastfed infants were observed in two out of the five reported cases [16]. If a mother is willing to breastfeed, the infant should be monitored for drowsiness, inadequate weight gain, and hyperexcitability. A measurement of the serum ethosuximide level can be performed when toxicity is suspected [16].

Felbamate

No studies of felbamate during breastfeeding have been published. There has been a report of felbamate toxicity in an adult by the manufacturer, including fatal aplastic anemia and acute liver failure. Therefore, breastfeeding is not recommended during felbamate treatment because of the lack of evidence-based safety data and the potential serious toxicity [8, 24].

Gabapentin

Maternal use of gabapentin is associated with relatively low levels in breastfed infant serum. The maximum estimated infant dose through milk is only 13% of the recommended therapeutic dose (Table 18.3). Both the maternal weight-adjusted infant dose and the Exposure Index are well below 10%. There have been eight cases of gabapentin treatment during breastfeeding published to date and none of the breastfed infants experienced any adverse effects [16]. Until more data are available, however, gabapentin should be used with caution during breastfeeding and the infant should be monitored for adverse effects [8].

Lamotrigine

Lamotrigine has increased in popularity for epilepsy treatment as well as some psychiatric conditions [25]. Its use during breastfeeding is of concern due to a relatively high concentration in breast milk, as it has low plasma protein-binding [25]. Moreover, breastfed infants have a limited ability to metabolize this drug by glucuronidation, posing a risk of accumulation. This may be further enhanced by precipitous rise of maternal lamotrigine plasma concentrations during the postpartum period if the dose remains the same as in pregnancy. Several studies reported the estimated infant dose through milk, and plasma lamotrigine concentrations in breastfed infants whose mothers were taking lamotrigine were relatively high, sometimes reaching therapeutic ranges [25]. The reported highest maternal weight-adjusted infant dose was 33%. The maximum Exposure Index was 74% (Table 18.3). Despite these facts, many infants are breastfed without problems while mothers are on lamotrigine. There is one case report of serious apnea, which is questionable in its causative link to the drug. Another case report described an infant who developed apparent withdrawal symptoms after an abrupt discontinuation of breastfeeding. Thrombocytosis without adverse clinical effects has also been reported in seven out of eight infants tested, although the causative link to the drug is unclear [16]. A long-term study of cognitive function of the infants exposed to lamotrigine through breastfeeding showed no difference in the average intelligence quotient between breastfed (n = 30) and non-breastfed infants (n = 36) at 3 years of age [22]. In summary, lamotrigine during breastfeeding is not contraindicated. However, breastfed infants should be carefully monitored for side effects such as apnea or poor suckling. If there is a concern, measuring the infant serum lamotrigine level can rule out toxicity.

Levetiracetam

Levetiracetam levels in breast milk are highly variable among individuals, leading to a wide range of the estimated infant dose through milk (Table 18.3). The reported maternal weight-adjusted infant dose is less than 10% (Table 18.3). Adverse effects in breastfed infants whose mothers were taking levetiracetam have been reported in two cases, which include poor suckling and withdrawal seizures. However, the causes of these adverse events are debatable as there were other concomitant antiepileptic drugs. Despite these, studies have shown that many infants are safely breastfed during levetiracetam treatment. A usual management plan is to allow breastfeeding with clinical observation for adverse effects such as poor suckling and inadequate weight gain [16].

Oxcarbazepine

Oxcarbazepine is metabolized mainly by a glucuronidation pathway, which is immature in neonates. Therefore, breastfed infants whose mothers take this drug are potentially at risk of drug accumulation. However, studies reveal the oxcarbazepine concentration in milk is relatively low [9]. The estimated infant dose through milk is well below the recommended therapeutic dose, and the maternal weight-adjusted infant dose is less than 10% (Table 18.3). Only six cases of breastfed infants exposed to oxcarbazepine in milk have been published to date, showing no adverse effects. As with other new antiepileptic drugs, monitoring of the breastfed infant for drowsiness, adequate weight gain, and developmental milestones is recommended [16].

Phenobarbital

Neonates and infants have very low phenobarbital clearance, which may cause drug accumulation and increase in a blood concentration to a potential therapeutic level. The maximum estimated infant dose through milk is also within the therapeutic range (Table 18.3). Both the maternal weight-adjusted infant dose and the Exposure Index are relatively high (Table 18.3). A number of adverse effects in breastfed infants have been reported, including drowsiness, poor weight gain, methemoglobinemia, withdrawal symptoms, as well as death (Table 18.3). Although not contraindicated, a decision on breastfeeding during phenobarbital therapy should take into consideration the mother's previous experience with breastfeeding, the infant's underlying conditions, if any, and the accessibility to health care providers [8]. If concerns arise, a measurement of the infant serum phenobarbital concentration is warranted.

Phenytoin

The estimated infant dose through milk is far below the recommended therapeutic dose (Table 18.3). The highest reported maternal weight-adjusted infant dose is 8.9% (Table 18.3). However, the clearance of phenytoin in neonates and infants is markedly variable and some infants may have a very low clearance [9]. As a result, the Exposure Index based on clearance estimates shows a high variability ranging from 2% to 110% of the therapeutic dose, although the average exposure is considered to be small. In breastfed infants whose mothers took phenytoin with other antiepileptic drugs, adverse effects have been reported, including drowsiness, poor suckling, methemoglobinemia, and withdrawal effects (Table 18.3). In general, phenytoin is considered compatible with breastfeeding by many experts [8, 9, 16, 24]. More importantly, the cognitive function at 3 years of age of infants whose mothers were exposed to phenytoin during pregnancy and breastfeeding showed no difference in the intelligence quotient between breastfed (n = 17) and non-breastfed infants (n = 23) [22].

Primidone

Primidone is converted to phenobarbital, and has low plasma protein-binding. Due to its low clearance, the maternal weight-adjusted infant dose is relatively high (Table 18.3). Adverse effects in breastfed infants have been reported, including sedation, inadequate weight gain, withdrawal seizure and even death. However, the causes of these adverse effects were complicated by other factors, including concomitant drug therapies with other anti-epileptic drugs [16]. Monitoring the infant for adverse effects is crucial and if any concerns arise, the measurement of an infant serum drug concentration is informative if the infant is symptomatic.

Tiagabine

No study regarding tiagabine concentrations in milk has been published. The recommendation of breastfeeding during tiagabine treatment cannot be made at this time because of lack of evidence-based safety data.

Topiramate

Excretion of topiramate into breast milk is minimal. Hence, the estimated infant dose through milk and infant serum drug concentration are well below the therapeutic range (Table 18.3). The maternal weight-adjusted infant dose ranges from 3% to 23% (Table 18.3). Only 1 out of 10 reported infants had an adverse event of diarrhea while the mothers took topiramate, although the causal relationship is not clear. Topiramate can be used during breastfeeding with the monitoring of the breastfed infant for any adverse effects [16].

Valproic acid

Valproic acid is considered compatible with breastfeeding because it is excreted into human milk in low concentrations and the maximum estimated infant dose through milk is well below the therapeutic range (Table 18.3). The highest reported maternal weight-adjusted infant dose was 7% (Table 18.3). Moreover, the reported plasma valproic acid concentrations of infants whose mothers were treated with this drug are all below the therapeutic range. However, a wide variation of the Exposure Index ranging from 0.77% to 30% (Table 18.3) is predicted because valproic acid is metabolized by glucuronidation, which is not fully developed in neonates and young infants. This suggests that greater than 10% of the therapeutic plasma level may be observed if clearance remains low in extreme circumstances. Although valproic acid is contraindicated in children less than 2 years of age due to the potential hepatotoxicity, no such case was reported in nursing infants whose mothers were taking this drug. There is, however, a case report of an infant exposed to valproic acid through breastfeeding who showed anemia and thrombocytopenia. Both abnormalities resolved fully after cessation of breastfeeding. Another case of drowsiness was reported while the mother was taking valproic acid in combination with primidone. One long-term study investigating the cognitive function at 3 years of age of infants whose mothers were exposed to valproic acid found no difference in the average intelligence quotient between breastfed (n = 11) and non-breastfed infants (n = 24) [22].

Vigabatrin

Only a small amount of vigabatrin is excreted into breast milk. The estimated infant dose through milk is far below the therapeutic range (Table 18.3). The maternal weight-adjusted infant dose is less than 0.1% (Table 18.3). Unfortunately, no data on infant serum concentration, infant drug clearance, and adverse effects reported in breastfed infants are available. The minimal amount of vigabatrin excreted to breast milk justifies breastfeeding [8].

Zonisamide

Zonisamide is excreted at relatively high levels in milk. The maternal weight-adjusted infant dose ranges from 23% to 28% (Table 18.3). Only one breastfed infant whose mother was taking zonisamide and other unspecified antipsychotics reported not having any adverse effects [16]. Zonisamide is metabolized by CYP3A4, which shows a steady increase in its expression throughout the infantile period. Therefore, zonisamide exposure levels of the infant through breast milk are likely to decrease continually. Given the limited information, however, monitoring of breastfed infants for any adverse effects is advisable.

Drug interaction with domperidone

Some epileptic mothers may take domperidone as a galactogogue during breastfeeding. As domperidone is a substrate of CYP3A4, it has the potential to interact with some antiepileptics that share the same CYP3A4 metabolizing pathway. However, there is no report of clinically significant interactions to date.

Summary

In conclusion, most antiepileptic drugs are not contraindicated during breastfeeding. The benefits of breastfeeding to both infants and their mothers need to be clearly communicated to patients. However, given the lack of extensive safety information, monitoring breastfed infants for any adverse effects is also crucial.

References

1. Tomson T and Battino D. Antiepileptic treatment in pregnant women: morphological and behavioural effects. In: Seyberth HW, Rane A and Schwab M, eds. *Pediatric clinical pharmacology, handbook of experimental pharmacology 205*. Berlin, Heidelberg: Springer Verlag, 2011; 295–315.

2. Pennell PB. 2005 AES annual course: evidence used to treat women with epilepsy. *Epilepsia* 2006; 47(Suppl 1):46–53.

3. Harden CL, Meador KJ, Pennell PB, et al. Practice parameter update: management issues for women with epilepsy-focus on pregnancy (an evidence-based review): teratogenesis and perinatal outcomes. *Neurology* 2009; 73:133–41.

4. Ip S, Chung M, Raman G, et al. A summary of the Agency for Healthcare Research and Quality's evidence report on breastfeeding in developed countries. *Breastfeed Med* 2009; 4:S17–S30.

5. Kramer MS, Aboud F, Mironova E, et al. Breastfeeding and child cognitive development: new evidence from a large randomized trial. *Arch Gen Psychiatry* 2008; 65:578–84.

6. Ilett KF and Kristensen JH. Drug use and breastfeeding. *Expert Opin Drug Saf* 2005; 4:745–68.

7. Ito S and Lee A. Drug excretion into breast milk-overview. *Adv Drug Deliv Rev* 2003; 55:617–27.

8. Bar-Oz B, Nulman I, Koren G, et al. Anticonvulsants and breast feeding: a critical review. *Paediatr Drugs* 2000; 2:113–26.

9. Hovinga CA and Pennell PB. Antiepileptic drug therapy in pregnancy II: fetal and neonatal exposure. *Int Rev Neurobiol* 2008; 83:241–58.

10. Stika C and Frederiksen M. Drug therapy in pregnant and nursing women. In: Atkinson AJ, Abernethy D, Daniels C, et al., eds. *Principles of clinical pharmacology.* Burlington, VT: Academic Press, 2007; 339–57.

11. Ito S. Drug therapy for breast-feeding women. *New Eng J Med* 2000; 343:118–26.

12. McNamara PJ and Abbassi M. Neonatal exposure to drugs in breast milk. *Pharm Res* 2004; 21:555–66.

13. Anker JN, Schwab M and Kearns GL. Developmental pharmacokinetics. In: Seyberth HW, Rane A and Schwab M, eds. *Pediatric clinical pharmacology, handbook of experimental pharmacology 205.* Berlin, Heidelberg: Verlag Springer, 2011; 51–75.

14. Kearns GL, Abdel-Rahman SM, Alander SW, et al. Developmental pharmacology-drug disposition, action, and therapy in infants and children. *New Eng J Med* 2003; 349:1157–67.

15. Anderson Gail D. Children versus adults: pharmacokinetic and adverse-effect differences. *Epilepsia* 2002; 43:53–9.

16. Drug and lactation database (LactMed). http://toxnet.nlm.nih.gov.

17. Ito S and Koren G. A novel index for expressing exposure of the infant to drugs in breast milk. *Br J Clin Pharmacol* 1994; 38: 99–102.

18. Bhutta ZA, Chopra M, Axelson H, et al. Countdown to 2015 decade report (2000–10): taking stock of maternal, newborn, and child survival. *Lancet* 2010; 375:2032–44.

19. Callen J and Pinelli J. Incidence and duration of breastfeeding for term infants in Canada, United States, Europe, and Australia: a literature review. *Birth* 2004; 31:285–92.

20. Ito S, Lieu M, Chan W, et al. Continuing drug therapy while breastfeeding. Part 1. Common misconceptions of patients. *Can Fam Physician* 1999; 45:897–9.

21 . Ito S, Moretti M, Liau M, et al. Initiation and duration of breast-feeding in women receiving antiepileptics. *Am J Obstet Gynecol* 1995; 172:881–6.

22. Meador KJ, Baker GA, Browning N, et al. Effects of breastfeeding in children of women taking antiepileptic drugs. *Neurology* 2010; 75:1954–60.

23. Abdel-Latif ME, Pinner J, Clews S, et al. Effects of breast milk on the severity and outcome of neonatal abstinence syndrome among infants of drug-dependent mothers. *Pediatrics* 2006; 117: e1163–e9.

24. Hagg S and Spigset O. Anticonvulsant use during lactation. *Drug Saf* 2000; 22:425–40.

25. Madadi P and Ito S. Perinatal exposure to maternal lamotrigine: clinical considerations for the mother and child. *Can Fam Physician* 2010; 56:1132–4.

Postpartum safety issues for women with epilepsy

Diane T. Sundstrom and Patricia Osborne Shafer

Key points:

- Women with epilepsy (WWE) may have a lower knowledge level in childrearing and postpartum concerns
- Having a well-established plan in the event of seizures is important for safety of a WWE and her newborn
- Plans should involve a WWE's partner, family members, and extended network of support
- Building confidence in a WWE's ability to safely care for her newborn is a key feature in postpartum safety counseling

Introduction

Becoming a parent is a challenge for any woman, yet these challenges may be magnified when the woman is also living with epilepsy. The parent with epilepsy should be competent in multiple self-management skills, have appropriate knowledge of epilepsy and parenting, and have access to supports for seizure management and safe childcare. A key predictor in successful self-management is self-efficacy, or confidence in one's abilities to carry out self-management tasks [1–4]. This finding, seen in many chronic diseases, emphasizes the need to incorporate strategies to enhance a person's self-confidence into health care interactions. Building on self-management approaches, this chapter will address postpartum safety issues for WWE to assist health care professionals in caring for WWE during this critical time.

Learning needs of women with epilepsy

While some information about learning needs of WWE has been documented [5, 6], very little has been written about safety practices in the postpartum phase. May and colleagues [7] found a number of pregnancy-related concerns in addition to safety and parenting needs. Of 365 women between 16 and 75 years old, 40.8% worried about the child's safety when the mother had a seizure and 36% worried that seizures would frighten their child. A prospective study in India of 85 WWE and 85 women without epilepsy matched for age, education, and parity, were evaluated for childrearing knowledge and practices [8]. Participant's baseline knowledge assessed in the first trimester was compared to

Women with Epilepsy, ed. Esther Bui and Autumn Klein. Published by Cambridge University Press.
© Cambridge University Press 2014.

childrearing practices assessed at 3–4 months after delivery. WWE were found to have lower knowledge scores than women without epilepsy, and were rated worse in the child-rearing practices evaluated, e.g., feeding, growth and development, cleaning, protection, and infant stimulation. However, health care professionals must realize that providing information to women about pregnancy and safety does not ensure that it is understood, remembered, or able to be used. Bell and colleagues [9] assessed the recall of 795 WWE who were given information about childrearing. Topics pertaining to safety in child care and breastfeeding were recalled at lower rates (24%) than topics pertaining to other women's health needs.

A pilot study of self-management behaviors in 45 WWE attending a tertiary epilepsy center found that the majority of respondents reported that they did not use any different safety practices, or care for their children differently, than a woman without epilepsy [10]. While these studies highlight potential safety gaps, findings cannot be generalized to all WWE. Different groups of people were sampled from different countries and backgrounds. However, these studies suggest that it is important to consider potential differences in the type and methods of patient/family education, support systems, and cultural differences when examining health practices.

Common self-management needs in the postpartum period

Self-management is defined as "the sum total of steps a person takes to control seizures and the effects of having a seizure disorder" [11]. Self-management in epilepsy includes both healthy living practices common to many chronic illnesses as well as epilepsy-specific tasks, for example managing seizures, treatments, lifestyle, safety, personal health needs and comorbid conditions, communication, information, stigma, and independent living needs [4, 12–16]. The self-management tasks for women with seizures who have just given birth may cover all these areas, but to varying degrees. For example, some women with well-controlled epilepsy may face little changes in life after pregnancy. However, safety risks, may be higher than pre-pregnancy, suggesting the need to monitor medications, side effects and triggers carefully. Women with persistent or uncontrolled seizures may experience more diverse problems or challenges from seizures, medication changes, and comorbidities.

All women, regardless of seizure control, will experience needs related to being a parent. For newborns and infant care, self-management may include, but are not limited to, feeding, bathing, changing diapers, interacting, stimulating, responding to and establishing sleep habits, carrying, transporting, and keeping a child safe. The following discussion highlights some of the major self-management components and strategies that women will face. Health care professionals should incorporate teaching about postpartum self-management and safety issues early in the course of pregnancy and even during family planning sessions pre-pregnancy.

Managing seizures
Tracking seizures

Since seizures may be different in the postpartum period, it is important that the mother and/or her family records events and shares them with the health care team. Descriptions should include what happened before and during the event, how long it lasted, behaviors involved, presence and description of postictal phase, and any safety concerns. If an intervention was needed (e.g., rectal diazepam, lorazepam, VNS magnet), the effectiveness, frequency of use, and any side effects should also be recorded. This information is important to know when determining the need for medication changes and assessing the safety of mother and child. Since new mothers are usually busy and may put their own needs last, women should have an easy system to use for tracking seizure information. Consider online epilepsy diaries with mobile applications so data can be constantly available and easy to access [17]: for example *My Epilepsy Diary* (www.epilepsy.com), *Seizure Tracker* (www.seizuretracker.com) and *Patients Like Me* (www.patientslikeme.com).

Developing seizure response plans

Ideally, every woman should have a seizure response plan which communicates information about her typical seizures, medications, first aid, when to intervene, and when and who to call for additional help. These documents can be used to communicate critical information during pregnancy, labor and delivery, and the postpartum period to people who may not be familiar with the woman's epilepsy and her management plans [13]. Plans usually work best when they can be individualized between the woman and her health care team and shared among pertinent people involved in her life at home. Family members and any people who may be in the home helping mother and baby should have access to this information and be taught what to do to prevent a potential emergency situation. It is imperative that the mother and her caregivers understand and agree to follow the seizure response and safety plans.

Responding to seizures

Basic seizure first aid for a woman with epilepsy in the postpartum period is the same for any person with epilepsy. However, one must take into consideration that seizures may be manifested or present differently in the postpartum period. First aid for all appropriate seizure types should be reviewed with the new mother and family or friends who may be helping her in the postpartum period. Since most seizures end within seconds to a few minutes, usually no further intervention is needed when a mother has a seizure. However, safety of the mother and child should be assessed, and what to do if another seizure occurs or the seizure or postictal period lasts longer than usual.

Special considerations

It's important for all women with seizures to consider what to do if they have a seizure when they are alone. Establishing a safe environment ahead of time and using appropriate safety precautions can be of tremendous help in these situations. If the woman has an aura, or is not feeling well, encourage her to limit time walking around with the baby by herself. She should have a safe place to put the baby if she feels a seizure beginning, and her home should be set up in a way that limits injury from falls or other movements.

For women with frequent seizures, it may be advisable to have supports available to help her. For example, setting up babysitters when the partner or spouse is out of the home, using daycare services, or family and friends are options to consider. When family supports are lacking, personal care attendants or health aides may help in the home when the mother is more likely to have seizures or when childcare needs are busiest. The length of time that additional help may be needed for mother and/or child will depend on the individual situation. While the first 6–8 weeks postpartum is a time of many changes, women with persistent seizures may need to establish long-term plans for home and childcare help.

Medication management

In the midst of giving birth to a child and preparing to care for a newborn, a mother must also maintain vigilance about her own health. Managing medications is one of the most important self-management tasks and involves multiple steps. With new stressors and competing health needs, women may need additional help to obtain medicines from pharmacies and reminders to take them on schedule, especially since her usual routines have been disrupted and her schedule likely focuses around her baby's needs. The health care professional can help her find new or additional ways to remember medicines, such as electronic reminders or alarms, epilepsy diaries, and pillboxes. The times of pill-taking should be tailored to her new routines. For example, instead of recommending that she take her medicines when she gets up or goes to bed, since this may change frequently, encourage her to take her AEDs after she eats breakfast and dinner, or at another routine time of day. Family and friends can offer reminders in helpful ways by calling at regularly scheduled intervals, helping fill or check a pillbox, picking up medicines at the pharmacy so she does not run out unexpectedly, or setting up mail-order prescriptions. How help is offered and implemented is important. The goal should be to work collaboratively with the mother and her partner and offer help in a way that will help her feel more confident and in control of her life.

During the postpartum phase, a woman's medicine levels will rise with changes in weight and metabolism. If doses were increased during pregnancy, careful attention must be given to proactively working with the woman to adjust AED doses and prevent toxicity and breakthrough seizures. She may have to get antiepileptic drug levels checked more frequently and be more cognizant of side effects or seizures. The health care professional should make sure that they review how to monitor and record side effects, when to make changes recommended by her health care provider, and when to call first and discuss symptoms or changes. Some women may be reluctant to seek help for side effects, misinterpreting symptoms to sleep deprivation, hormonal changes, or stress. They may fear that the provider questions her parenting abilities if she reports problems. Frequent check-in periods, by phone or clinic visits, will provide the mother a chance to talk directly with her provider, explore how she feels and contributing factors, and assess for toxicity and medication changes.

Lifestyle management for triggers

Many people report lifestyle or environmental factors that can increase the likelihood of having a seizure. Some people may have predictable triggers or precipitants, while others may notice that seizures increase or change when a number of variables or precipitants happen at the same time. Sleep deprivation, stress, and anxiety are frequently reported triggers by people with epilepsy, with some people able to self-predict their seizures when sleep deprivation has occurred [18]. WWE after childbirth are theoretically at high risk for seizures, as multiple precipitants are culminating at the same time, e.g., hormonal changes, medication changes, sleep deprivation, stress, and changes in diet, activity, and other routines. Seizure triggers in the postpartum period should be discussed in detail with the mother and her caregivers as a way to reduce seizure risk and maintain the safety of both mother and baby.

Once possible triggers are identified, women should be taught how to modify their lifestyle and environment to lessen the risk of seizure occurrence. For WWE, lifestyle changes and additional supports may be needed to incorporate healthy living strategies. The mother's pre-existing lifestyle will need to be taken into consideration as well as any other neurological problems or comorbid health conditions that may affect her health and lifestyle.

Epilepsy-specific lifestyle modifications may include strategies that the mother takes in addition to general healthy living tips [19, 20]. For example, getting adequate rest is crucial for all mothers, but the consequences for a mother with epilepsy is much different than for a woman without seizures. In WWE during the postpartum period, 8 hours of sleep within a 24-hor period is recommended. Typical strategies for a mother who is not getting enough sleep due to breastfeeding or waking up frequently may be for her to rest when the baby sleeps [21]. However, for the woman with epilepsy who is sensitive to sleep deprivation, short frequent naps can lead to poor quality of sleep and aggravate seizures. Recommendations for the mother with epilepsy may include encouraging the spouse/partner to do the nighttime feedings, hire babysitters, or use family/friends to help if needed, to allow longer periods of uninterrupted sleep [21]. Managing stress and mood are other areas that may need extra attention as seizure triggers. Establishing plans ahead of time can help the mother and her partner identify stressors and have a plan and resources for managing them.

Managing mood changes

Changes in mood are an important consideration for every new mother. Health professionals caring for WWE must take into account comorbid conditions, such as developmental delay or pre-existing mood or cognitive problems. Depression and anxiety are frequently reported problems in people with epilepsy and have been found to be a significant factor affecting functional status of people with epilepsy [22]. Assessing mood should therefore be incorporated into the care of all WWE, particularly at high-risk times, such as the postpartum period. Asking about mood and coping may help identify problems early, detect if pre-existing problems are worsening over time, or if a change in mood is typical in the postpartum period. If mood problems are present, referring the mother and partner to appropriate supports, for example psychiatrists, counselors, or support groups, is critical. Home care services by a visiting nurse or social worker may assist in monitoring mood and providing in-home counseling for the homebound mother without other supports, or to provide assistance with other family stressors and childcare.

Parenting safely

Parenting safety is more than just assessing and monitoring the mother's safety; it also includes assessing and monitoring the newborn. This is an ongoing process as the newborn grows and the parents adapt to these changes. Developing safety plans and teaching safety skills is often easiest if done collaboratively, just like seizure response plans, and takes into consideration the mother's seizure characteristics, frequency, and the impact on safety and family.

Developing safety plans

When developing safety plans, a careful assessment of the mother's daily life, activities, seizure type and frequency, triggers, history of injury, or other safety concerns should be obtained [23, 24]. This information will help the health professional, mother, and family identify potential dangers or risks. The following sections include examples of self-management strategies and resources that may make parenting easier and safer for WWE [23, 24, 25].

Preparing meals

To lessen the risk of burns or injuries from cooking, the mother and family may make meals ahead of time that can be frozen, easily thawed, and cooked for mealtimes. Stovetop cooking may be discouraged for a woman if she is having frequent seizures and is alone, or who may be at risk for falling. Using a microwave or crockpot may lessen the risk of burns. Encourage the family to keep the kitchen well stocked with quick and easy food items that can be prepared safely with a minimum amount of time or fuss.

Adequate hydration is more than just a healthy living strategy. It is a critical task for women who have just given birth, but often one that is hard to accomplish. Mothers should be reminded to drink adequate amounts of water, and possibly more if breastfeeding. However, women who are taking AEDs that may cause hyponatremia (e.g., oxcarbazepine, zonisamide) should monitor their sodium levels at appropriate intervals, or if feeling symptomatic. Avoiding beverages or products that contain caffeine, alcohol, or other foods/fluids that may affect seizures, sleep, or breastfeeding is important to convey.

Feeding newborns

The most common reason for sleep deprivation is being up at night to feed the baby. For various health reasons, women in general are encouraged to try breastfeeding their baby for a period of time. Whether or not this is right for each woman should be assessed individually, considering their seizures, medications, triggers, sleep habits, personal preferences and beliefs, other health conditions, and available supports. Health care professionals should consider referring women to lactation specialists for guidance in this area.

Regardless of how the baby is fed, getting adequate sleep is important for the mother's health. It may be possible for the mother to sleep in a separate room or part of the house at times and allow the spouse/partner or family to attend to the baby's needs at night. If the mother is breastfeeding, she may pump and store breast milk to use later in a bottle. Another alternative is to supplement breastfeeding with bottle-feeding as the child grows. Even if it were not possible to be in a quiet or separate area, letting another person take primary night duty would allow the mother to get more uninterrupted sleep.

Home maintenance

Home chores should be re-examined to see which ones may not be safe for the mother to do alone for a while. For example, if a woman has had a seizure recurrence during pregnancy or experiencing medicine side effects during the postpartum period, she may be at greater risk of falling or injury with some household chores. Safety plans may need to include splitting up chores among family members differently, using friends, or seeking paid help for some chores.

Table 19.1: Home safety strategies

- Organize baby care items on all levels to lessen need to climb stairs
- Change baby on the floor or use portable changing pads on floor
- Keep commonly used rooms free of clutter, avoid throw rugs and other fall risks
- Remove or pad objects with hard or sharp edges, avoid glass furniture
- Use safety locks on cupboards and closets, electrical outlet covers, keep cords out of reach
- Feed baby when sitting on a couch, padded floor, or middle of bed
- Bathe baby when someone else is around. Use baby-sized bathtub to provide support and safety with minimum amount of water, rather than the regular bathtub
- Use safety gates on stairs and between rooms when the baby starts to crawl
- Use playpens or enclosed play areas where the baby can stay safe
- Women with frequent seizures or those with falls may consider using a stroller in the house and limit walking around alone with the baby
- Use strollers/carriages walking outside, and take walks with a friend or family member
- Carry personal identification, medical information and, ideally, a cellphone at all times with emergency contact numbers
- Have a system to call for help – pagers, alert systems on phones, or new devices that are able to alert someone if a person falls or has a seizure
- Give a house key to a close friend or family member in case of emergency
- Parents with frequent seizures should speak to their local first responders about their needs and seizure response
- Teach older children what to do in case the mother has a seizure, and how to call for help
- Keep all medications out of reach of children in childproof bottles

Environmental/home safety

Taking stock of the mother and baby's home environment is necessary to identify risks and help her implement reasonable accommodations or changes for safety. Even though the baby is still an infant, the parents should be encouraged to start thinking about "childproofing" the living space right from the beginning. Consider this as a way of assessing the mother's and baby's safety should the mother have a seizure in the home [25]. Table 19.1 suggests some safety strategies to share with women. These ideas are not all inclusive, and health care professionals are encouraged to have women explore parenting safety materials and consider a home safety evaluation by a visiting nurse for individualized onsite help [23, 25].

Getting around

After delivery, it's crucial that health care providers reassess the woman's ability to drive and counsel her and her family about recommendations and laws where she lives. If she had seizures only during pregnancy, the health care provider should be very clear about her ability to drive after the baby is born. A new risk assessment should be conducted considering medication changes, and presence of side effects, seizures, or other safety concerns.

Impact and involvement of family

Parenting is a family affair, and so too is living with epilepsy. In this sense, the term "family" may include partners, children, grandparents, close friends, and other relatives. Involving family and friends is paramount in assisting the mother and her partner to adjust to new roles, and provide for the safety of herself and the baby. It is imperative to assess these resources as soon as possible prior to or during the pregnancy and actively involve family or designated supports. Family meetings or specific visits are often helpful to explore this topic, determining what type of help may be needed, who should be involved, and to what extent.

Family members and close friends may also need assistance in coping with epilepsy. Since epilepsy is often a hidden disorder, people may not have witnessed the mother having seizures prior to pregnancy. They may be frightened, not know what to do, or have fears and misinformation about how seizures affect the woman and her baby. Fears and misinformation need to be addressed early to avoid stigmatizing communications and behaviors that are detrimental to the mother and her child. However, family members may also have important insight about the parent's seizures or parenting issues that the woman does not recall, thus incorporating family into the care of women during the postpartum period and beyond can be helpful for all involved.

Summary

Having a baby opens a new chapter in every woman's life, bringing both opportunities and challenges for the mother and her family. Living with epilepsy may magnify challenges or pose new ones, but early identification and planning can prepare the woman and her family to tackle these issues and use support appropriately. A self-management approach to working with mothers with epilepsy can foster collaborative patient-centered care and assist in devising strategies for managing seizures, treatments, and parenting safely.

References

1. DiIorio C, Faherty B and Manteuffel B. Self-efficacy and social support in self-management of epilepsy. *West J Nurs Res* 1992; 14:292–307.

2. DiIorio C, Faherty B and Manteuffel B. Epilepsy self-management: partial replication and extension. *Res Nurs Health* 1994; 17:167–74.

3. DiIorio C, Hennessy M and Manteuffel B. Epilepsy self-management: a test of a theoretical model. *Nurs Res* 1996; 45:211–17.

4. DiIorio C, Shafer, P, Letz R, et al. Project EASE: A study to test a psychosocial model of epilepsy medication management. *Epilepsy Behav* 2004; 5(6):926–36.

5. Crawford P and Hudson S. Understanding the information needs of women with epilepsy at different lifestages: results of the "Ideal World" survey. *Seizure* 2003; 12(7):502–7.

6. Vazquez B, Gibson P and Kustra R. Epilepsy and women's health issues: unmet needs – survey results from women with epilepsy. *Epilepsy Behav* 2007: 10(1):163–9.

7. May TW, Pfafflin M, Coban I, et al. Fears, knowledge and need of counseling for women with epilepsy. Results of an outpatient study. *Nervenarzt* 2009: 80 (2):174–83. (German)

8. Saramma PP, Sarma PS and Thomas SV. Women with epilepsy have poorer knowledge and skills in childrearing than women without epilepsy. *Seizure* 2011; 20(7):575–9.

9. Bell GS, Nashef L, Kendall S, et al. Information recalled by women taking anti-epileptic drugs for epilepsy: a questionnaire study. *Epilepsy Res* 2002; 52(2):139–46.

10. Shafer PO, DiIorio C, Yeager K, et al. Self-management practices and health behaviors of women with epilepsy. *Epilepsia* 2003; Suppl. 9:285 (Abst 2.320).

11. DiIorio C. Epilepsy self-management. In: Gachman DS, eds. *Handbook of health behavior research II: provider determinants*. New York, NY: Plenum Press, 1997; 213–30.

12. Buelow JM. Epilepsy management issues. *J Neursc Nsg* 2001; 33(5):260–69.

13. Shafer PO. Counseling women with epilepsy. *Epilepsia* 1998; 39(Suppl. 8):S38–S44.

14. Shafer PO and DiIorio C. Managing life issues in epilepsy. *Continuum (mimcocrp mim)* 2004; 10(4):138–56.

15. Shope JT. Intervention to improve compliance with pediatric anticonvulstant therapy. *Patient Coun Health Educ* 1980; 2 (3):135–41.

16. IOM (Institute of Medicine). *Epilepsy across the spectrum: promoting health and understanding.* Washington, DC: The National Academies Press, 2012; Ch.7.

17. Le S, Shafer PO, Bartfeld E, et al. An online diary for tracking epilepsy. *Epil Behav* 2011; 22(4):704–9.

18. Haut SR, Hall CB, Masur J, et al. Seizure occurrence: precipitants and prediction. *Neurology* 2007; 69(20):1905–10.

19. Shafer PO. Nursing support of epilepsy self-management. *Clin Nurs Pract Epilepsy* 1994; 2(1):11–13.

20. Epilepsy Therapy Project. Managing seizure triggers: tips for lifestyle modifications. www.epilepsy.com/pdfs/Lifestyle_modifications_tips.pdf.

21. Callanan M. Parenting for women with epilepsy. In: Morrell MJ and Flynn K, eds. *Women with epilepsy: a handbook of health and treatment issues.* New York, NY: Cambridge University Press, 2003; 228–36.

22. Gilliam F, Hecimovic H and Sheline Y. Psychiatric comorbidity, health and function in epilepsy. *Epilepsy Behav* 2003; 4(Suppl. 4):S26–S30.

23. Dean P. Safety issues for women with epilepsy. In: Morrell MJ and Flynn K, eds. *Women with epilepsy: a handbook of health and treatment issues.* New York: Cambridge University Press, 2003; 263–8.

24. Callanan M and Stalland N. Issues for women with epilepsy. In: Santilli N, ed. *Managing seizure disorders: a handbook for health care professionals.* Philadelphia, PA: Lippincott-Raven Publishers, 1996.

25. Stalland N and Shafer PO. When the parent has epilepsy. In: Santilli N, ed. *Managing seizure disorders: a handbook for health care professionals.* Philadelphia: Lippincott-Raven Publishers, 1996.

Management of the neonate: clinical examination and surveillance

Eugene Ng

Key points:

- When deciding to initiate or continue antiepileptic drugs (AEDs) for seizures during pregnancy, clinicians must balance the risk of potential health and developmental effects on the fetus against the risk of fetal compromise due to inadequate seizure control
- Prenatal consultation with a neonatal practitioner may be beneficial in understanding the potential risks of epilepsy and AEDs on the fetus and newborn
- In the immediate postnatal period, management of newborns exposed to AED in utero should be focused on facilitation of neonatal adaptation and transition, and monitoring for symptoms of drug withdrawal
- The initial assessments of these newborns must include a full physical examination to identify any congenital malformation and detailed anthropometric assessment
- Longitudinal follow-up of these infants must also include assessment for physical and developmental problems based on current understanding of the potential long-term effects from in utero exposure to AEDs

Introduction

Epilepsy requiring ongoing medical treatment is the most common neurologic disorder in pregnancy [1]. Data from a number of population-based studies estimated an incidence between 0.3% and 0.8% of all pregnancies [2, 3]. A significant number of these pregnant women are required to continue on AEDs. The incidence of AED use is estimated between 0.3% and 0.4% of all pregnancies, which includes those who are maintained on AEDs for non-epileptic conditions, such as bipolar affective disorders [3–5]. The effect of epilepsy and in utero AED exposure on the developing fetus has been studied extensively, and although the fetal effects of certain AEDs such as carbamazepine and valproic acid are better known [6–8], the effects of some of the newer AEDs such as lamotrigine, topiramate, and gabapentin are less well understood [3, 4].

When considering the care of the newborn whose mother was maintained on an AED through pregnancy and lactation, clinicians must first have a thorough understanding of the potential effects of an AED on fetal growth and development, on neonatal adaptation and transition, and their potential long-term health and developmental effects. Table 20.1 summarizes these currently known potential adverse effects of the commonly used AEDs.

Table 20.1: Summary of potential adverse effects from in utero exposure to AED in infants and children

Potential adverse effects	VPA	CBZ	PHT	PB	TPM	LTG	Prim	Any	No Rx	Poly	Reference
Pregnancy and delivery											
Pre-term labor	–	•	–	–	–	–	–	•	–	•	3
Pre-eclampsia	•	•	–	–	–	–	–	•	–	–	3, 5
Third trimester vaginal bleeding	–	•	–	–	–	–	–	•	–	–	3
Placental complications	–	–	–	–	–	–	–	•	–	–	5
Emergency cesarean section	–	–	–	–	–	–	–	•	–	–	3, 5
Newborn											
Prematurity	–	•	–	–	–	–	–	•	–	•	3
Low 5-minute Apgar score	–	–	–	–	–	–	–	–	–	–	3, 5
Respiratory distress	–	–	–	–	–	–	–	–	–	–	5
Postnatal											
Hemorrhagic disease of newborn (disputed)	–	•	•	•	•	–	•	–	–	–	7, 9, 10
Intracranial hemorrhage	–	–	–	–	–	–	–	–	–	–	3
Neonatal seizure	–	–	–	–	–	–	–	•	–	–	3
Neonatal abstinence syndrome	•	•	•	•	–	–	–	–	–	•	7, 8, 20, 21
Neonatal hypoglycemia	•	–	–	–	–	–	–	•	–	–	21
Transient liver toxicity	•	–	–	–	–	•	–	–	–	–	8, 22
Long term											
Cognitive delay	•	•	–	–	–	–	–	–	–	–	24, 25
Motor delay	•	–	•	–	–	–	–	–	–	•	23
Speech delay	•	•	–	–	–	–	–	–	–	•	23, 24
Behavioral problems	•	•	–	–	–	–	–	–	–	•	23
Developmental delay (general)	•	•	•	–	–	–	–	–	–	•	23, 25

VPA, valproic acid; CBZ, carbamazepine; PHT, phenytoin; PB, phenobarbital; TPM, topiramate; LTG, lamotrigine; Prim, primidone; Any, any AED; No Rx, mothers not on AED during pregnancy; Poly, polytherapy. Solid circles (•): known effects; small dashes (–): effect unknown or not studied/reported.

While exposing fetuses to potentially teratogenic drugs may generate anxiety and apprehension, the potential developmental effect on the fetus must be weighed against complications related to inadequately controlled epileptic seizures which may, in turn, compromise fetal wellbeing.

The objective of this review is to guide clinicians involved in the care of these infants and children, focusing on delivery room stabilization, newborn assessment, and ongoing surveillance in the neonatal and infancy period and beyond.

Care of the newborn in the delivery room

In a study of the Norwegian birth registry involving 2,900 deliveries by epileptic mothers [3], the risk of pre-term births (<37 weeks) was significantly increased, particular in those on multiple AEDs or carbamazepine. Although it is difficult to identify the reasons for premature deliveries, some of the known factors leading to pre-term births, including pre-eclampsia, third trimester vaginal bleeding, and a marginal risk of placental complications, have been reported in mothers treated with AED; there was also a significant increase in the rate of emergency cesarean sections and a trend towards lower 5-minute Apgar score [3, 5].

In terms of immediate neonatal complications, besides those related to prematurity, there is also a significantly increased risk of respiratory distress. In a population-based study from the Swedish Medical Birth Registry, respiratory distress was unrelated to the mode of delivery or the presence of premature rupture of membranes [5]. In the immediate newborn period, older studies suggest that there may be an increased risk of bleeding in the neonate, as a result of altered vitamin K metabolism by exposure to hepatic enzyme-inducing AEDs (such as carbamazepine and phenobarbital) [7, 9]. However, the most recent and best available evidence does not support this hypothesis [10, 11].

The neonatal clinicians must always be prepared for the birth of infants of epileptic mothers, especially those maintained on AEDs. A prenatal consultation is often helpful so that the pregnancy and medical history can be reviewed, and the birth plan devised in the context of potential medical problems that may be encountered in the delivery room and the postnatal period. At the time of delivery, a full neonatal resuscitation team should be available in anticipation of any neonatal complication at birth. For term and pre-term deliveries, the neonatal practitioners must be prepared for neonatal depression, as well as the occurrence of respiratory distress. The clinician must also ensure that vitamin K injection, a routine common practice in many countries, is given to the newborn, particularly if the mother has a history of enzyme-inducing AED use.

Physical examination of the newborn

There have been many published reports describing the effects of AEDs on fetal development. The rate of major congenital malformation varies from 4% to 10% in infants of epileptic mothers [2, 3, 7, 12, 13], which is significantly higher than the general population rate of 2–3% [4].

It is somewhat unclear as to the relative contribution of maternal epilepsy versus the use of AED in the development of congenital anomalies. In the Norwegian population study [3] where the majority (66%) of pregnant epileptic women did not take an AED throughout gestation, the risk of major and minor congenital malformation were similar in the AED-treated and the untreated groups. However, certain AEDs, such as carbamazepine and valproic acid, as well as polytherapy, were associated with a significantly increased risk of malformations. Compared with controls, the untreated epilepsy group had a significantly higher risk of chromosomal abnormality (0.6 vs. 0.3% for Trisomy 21) and genitourinary malformations (1.2 vs. 0.6%), suggesting the potential effects of other factors such as genetic, socioeconomic status, and maternal health on the development of congenital malformations in these infants.

There is a plethora of reported congenital malformations in the literature, including major and minor anomalies [3, 4, 7, 8, 13–16]. The majority of these anomalies reported were associated with carbamazepine, valproic acid, and phenytoin, particularly in combination with other AED (polytherapy) use during pregnancy, and discussed in greater detail in Chapter 12. The relatively low frequency of congenital malformations reported for the newer AEDs may imply that they indeed have a better safety profile for pregnant women and their fetuses. Furthermore, some of the older studies were uncontrolled and not population-based, so that the strength of association may actually be relatively poor.

In terms of fetal growth, there are a number of studies suggesting that the incidence of intrauterine growth restriction is higher in pregnancies of epileptic women compared with controls [3, 7, 13, 14]. These effects were not necessarily related to a diagnosis of placental disorders, but would indicate that the growth environment in utero may be suboptimal. It may also be related to a direct or indirect effect of AED on the growing fetus. Poor head growth has been associated with a number of AEDs used in pregnancy [3, 4, 7, 14], which may have significant impact on long-term development.

In summary, the initial assessment of newborns of epileptic mothers must include a complete and detailed physical examination, with particular focus on the common congenital malformations associated with AED use. Clinicians must also include anthropometric assessment to identify those small for gestational age and those with microcephaly, both of which may have long-term growth and developmental implications. Table 20.2 summarizes the congenital malformations associated with various AEDs as reported in the literature, so it may serve as a guide for clinicians during assessment of newborns and infants of epileptic mothers. Efforts should be made in diagnosing and confirming abnormal physical findings so that appropriate management, including relevant referrals to subspecialists, can be made in a timely fashion.

Immediate postnatal management and pre-discharge assessment

During the initial birth hospitalization, the care of newborns of epileptic mothers should primarily be focused on transition and adaptation. Because of the potential challenges in these areas, early hospital discharge (≤24 hours), in general, should not be recommended. Since the physical and emotional health benefits of breastfeeding for mothers and their infants are clear, these must be weighed against the potential risks of drug exposure by breastfeeding. In the majority of mothers on AEDs, though, breastfeeding is not contraindicated, mainly because of the low level of drug excreted in breast milk, or that adverse effects have not been reported [8]. Some AEDs, such as gabapentin, have been associated with decrease in milk production [8].

Clinicians must also be aware of the potential neurologic effects of AED exposure on the newborns in the immediate postnatal period. There have been rare reports of intracranial hemorrhage in neonates born to epileptic mothers, particular in those with inadequate seizure control during pregnancy [17, 18]. Seizure-like activity has also been reported from in utero exposure to carbamazepine [8]. Drug withdrawal has also been described in

Table 20.2: Summary of congenital malformations associated with in utero exposure to AED in infants and children

	Congenital malformation	VPA	CBZ	PHT	Vig	Clob	PB	Gaba	LTG	Prim	Any	Poly	Reference
Nervous system	Neural tube defect	•	–	–	–	–	–	–	–	–	–	–	3, 4, 7, 14
	Hydrocephalus	•	–	–	–	–	–	–	–	–	–	–	4, 14
Cardiovascular	Any cardiac defect	•	–	•	–	•	•	–	•	–	•	•	3, 4, 7
	Septal defects	•	–	–	–	–	–	–	–	–	•	–	3, 14
	Patent ductus arteriosus	–	–	–	–	–	–	–	•	–	–	–	3
	Aortic root dilatation	–	–	•	–	–	–	–	–	–	–	•	14
Genitourinary	Cryptorchidism	•	–	–	–	–	–	–	–	–	–	–	14
	Hypospadias	•	–	–	–	–	–	–	–	–	•	•	4, 14
	Renal pelviectasis	•	–	–	–	–	–	–	–	–	–	–	14
Skin	Nail hypoplasia	•	•	–	–	•	–	–	–	–	•	•	14
	Hemagiomata	•	•	•	–	•	–	–	–	–	•	•	14
Musculoskeletal	Digit hypoplasia	•	–	•	–	•	–	–	–	–	•	•	14, 15
	Polydactyly	–	–	–	–	–	–	–	–	–	–	–	14
	Syndactyly	–	–	–	–	•	–	–	–	–	•	•	4, 14
	Joint laxity	–	–	•	–	•	–	–	–	–	–	–	14
	Hip dysplasia	–	–	–	–	•	–	–	–	–	•	–	14
	Talipes equinovarus	•	•	•	–	–	–	–	•	–	•	•	4, 14
	Distal limb hypoplasia	–	•	•	–	•	–	–	–	–	•	•	4
Craniofacial	Facial dysmorphism	•	•	•	–	•	•	–	•	–	•	•	3, 14, 15
	Cleft lip and palate	•	•	•	–	–	•	–	–	–	•	•	4, 7
	Craniosynostosis	•	–	–	–	–	–	–	–	–	–	•	16
	Narrow/high palate	•	–	•	–	–	•	–	•	–	–	•	14
	Subglottic stenosis	•	–	–	–	–	–	–	–	–	–	–	14
	Bifid uvula	•	–	–	–	–	–	–	–	–	–	–	14
	Peg/notched teeth	•	–	–	–	–	–	–	–	–	–	•	14
	Delayed dentition	•	–	–	–	–	–	–	–	–	–	•	14
	Congenital cataracts	•	–	–	–	–	–	–	–	–	–	–	14
Gastrointestinal	Hernias	•	–	–	–	–	–	–	–	–	–	–	14
	Diastasis recti	•	–	–	–	–	–	–	–	–	–	–	14
	Diaphragmatic hernia	–	–	–	–	–	–	–	–	–	–	–	3

VPA, valproic acid; CBZ, carbamazepine; PHT, phenytoin; Vig, vigabatrin; Clob, clobazam; PB, phenobarbital; Gaba, gabapentin; LTG, lamotrigine; Prim, primidone; Any, any AED; Poly, polytherapy. Solid circles (•): known effects; small dashes (–): effect unknown or not studied/reported.

relation to maternal AED use of valproic acid, carbamazepine, phenytoin, alone or in combination with other AEDs during pregnancy [7, 8, 19, 20]. Symptoms have been reported to occur between 12 to 72 hours after birth, and the severity may be dose-dependent. Symptoms of withdrawal include drowsiness, irritability, high-pitched cry, jitteriness, tremors, excitability, hypertonia, hyperreflexia, and feeding difficulties [19, 20], which are not dissimilar to that of abstinence from narcotics.

Ebbesen et al. reported a significantly increased risk of asymptomatic neonatal hypoglycemia not related to prematurity, growth restriction, or hyperinsulinemia, in those exposed to valproic acid and carbamazepine in utero [20]. Speculated mechanisms include impaired ketogenesis and decreased liver glycogen synthesis. There were also reports of transient liver toxicity, manifested by cholestasis and transaminitis, associated with maternal use of carbamazepine and lamotrigine [8, 21]. Interestingly, hepatic enzyme-inducing AEDs such as phenobarbital may reduce the risk of neonatal unconjugated hyperbilirubinemia [5].

In summary, infants born to epileptic mothers on AED during pregnancy may face a number of challenges in the immediate postnatal period. Anticipating the potential problems with feeding and reduced breast milk supply, the mother-infant dyad should be provided with ample breastfeeding support even beyond the birth hospitalization. To adequately observe the newborns for neurologic symptoms such as drug withdrawal or seizures, it is the author's opinion that they should remain in hospital for a minimum of 48 hours after birth. Other workup, such as neuroimaging studies, might be performed where indicated (e.g., suspected intracranial hemorrhage, neonatal seizures). For newborns exposed to carbamazepine or valproic acid in utero, routine checks of serum glucose should be performed in the first days of life, especially while feeding is being established.

Long-term follow-up

Large international registries have shown that congenital malformations in offspring of mothers exposed to AED during pregnancy may be diagnosed up to 12 months after birth [22], suggesting that periodic health examination by primary care providers must include complete physical assessment to ensure late manifestations of any anomaly be identified and managed.

In terms of overall health status in childhood, one study showed that in utero exposure to carbamazepine, valproic acid, or polytherapy was associated with a higher incidence of medical problems in childhood. There was also a trend toward more myopia in the AED-exposed group [23].

The developing neonatal brain is particularly vulnerable to injury, not only during the process of neuronal migration and organization of synaptic connections but also throughout the maturation process, which may extend well beyond the neonatal period [24]. Longitudinal follow-up studies to date suggest in utero AED exposure has potential adverse neurodevelopmental effects in these infants. In earlier studies, exposure of AED in utero was inconsistently shown to be associated with lower scores in developmental and language skills, and impairment in specific areas of cognitive development such as visual-spatial skills [4, 24].

Other studies examined AED-exposed children at a broader age range. In a retrospective cohort study, 255 children whose mothers were treated with AEDs during their pregnancy were assessed between 2 days and 39 years (mean of 9 years). Compared with non-exposed controls, the incidence of neurodevelopmental impairment, including speech, motor, or global developmental delay, was significantly increased (10.5% in non-exposed controls versus 24% in children exposed to any form of AED) [23]. Speech delay and other behavioral disorders were more prevalent in those exposed to carbamazepine, valproic acid, or polytherapy [23]. In a similar study, 163 epileptic mothers and their children between the ages of 6 and 16 years were prospectively assessed by neuropsychological tests. Exposure to valproic acid in utero was associated with a significantly lower verbal IQ score compared with those not exposed to AED, or with those exposed to other AEDs; these same children were also more likely to score with IQ less than 69 and within the "impaired" category in memory functioning. Other significant predictors of poor verbal IQ in this cohort include mother's IQ score and the number of tonic-clonic seizures during pregnancy, suggesting that in utero and postnatal environmental factors in those already exposed to AED may have an additional influence on their long-term cognitive outcomes [24]. In a more recent prospective cohort study of younger children between the ages of 16 and 49 months whose mothers received AED monotherapy during pregnancy, valproic acid and carbamazepine, but not lamotrigine, were significantly associated with delays in development compared with non-exposed controls [25].

In summary, there is still a paucity of literature on the long-term developmental outcome of children exposed to AED in utero. Longitudinal follow-up studies focusing mainly on older AEDs such as carbamazepine, valproic acid, and phenytoin showed a potentially increased risk of cognitive, language, and behavioral problems in childhood. Information on long-term effects of newer AEDs is lacking, although limited data on lamotrigine seems to suggest its relative safety. Primary care clinicians should consider any children who were exposed to AED in utero at risk of neurodevelopmental impairment; if there is any developmental concern identified, prompt referral for detailed developmental and neuropsychological assessment is warranted.

Conclusion

This chapter summarized the clinically relevant effects of maternal epilepsy and, more specifically, maternal treatment with AED on their offspring. Amongst the vast number of AEDs used, there are a large number of congenital malformations associated with these potential teratogens. Specific care and surveillance of these infants should begin from the time of birth, through the period of neonatal transition, long until childhood and beyond, paying particular attention to issues with growth, cognitive, and behavioral development. With accumulating experience in use of the newer classes of AED, future research in this area must focus on studying the short- and long-term effects from in utero and postnatal exposure of these drugs, so clinicians may gain a better understanding of how individualized care may be provided to optimize the health and developmental potentials of these children.

References

1. Pennell PB. Pregnancy in women who have epilepsy. *Neurol Clin* 2004; 22:799–820.

2. Olafsson E, Hallgrimsson JT, Hauser WA, et al. Pregnancies of women with epilepsy: a population-based study in Iceland. *Epilepsia* 1998; 39:887–92.

3. Veiby G, Daltveit AK, Engelsen BA, et al. Pregnancy, delivery, and outcome for the child in maternal epilepsy. *Epilepsia* 2009; 50:2130–9.

4. Stoler JM. Maternal antiepileptic drug use and effects on fetal development. *Curr Opin Pediatr* 2001; 13:566–71.

5. Pilo C, Wide K and Winbladh B. Pregnancy, delivery, and neonatal complications after treatment with antiepileptic drugs. *Acta Obstet Gynecol Scand* 2006; 85:643–6.

6. ACOG Practice Bulletin No. 87 November 2007. Use of psychiatric medications during pregnancy and lactation. *Obstet Gynecol* 2007; 110:1179–98.

7. Burja S, Rakovec-Felser Z, Treiber M, et al. The frequency of neonatal morbidity after exposure to antiepileptic drugs in utero: a retrospective population-based study. *Wien Klin Wochenschr* 2006; 118(Suppl 2):12–16.

8. Iqbal MM, Gundlapalli SP, Ryan WG, et al. Effects of antimanic mood-stabilizing drugs on fetuses, neonates, and nursing infants. *South Med J* 2001; 94:304–22.

9. Kazmin A, Wong RC, Sermer M, et al. Antiepileptic drugs in pregnancy and hemorrhagic disease of the newborn: an update. *Can Fam Physician* 2010; 56:1291–2.

10. Kaaja E, Kaaja R, Matila R, et al. Enzyme-inducing antiepileptic drugs in pregnancy and the risk of bleeding in the neonate. *Neurology* 2002; 58:549–53.

11. Harden CL, Pennell PB, Koppel BS, et al. Practice parameter update: management issues for women with epilepsy–focus on pregnancy (an evidence-based review): vitamin K, folic acid, blood levels, and breastfeeding: Report of the Quality Standards Subcommittee and Therapeutics and Technology Assessment Subcommittee of the American Academy of Neurology and American Epilepsy Society. *Neurology* 2009; 73:142–9.

12. Canger R, Battino D, Canevini MP, et al. Malformations in offspring of women with epilepsy: a prospective study. *Epilepsia* 1999; 40:1231–6.

13. Fonager K, Larsen H, Pedersen L, et al. Birth outcomes in women exposed to anticonvulsant drugs. *Acta Neurol Scand* 2000; 101:289–94.

14. Holmes LB, Harvey EA, Brown KS, et al. Anticonvulsant teratogenesis: I. A study design for newborn infants. *Teratology* 1994; 49:202–7.

15. Moore SJ, Turnpenny P, Quinn A, et al. A clinical study of 57 children with fetal anticonvulsant syndromes. *J Med Genet* 2000; 37:489–97.

16. Chabrolle JP, Bensouda B, Bruel H, et al. Metopic craniosynostosis, probable effect of intrauterine exposure to maternal valproate treatment. *Arch Pediatr* 2001; 8:1333–6.

17. Minkoff H, Schaffer RM, Delke I, et al. Diagnosis of intracranial hemorrhage in utero after a maternal seizure. *Obstet Gynecol* 1985; 65:22S–4S.

18. Sherer DM, Anyaegbunam A and Onyeije C. Antepartum fetal intracranial hemorrhage, predisposing factors and prenatal sonography: a review. *Am J Perinatol* 1998; 15:431–41.

19. D'Souza SW, Robertson IG, Donnai D, et al. Fetal phenytoin exposure, hypoplastic nails, and jitteriness. *Arch Dis Child* 1991; 66:320–4.

20. Ebbesen F, Joergensen A, Hoseth E, et al. Neonatal hypoglycaemia and withdrawal symptoms after exposure in utero to valproate. *Arch Dis Child Fetal Neonatal Ed* 2000; 83:F124–F9.

21. Dubnov-Raz G, Shapiro R and Merlob P. Maternal lamotrigine treatment and elevated neonatal gamma-glutamyl transpeptidase. *Pediatr Neurol* 2006; 35:220–2.

22. Tomson T, Battino D, Bonizzoni E, et al. Dose-dependent risk of malformations with antiepileptic drugs: an analysis of data from the EURAP epilepsy and pregnancy registry. *Lancet Neurol* 2011; 10:609–17.

23. Dean JC, Hailey H, Moore SJ, et al. Long term health and neurodevelopment in children exposed to antiepileptic

drugs before birth. *J Med Genet* 2002;
39:251–9.

24. Vinten J, Adab N, Kini U, et al.
Neuropsychological effects of exposure to
anticonvulsant medication in utero.
Neurology 2005; 64:949–54.

25. Cummings C, Stewart M, Stevenson M,
et al. Neurodevelopment of
children exposed in utero to
lamotrigine, sodium valproate and
carbamazepine. *Arch Dis Child* 2011;
96:643–7.

Menopause and HRT in women with epilepsy

Cynthia L. Harden

Key points:

- Discuss with the patient whether she has had a catamenial seizure pattern; this may be particularly associated with increased seizures at perimenopause
- Counsel women when appropriate that epilepsy may be associated with early onset perimenopause and menopause
- Determine whether the patient is perimenopausal and this should prompt consideration for monitoring levels of appropriate antiepileptic drugs (AEDs) to maintain robust therapeutic levels
- Advise perimenopausal women with epilepsy to be especially vigilant with taking AEDs and getting adequate sleep
- If vasomotor symptoms disrupt sleep, CEE/MPA should not be used, and other regimens should be considered, such as estradiol plus natural progesterone

Menopause is a time of transition for women. It occurs when the ovarian follicles are depleted, therefore women who bear children tend to have later menopause, due to the ovulation-sparing months of pregnancy. This transition occurs gradually over several years and is a normal aging process. It marks the end of reproductive years, and usually occurs during the late 40s or early 50s. The mean age at menopause is 50–51 years and is remarkably stable across populations and generations. Menopausal age has been stated to be 50 years by observers for centuries, including Aristotle in the third century BC, Paulus Aeginata in the seventh century AD, and Gilberts Anglicus in the thirteenth century AD [1]. Ovarian follicles secrete estrogen and progesterone to promote ovulation and endometrial proliferation. Hormonally, as menopause approaches (perimenopause), estrogen levels remain unchanged, may rise steadily, or can surge erratically in response to the elevated FSH levels. The cyclic progesterone elevation, which normally occurs during the luteal phase of the menstrual cycle gradually, becomes less frequent throughout perimenopause, thus causing increased occurrence of anovulatory cycles [2, 3]. Estrogen and progesterone stabilize at low levels with complete ovarian failure at menopause; when a woman has not had menses for 12 months, she is considered postmenopausal.

What makes perimenopause and menopause interesting from the epilepsy viewpoint is that estrogen and progesterone are neurosteroids. These are steroid molecules that modulate brain excitability, and can influence seizure occurrence. Estrogen and progesterone have opposing effects on neuronal excitability [4, 5], which has been demonstrated in

Women with Epilepsy, ed. Esther Bui and Autumn Klein. Published by Cambridge University Press. © Cambridge University Press 2014.

experimental models of epilepsy [6]. Estrogen exerts neuroexcitatory effects by modulating gene expression. Like other steroid hormones, estrogen enters passively into neurons where it binds to and activates the estrogen receptor, a dimeric nuclear protein that binds to DNA and controls gene expression. After estrogen-binding, the receptor complex forms a transcription factor that binds to hormone receptor elements on genes to modify cellular responses. An example is the estradiol-induced increased density of agonist-binding sites on the N-methyl D-aspartate (NMDA) receptor complex in hippocampal cells [7]. However, this neuroexcitatory effect is not without complexity; estrogen dose, route of administration, acute versus chronic administration, natural hormonal milieu, and estrogenic species affects whether estrogen is proconvulsant or anticonvulsant [8].

Progesterone promotes neuroinhibitory effects primarily through the action of its reduced metabolite, allopregnanolone, a positive allosteric modulator of gamma-amino-butyric acid (GABA) conductance [6, 9]. The neuroinhibitory effect of allopregnanolone is also complicated by its being subject to a feedback mechanism within the receptor. The GABA-A receptor subunit components undergo compensatory alterations in response to changes in the endogenous hormonal neurosteroid milieu and to pharmacological agents that modulate GABA-A receptors, such as benzodiazepines [10, 11].

Seizures at menopause and perimenopause

What happens at menopause then, when the cyclic hormonal fluctuations of the reproductive years cease? Unlike puberty and young adulthood, menopause and perimenopause do not appear to be a time of increased epilepsy onset. The incidence of epilepsy is stable across young and middle-age adult age groups, but increases with age after 59 years [12]. Further, the onset is always slightly more frequent in men than in women. However, women with epilepsy (WWE) may encounter changes in their seizure disorder with perimenopause and menopause.

No prospective information is available on the course of epilepsy as WWE progress through the menopausal transition. However, a cross-sectional evaluation using mailed questionnaires, queried women with epilepsy to recall the course of their epilepsy from their reproductive years through perimenopause and menopause [13]. Two-thirds of these perimenopausal WWE reported an increase in seizures during perimenopause. Remarkably, history of a catamenial seizure pattern was significantly associated with an increase in seizures at perimenopause. These findings are consistent with postulated mechanisms for women with hormonally sensitive seizures; the elevated estrogen-to-progesterone ratio may contribute to the increase in seizure frequency at perimenopause. Further, a history of a catamenial seizure pattern, defined as seizures in the week prior to menses, was associated with a decrease in seizures at menopause. A high percentage of women in the perimenopausal group took synthetic hormone replacement therapy (HRT), and HRT was significantly associated with an increase in seizures (p = 0.001) [13].

Hormone replacement and epilepsy

These questionnaire findings prompted the exploration as to whether HRT itself could alter seizure frequency in women with epilepsy, due to a possible neurosteroid effect. In a randomized, double blind, placebo-controlled trial of Prempro (0.625 mg of conjugated equine estrogens plus 2.5 mg of medroxyprogesterone acetate (CEE/MPA) daily, or double-dose CEE/MPA daily for three months), seizure frequency significantly increased with the use of CEE/MPA in a dose-related manner [14]. This is a clinical example of an adverse exogenous neurosteroid effect on seizures in menopausal WWE. This finding also implies that the low and stable hormonal milieu for menopausal WWE is physiologically vulnerable to neuroexcitatory influence. No such data are available for other HRT regimens [15].

Early menopause for women with epilepsy

Epilepsy is an endocrine disruptor, causing hypothalamic-pituitary-gonadal axis dysfunction, which in turn produces dysregulation of maturation of ovarian follicles and early loss of follicles available for ovulation. Therefore, through this mechanism of follicle wasting, WWE are at risk for early onset of the menopausal transition. Klein et al. provided the first report of early perimenopausal symptoms and premature menopause in WWE, in which 14% of 50 WWE in an epilepsy clinic population had premature ovarian failure (POF) compared with 3.7% of healthy control women (p = 0.04) [16]. Consistent with the concept that a portion of WWE has specific reproductive hormone sensitivity, women with POF were more likely to have had catamenial exacerbation of their seizures during earlier reproductive years. The risk for earlier menopause appears to be related to seizure frequency, with increased seizure frequency perhaps indicating a stronger "dose" of endocrine disruption. Harden et al. reported a negative correlation between the age at menopause and seizure frequency (p = 0.014) [17]. For example, the women with only rare seizures had a normal age at menopause of 50–51 years, while women with frequent seizures experienced earlier menopause at 46–47 years. In this study, there was no relationship between early menopause and specific AED treatments.

The implications for management during perimenopause and menopause generally encompass having an understanding of the patient in terms of her history of catamenial seizure patterns, ongoing reproductive state, and whether vasomotor symptoms are interfering with sleep, since this may be an important factor for seizure increase as well [11]. Management should include increased vigilance for seizure occurrence at perimenopause, and a low threshold for relieving vasomotor symptoms that interfere with sleep, although not with the use of CEE/MPA. A simplified regimen of estradiol only (without the multiple estrogenic compounds in CEE), plus natural progesterone may be a reasonable alternative, especially considering the anti seizure potential of natural progesterone. Seizure freedom is always a goal of treatment, and for WWE, this may prolong the period of reproductive years to a normal duration.

References

1. Brincat M, Baron YM and Ray Galea R. The menopause. In: Shaw R, Soutter P and Stanton S, eds. *Gynaecology*, 2nd edn. London: Churchill Livingstone 1997; 374.

2. Prior JC and Hitchcock CL. The endocrinology of perimenopause: need for a paradigm shift. *Front Biosci (Schol Ed)* 2011; 3:474–86.

3. Burger HG, Dudley EC, Robertson DM, et al. Hormonal changes in the menopause transition. *Recent Prog Horm Res* 2002; 57:257–75.

4. Reddy DS. Neurosteroids: endogenous role in the human brain and therapeutic potentials. *Prog Brain Res* 2010; 186: 113–37.

5. Majewska MD, Harrison NL, Schwartz RD, et al. Steroid hormone metabolites are barbiturate-like modulators of the GABA receptor. *Science* 1986; 232 (4753):1004–7.

6. Reddy DS, Gould J and Gangisetty OA. Mouse kindling model of perimenstrual catamenial epilepsy. *J Pharmacol Exp Ther* 2012; 341(3): 784–93.

7. Pack M, Reddy DS, Duncan S, et al. Neuroendocrinological aspects of epilepsy: important issues and trends in future research. *Epilepsy Behav* 2011; 22(1): 94–102.

8. Velísková J. Estrogens and epilepsy: why are we so excited. *Neuroscientist* 2007; 13:77.

9. Frye CA. Effects and mechanisms of progestogens and androgens in ictal activity. *Epilepsia* 2010; 51(Suppl 3):135–4.

10. Smith SS, Shen H, Gong QH, et al. Neurosteroid regulation of GABAA receptors: focus on the α4 and δ subunits. *Pharmacol Ther* 2007; 116:58–76.

11. Gulinello M, Gong QH and Li Xand Smith SS. Short-term exposure to a neuroactive steroid increases α4 GABAA receptor subunit levels in association with increased anxiety in the female rat. *Brain Res* 2001; 910:55–66.

12. Kotsopoulos IA, van Merode T, Kessels FG, et al. Systematic review and meta-analysis of incidence studies of epilepsy and unprovoked seizures. *Epilepsia* 2002; 43 (11):1402–9.

13. Harden CL, Pulver MC and Jacobs AR. The effect of menopause and perimenopause on the course of epilepsy. *Epilepsia* 1999; 40:1402–07.

14. Harden CL, Herzog AG, Nikolov BG, et al. Hormone replacement therapy in WWE: a randomized, double-blind, placebo-controlled study. *Epilepsia* 2006; 47 (9):1447–51.

15. North American Menopause Society. Estrogen and progestogen use in postmenopausal women: 2010 position statement of The North American Menopause Society. *Menopause* 2010; 17 (2):242–55.

16. Klein P, Serje A and Pezzullo JC. Premature ovarian failure in WWE. *Epilepsia* 2001; 42:1584–9.

17. Harden CL, Koppel BS, Herzog AG, et al. Seizure frequency is associated with age of menopause in WWE. *Neurology* 2003; 61:451–5.

Chapter 22

Bone health in adolescent girls and postmenopausal women with epilepsy

Alison M. Pack

Key points:

- Adolescent girls and postmenopausal women with epilepsy treated with antiepileptic drugs (AEDs) may be at increased risk for low bone mineral density (BMD). Adolescence is a critical time of bone development and AED exposure may impact bone accrual. Postmenopausal women are at increased risk because of effects of AED exposure superimposed on estrogen-deficient bone loss
- Cytochrome P450 enzyme-inducing AEDs are most consistently associated with abnormalities in bone. Cytochrome P450 enzyme-inducing AEDs include phenytoin, carbamazepine, and phenobarbital
- There are multiple proposed mechanisms to explain why AEDs are associated with low BMD. The principal mechanism proposed relates to induction of the hepatic cytochrome P450 enzyme system leading to accelerated vitamin D metabolism and subsequent less biologically active or inert vitamin D
- Official recommendations for screening bone health in persons with epilepsy treated with AEDs are not available. Obtaining BMD measurements using DXA in persons at risk should be considered. Routine screening of 25 hydroxyvitamin D, particularly in persons treated with enzyme-inducing AEDs, should also be considered
- Among the available treatment options for low BMD only vitamin D supplementation has been studied in persons with epilepsy treated with AEDs. The current recommended daily allowance of vitamin D is 600 IU per day. Persons taking enzyme-inducing AEDs will likely need higher doses

Introduction

Poor bone health, including low BMD and fractures, are increasingly common and contribute to significant comorbidities and health care expenditures. Recognized risk factors include menopause, glucocorticoid exposure, and family history. Studies suggest that people with epilepsy are at increased risk. Adolescent girls may be particularly susceptible because of AED exposure during a critical time of bone development. As well, postmenopausal women are at increased risk because of effects of AED exposure superimposed on estrogen-deficient bone loss.

Women with Epilepsy, ed. Esther Bui and Autumn Klein. Published by Cambridge University Press.
© Cambridge University Press 2014.

Bone physiology

Bones are vital to our metabolic homeostasis and functioning. Bones are repositories for important minerals,including calcium, and play an integral role in the regulation of these minerals. Bones, as part of our skeletal network, allow us to move. In addition, they protect vital organs, including the heart and lungs, and the central nervous system.

Among women, the lifespan of bone has distinct phases. During childhood, bone elongates and increases in diameter, with the most dramatic changes occurring in infancy and adolescence [1]. At birth, skeletal mass is on average 70 g in girls with very little mineralization. Skeletal mass then increases dramatically through to the end of puberty. Peak BMD is obtained between the second and third decade of life, with young women having an average mass of 2,400 g. Women after age 30 typically steadily lose BMD until menopause. During the early menopausal years more significant bone loss occurs.

Increasing and maintaining BMD is the result of bone resorption and formation mediated by bone cells. The cells responsible for resorption are osteoclasts, whereas those responsible for formation are osteoblasts. An uncoupling of these processes and cells results in either high or low bone turnover. In childhood, uncoupling of osteoblasts and osteoclasts affects accumulation of peak BMD. In adulthood, the uncoupling results in accelerated bone loss. High turnover bone loss occurs in the early postmenopausal years. Low turnover bone loss occurs in advanced age.

Calcium homeostasis is a highly regulated process of which bone is integral. The ionized fraction of calcium is tightly maintained. As the concentration of this fraction changes, parathyroid hormone (PTH) levels change. For example, if the ionized fraction is low, PTH rises. PTH acts to restore the ionized calcium concentration by increasing distal renal tubule reabsorption and facilitating bone resorption.

Vitamin D plays a critical role in calcium homeostasis and has direct effects on bone, such as promoting differentiation of osteoclasts. Vitamin D metabolism occurs through a series of oxidative pathways involving multiple hepatic and renal cytochrome p450 isoenzymes [2]. Vitamin D is hydroxylated to 25 hydroxyvitamin D (25OHD), the major circulating form of vitamin D, in the liver. 25OHD is the most commonly used index of vitamin D status. 25OHD is further hydroxylated to 24, 25 dihydroxyvitamin D (24, 25(OH)2D) and 1,25(OH)2D. 24, 25(OH)2D also has little effect in bone whereas 1,25(OH)2D is responsible for the majority of the biological effects of vitamin D.

Reproductive hormones directly and indirectly impact bone. Estrogen reduces bone resorption by both inhibiting the formation and function of osteoclasts [3]. Estrogen receptors have been identified on both osteoclasts and osteoblasts, suggesting direct effects on these bone cells [3].

Increasing evidence supports nervous system control of bone remodeling [4, 5], mediated both centrally and peripherally by neurotransmitters and neuropeptides. Prolactin, norepinephrine, leptin, serotonin, and inflammatory cytokines have all been documented to influence bone resorption and/or formation. Prolactin receptors are expressed on osteoblasts and high prolactin concentrations up-regulate multiple osteoblast-derived osteoclastogenic mediators, promoting increased bone resorption [6, 7]. Genetic and pharmacologic studies demonstrate that norepinephrine controls bone cell function by binding to ß2-adrenergic receptors on osteoblasts [5, 8]. Leptin is highly expressed in the hypothalamus and is a powerful inhibitor of bone formation [4, 9]. Its anti-osteogenic function is secondary to its effect on hypothalamic neurons, the autonomous nervous system, and β2-adrenergic receptors on osteoblasts

[10]. Serotonin, both gut- and CNS-derived, affects bone remodeling. In the gut, serotonin inhibits bone formation [11], whereas CNS serotonin has the opposite effect [12]. The action of leptin on bone may be mediated through serotonin, as leptin inhibits bone accrual by inhibiting serotonin synthesis [12]. The inflammatory cytokines, IL-6 and TNF-α, stimulate osteoclastogenesis, promoting bone loss [13].

Fracture

Children and adults with epilepsy treated with AEDs have a 2–6-fold increased risk of fracture. Multiple factors including increased risk of falling and reduced BMD contribute to the increased risk. The impact of multiple factors is demonstrated by meta-analysis findings. In this analysis, although BMD was reduced among persons with epilepsy taking AEDs [14], the reduction in BMD was not enough to explain the elevated fracture risk.

Persons with epilepsy are more likely to fall because of seizures, as well as direct effects of AEDs. Increased risk of falling can contribute to fracture risk. In a population-based study of older women, those prescribed AEDs had an increased risk for frequent falls (multivariate odds ratio = 2.56, 95% confidence interval (CI) = 1.49–4.41) [15]. This increased risk of falls may be explained in part by balance impairment secondary to AED exposure. In a study of 29 ambulatory community-dwelling twin and sibling pairs, balance performance was found to be impaired in the AED users compared to the siblings not taking AEDs [16].

Seizures themselves may result in fractures. In a large case-control study of 3,478 patients with epilepsy [17], seizure severity was associated with fracture. The type of seizure may influence the fracture risk. Generalized tonic-clonic seizures are found to be associated with a higher fracture risk than partial seizures [18]. Population-based studies, however, find that trauma related to seizures is not associated with fractures [19, 20]. Although seizures likely contribute to the risk of fracture, studies evaluating the direct effect do not reveal consistent findings.

AED exposure potentially increases fracture risk. Using the General Practice Research Database (GPRD) from the UK and a nested case-control study design, long-term AED use was associated with an increased fracture risk, particularly in women [21]. Similarly, a case-control study using data from the Funen County, Denmark hip register found that AED use increased fracture risk [22]. Independent predictors of fracture included the use of cytochrome P450 enzyme-inducing AEDs as well as higher daily doses of current and recent AEDs. Results from a pharmacoepidemiologic, population-based case-control study, also in Denmark, suggests that AEDs differentially affect fracture risk [23]. Carbamazepine, clonazepam, phenobarbital, and valproate were all associated with an increased fracture risk after adjusting for significant confounders, such as a diagnosis of epilepsy. A dose relationship was found for these specific AEDs.

Bone mineral density

Adolescent girls

Peak BMD achieved by the end of adolescence determines the risk for later pathological fractures and osteoporosis [1]. Factors that determine bone mass include genetics, sex, and ethnicity. Chronic disease and medications that interfere with bone mineralization can have significant long-term implications for bone health. Epilepsy and AED exposure are among potential factors that may adversely affect bone.

BMD has been reported to be lower in children and adolescents with epilepsy when compared to controls without epilepsy not taking AEDs. A cross-sectional study compared 82 ambulatory children with epilepsy (aged 6–18) to a control group of healthy children [24]. The children with epilepsy were classified by length of time with the diagnosis (less than a year, 1–5 years, or ≥ 6 years). Age- and sex-corrected BMD Z-scores were used in the analysis. Total BMD Z-score was lower in children with epilepsy. Increasing duration of epilepsy was associated with a progressive reduction in BMD compared to controls. Another cross-sectional study examined BMD among 108 ambulatory children between the ages 6 and 18 and compared findings to healthy controls who were first-degree cousins [25]. BMD was significantly reduced among males and females. Interestingly, in this cohort the young males and not the females had the lowest BMD. In contrast, another pediatric study did not find reduced BMD at multiple sites among healthy children. Overall, multiple studies do report reduced BMD among children with epilepsy, but this is not a consistent finding.

Comorbidities are important to consider when addressing bone health in adolescence. For example, cerebral palsy and mental retardation are independently associated with low BMD. Table 22.1 outlines factors that lower BMD. Among a cohort of 117 children and adolescents with moderate-to-severe cerebral palsy, 77% of studied patients had evidence of low BMD [26]. Of significance, AED use correlated with low BMD. Another study assessed BMD in 96 children, adolescents, and young adults with either epilepsy alone or in combination with cerebral palsy and/or mental retardation [27]. Results were compared to 63 healthy controls. Abnormal BMD was found in almost 60% of studied subjects with cerebral palsy (n = 47). Among the total group, lack of autonomous gait, severe mental retardation, prolonged AED therapy, adjunctive topiramate therapy, and less physical activity all significantly correlated with abnormal BMD. Similarly, three groups of subjects (40 patients affected by cerebral palsy and mental retardation; 47 with cerebral palsy, mental retardation, and epilepsy; 26 with epilepsy alone) had BMD evaluations [28]. Thirty-three of the subjects (70.2%) with cerebral palsy, mental retardation, and epilepsy had abnormally low BMD compared with 42.5% of those with cerebral palsy and mental retardation, and 11% of subjects with epilepsy alone. These results all support the theory that although subjects with cerebral palsy and mental retardation are at risk for low BMD, those who also have epilepsy are at even greater risk.

Table 22.1: Factors associated with low bone mineral density

- Ethnicity (Caucasian or Asian)
- Family history of osteoporosis
- Small frame
- Menopause
- Poor nutrition
- Smoking history
- Alcohol use
- Eating disorder history
- Mental retardation
- Cerebral palsy
- Hyperthyroidism
- Hyperparathyroidism
- Liver disease
- Medication use: antiepileptic drugs; glucocorticosteroids; heparin

Postmenopausal women

Postmenopausal women with epilepsy receiving AEDs are likely at greater risk for adverse effects on bone than the general population, as the effects of AEDs are superimposed upon estrogen-deficient bone loss. Significantly reduced BMD at the femoral neck has been described in postmenopausal women on AEDs as compared to drug-naïve controls [29]. One population-based study confirmed that women older than 65 years receiving anticonvulsants have a very high risk of hip fracture [30]. The Study of Osteoporotic Fractures [31] is a population-based study that measured serial BMD determinations at both the hip and calcaneus, together with many clinical risk factors for low BMD, in more than 6,000 postmenopausal women. After adjustment of multiple confounders, including health status, walking for exercise, smoking status, and estrogen status, the average rate of decline in total hip BMD steadily increased from −0.70%/year in non-AED users, to −0.87%/year in partial AED users, to −1.16%/year in continuous AED users (p value for trend = 0.015) [31].

Specific antiepileptic drugs

Carbamazepine: Carbamazepine treatment increases fracture risk and may reduce BMD [23, 32]. In a Danish pharmacoepidemiologic study, the adjusted risk of fracture among carbamazepine users was elevated (OR 1.18, 1.10–1.26) [23]. Two pediatric studies reveal differing results regarding the impact of carbamazepine treatment on BMD. In a cross-sectional study, 13 otherwise healthy children with epilepsy treated with carbamazepine did not have significantly reduced BMD at either the radius or lumbar spine when compared to controls [33], whereas BMD at the lumbar spine in another cross-sectional study was significantly lower in subjects on carbamazepine when compared to controls [34]. Adult studies also reveal conflicting results. BMD was significantly reduced at the right calcaneus in 10 adults [35] who were followed longitudinally. In contrast, 21 outpatients treated with carbamazepine did have reduced BMD [36]. Carbamazepine is associated with increased risk of fracture, but there are conflicting reports in both pediatric and adult studies regarding the effect of carbamazepine on BMD.

Gabapentin: Gabapentin use resulted in increased fracture in a Canadian population-based study [32]. Several studies have evaluated BMD among adults taking multiple AEDs including gabapentin [37, 38, 39], finding that gabapentin may cause bone loss. In a population-based epidemiologic study, older men prescribed gabapentin had significant hip bone loss (25). There has not been a similar effect described specifically in adolescent girls or older postmenopausal women.

Lamotrigine: No studies support an effect of lamotrigine on fracture risk, whereas there are studies evaluating BMD among lamotrigine users. The data regarding lamotrigine's effects on BMD are mixed. Lamotrigine treatment in children and more than 2 years was associated with shorter stature and lower BMD [40]. Physical inactivity, however, was the major predictor of lowered BMD. Another study among children found no difference in BMD between controls and those with epilepsy treated with lamotrigine (17). Similarly, premenopausal women treated with lamotrigine did not have significant reductions in BMD at baseline [41] or after 1 year of follow-up [42].

Levetiracetam: There is limited study on the effects of levetiracetam on bone. Results from an animal study found that levetiracetam therapy may affect bone quality [43].

Rats treated with low-dose levetiracetam had reduced bone strength and bone formation and no changes in bone mass. Among drug-naïve subjects (mean age 31.0 ±13.1 years), there were no reductions in BMD after approximately 1 year of levetiracetam treatment [44].

Oxcarbazepine: Oxcarbazepine has been found to increase fracture risk and may decrease BMD. In a Danish fracture study [23] oxcarbazepine was associated with a significantly elevated risk of fracture (OR 1.14, 1.03–1.26). BMD was significantly lower among 14 healthy children with idiopathic epilepsy treated with oxcarbazepine for at least a year when compared to healthy controls [45, 46, 47]. In another study of 34 newly diagnosed subjects treated with oxcarbazepine for 18 months, BMD was decreased by 8% at the lumbar spine and femoral neck [46]. A Turkish study of 28 subjects did not, however, find any differences in oxcarbazepine-treated subjects in BMD when compared to controls [47]. These studies suggest that oxcarbazepine may be associated with a limited increase in fracture. Findings are not consistent regarding effects of oxcarbazepine on BMD.

Phenobarbital: Phenobarbital is associated with increased fracture risk and reduced BMD. A Danish pharmacoepidemiological, population-based case-control study found an adjusted increased fracture risk (OR 1.79, 1.64–1.95) [23] among those taking phenobarbital. A Canadian population-based, retrospective, matched cohort study of adults older than age 50 also reported increased fracture risk in association with phenobarbital use. Reduced BMD was seen among 130 evaluated consecutive subjects in a tertiary care epilepsy center treated with phenobarbital [48]. These studies support the theory that phenobarbital use results in poor bone health.

Phenytoin: Phenytoin use results in increased fracture risk and reduced BMD. In the Canadian population-based study of older persons [32], phenytoin was associated with the highest risk of fracture among the studied AEDs (1.91 (95% CI, 1.58–2.30)). Cross-sectional and longitudinal studies have found reduced BMD at multiple sites. Among the cohort of over 6,000 postmenopausal women who were continuous users of phenytoin, they had an adjusted 1.8-fold greater mean rate of loss at the calcaneus compared to non-AED users, and had an adjusted 1.7-fold greater mean loss at the total hip compared with non-AED users [31]. Phenytoin is consistently associated with adverse effects on bone, including increased fracture risk and low BMD.

Topiramate: There are no studies evaluating the association between topiramate and increased fracture risk. A single study investigated the effects of topiramate on BMD. Thirty-six women on long-term (at least 1 year) topiramate monotherapy were compared with women taking carbamazepine, valproate, and age- and sex-matched controls [49]. In this study, there were no significant reductions in BMD among topiramate-treated women.

Valproate: Findings regarding effects of valproate on fracture risk and BMD are contradictory. One study found a limited increased risk of fracture in association with valproate therapy [23], whereas another study did not find an increased risk [32]. Cross-sectional studies in adults and children treated with valproate find decreased BMD in some studies but not in others. One prospective study of 14 premenopausal women treated with valproate monotherapy demonstrated no bone loss after 1 year of treatment [42]. These studies reveal mixed findings regarding the association between valproate and an effect on bone.

Zonisamide: The effects of zonisamide on fracture risk and BMD have not been investigated in human studies. In rats, administration of zonisamide significantly decreased BMD at the tibial metaphysis and the diaphysis [50].

Mechanisms

There are multiple proposed mechanisms to explain why AEDs are associated with low BMD. The principal mechanism relates to induction of the hepatic cytochrome P450 enzyme system. Cytochrome P450 enzyme-inducing AEDs are most consistently associated with abnormalities in bone. Treatment with liver cytochrome P450-inducing AEDs increases activity of hepatic mixed-function oxidases, resulting in accelerated vitamin D metabolism and subsequent less biologically active or inert vitamin D. Reduced active vitamin D leads to decreased intestinal calcium absorption, decreased serum ionized calcium concentration, and increased serum PTH concentration. If hyperparathyroidism persists, bone turnover increases and BMD decreases. Basic studies evaluating the effect of enzyme-inducing AEDs on the expression of cytochrome P450 isoenzymes involved in vitamin D metabolism, support these clinical observations. Phenobarbital, phenytoin, and carbamazepine are xenobiotics which activate a nuclear receptor known as either the steroid and xenobiotic receptor (SXR) or pregnane X receptor (PXR). One study found that xenobiotics up-regulate 25 hydroxyvitamin D3 -24-hydroxylase (CYP24) in the kidney through activation of PXR. This enzyme catalyzes the conversion of 25(OH)D to its inactive metabolite, 24,(25 OH)2D, rather than to its active metabolite, 1,25(OH)2D [51]. Other investigators found that xenobiotic activation of PXR did not up-regulate CYP24 but did increase expression of a different isoenzyme, CYP3A4, in the liver and small intestine [52]. This enzyme converts vitamin D to inactive metabolites. Although valproate is typically considered a cytochrome P450 enzyme-inhibiting AED, in vitro studies find that valproate induces the cytochrome P450 isoenzyme CYP3A4 at clinically relevant concentrations, as well as CYP24, leading to disturbances in vitamin D and calcium homeostasis [53, 54].

Although some studies support this hypothesis, not all observations are consistent. Carbamazepine, a known inducer of cytochrome P450 enzymes, is not always associated with decreased BMD [33, 41, 55]. Although in vitro studies suggest that valproate may also be an inducer of the cytochrome P450 isoenzymes CYP3A4 and CYP24, low active vitamin D metabolites are not consistently described in association with valproate use [41, 56, 57]. In addition, significant osteopenia and other convincing evidence of increased bone turnover has been found in a series of persons treated with AEDs, even though 25(OH)D and PTH levels were normal [58, 59].

Other mechanisms have been proposed and investigated [2]. These include impaired calcium absorption, impaired response to PTH, vitamin K reduction, hyperparathyroidism, calcitonin deficiency, elevated homocysteine, reduced reproductive hormones, genetic predisposition, and a direct effect of epilepsy and seizures on bone.

Screening

Official recommendations for screening bone health in persons with epilepsy treated with AEDs are not available. Currently, the most sensitive predictor of fracture is BMD; it is therefore reasonable to consider obtaining BMD measurements using DXA in persons at risk. The WHO developed the fracture risk assessment tool, FRAX®, to calculate a 10-year fracture probability [60]. This tool combines BMD with clinical risk factors known to increase one's risk of low BMD to determine this risk. A prior history of fracture, family history of osteoporosis and fracture, glucocorticoid steroid use, history of rheumatoid arthritis, tobacco use, and chronic alcohol use are among the factors addressed in this tool. In practice, these risk factors should be addressed in addition to the potential impact of having epilepsy and AED treatment. Routine screening of 25 hydroxyvitamin D, particularly in persons treated with enzyme-inducing AEDs, should be considered. Enzyme-inducing AEDs (carbamazepine, phenobarbital, phenytoin, and oxcarbazepine) increase the activity of hepatic mixed-function oxidases, potentially accelerating metabolism of vitamin D and decreasing biologically active vitamin D. Decreased active vitamin D results in decreased intestinal calcium absorption, decreased serum ionized calcium concentration, and a subsequent compensatory increased serum PTH concentration. If hyperparathyroidism persists, bone turnover increases and BMD decreases.

Treatment

Among the available treatment options for low BMD, only vitamin D supplementation has been studied in persons with epilepsy treated with AEDs. Bisphosphonates, selective estrogen receptor modulators, and PTH have not been evaluated. A randomized double blind trial over 1 year compared low-dose (400 IU/day for adults and children) and high-dose (4,000 IU/day for adults and 2,000 IU/day for children) vitamin D supplementation [61]. In the adults, the baseline BMD was reduced at all sites when compared to age- and gender-matched controls. After 1 year, there were significant increases in BMD at all sites in those receiving high-dose, but not low-dose, vitamin D. The children had normal BMD when compared to age- and gender-matched controls, and had significant and comparable increases in BMD in both treatment groups. Persons with epilepsy treated with AEDs should be counseled about adequate vitamin D intake, particularly in persons taking enzyme-inducing AEDs. An Institute of Medicine report in 2011 [62] states the recommended daily allowance of vitamin D is 600 IU per day. Persons taking enzyme-inducing AEDs will likely need higher doses. The report cautions that the use of more than 4,000 IU per day may increase the risk of potential harm, including renal and tissue damage.

References

1. Bachrach L. *Skeletal development in childhood and adolescence*, 7th edn. Washington, DC: American Society for Bone and Mineral Metabolism, 2008.

2. Pack AM and Walczak TS. Bone health in women with epilepsy: clinical features and potential mechanisms. *Int Rev Neurobiol* 2008; 83:305–28.

3. Waters KS. Gonadal steroids and receptors. In: Favus M, ed. *Primer on the metabolic bone diseases and disorders of bone and mineral metabolism*, 4th edn. New York, NY: Lippincott Williams and Wilkins, 2006; 104–10.

4. Karsenty G and Oury F. The central regulation of bone mass, the first link between bone remodeling and energy metabolism. *J Clin Endocrinol Metab* 2010; 95(11):4795–801.

5. Qin W, Bauman WA and Cardozo CP. Evolving concepts in neurogenic osteoporosis. *Curr Osteoporos Rep* 2010; 8(4):212–18.

6. Nicks KM, Fowler TW and Gaddy D. Reproductive hormones and bone. *Curr Osteoporos Rep* 2010; 8(2):60–7.

7. Wongdee K, Tulalamba W, Thongbunchoo J, et al. Prolactin alters the mRNA expression of osteoblast-derived osteoclastogenic factors in osteoblast-like UMR106 cells. *Mol Cell Biochem* 2011; 349(1–2):195–204.

8. Elefteriou F. Regulation of bone remodeling by the central and peripheral nervous system. *Arch Biochem Biophys* 2008; 473(2):231–6.

9. Ducy P, Amling M, Takeda S, et al. Leptin inhibits bone formation through a hypothalamic relay: a central control of bone mass. *Cell* 2000; 100(2): 197–207.

10. Elefteriou F, Takeda S, Ebihara K, et al. Serum leptin level is a regulator of bone mass. *Proc Natl Acad Sci USA* 2004; 101(9):3258–63.

11. Yadav VK, Ryu JH, Suda N, et al. Lrp5 controls bone formation by inhibiting serotonin synthesis in the duodenum. *Cell* 2008; 135(5):825–37.

12. Yadav VK, Oury F, Suda N, et al. A serotonin-dependent mechanism explains the leptin regulation of bone mass, appetite, and energy expenditure. *Cell* 2009; 138(5):976–89.

13. Zhao B and Ivashkiv LB. Negative regulation of osteoclastogenesis and bone resorption by cytokines and transcriptional repressors. *Arthritis Res Ther* 2011; 13(4):234.

14. Vestergaard P. Epilepsy, osteoporosis and fracture risk – a meta-analysis. *Acta Neurol Scand* 2005; 112(5):277–86.

15. Ensrud KE, Blackwell TL, Mangione CM, et al. Central nervous system-active medications and risk for falls in older women. *J Am Geriatr Soc* 2002; 50(10):1629–37.

16. Petty SJ, Hill KD, Haber NE, et al. Balance impairment in chronic antiepileptic drug users: a twin and sibling study. *Epilepsia* 2010; 51(2), 280–8.

17. Souverein PC, Webb DJ, Weil JG, et al. Use of antiepileptic drugs and risk of fractures: case-control study among patients with epilepsy. *Neurology* 2006; 66(9):1318–24.

18. Persson HB, Alberts KA, Farahmand BY, et al. Risk of extremity fractures in adult outpatients with epilepsy. *Epilepsia* 2002; 43(7):768–72.

19. Annegers JF, Melton, III LJ, Sun, CA, et al. Risk of age-related fractures in patients with unprovoked seizures. *Epilepsia* 1989; 30(3):348–55.

20. Grisso JA, Chiu GY, Maislin G, et al. Risk factors for hip fractures in men: a preliminary study. *J Bone Miner Res* 1991; 6(8):865–8.

21. Souverein PC, Webb, DJ, Petri H, et al. Incidence of fractures among epilepsy patients: a population-based retrospective cohort study in the General Practice Research Database. *Epilepsia* 2005; 46(2):304–10.

22. Tsiropoulos I, Andersen M, Nymark T, et al. Exposure to antiepileptic drugs and the risk of hip fracture: a case-control study. *Epilepsia* 2008; 49(12):2092–9.

23. Vestergaard P, Rejnmark L and Mosekilde L. Fracture risk associated with use of antiepileptic drugs. *Epilepsia* 2004; 45(11): 1330–37.

24. Sheth RD, Binkley N and Hermann BP. Progressive bone deficit in epilepsy. *Neurology* 2008; 70(3):170–76.

25. Sheth RD, Binkley N and Hermann BP. Gender differences in bone mineral density in epilepsy. *Epilepsia* 2008; 49(1):125–31.

26. Henderson RC, Lark RK, Gurka MJ, et al. Bone density and metabolism in children and adolescents with moderate to severe cerebral palsy. *Pediatrics* 2002; 110(1 Pt 1):e5.

27. Coppola G, Fortunato D, Auricchio G, et al. Bone mineral density in children, adolescents, and young adults with epilepsy. *Epilepsia* 2009; 50(9):2140–46.

28. Coppola G, Fortunato D, Mainolfi C, et al. Bone mineral density in a population of children and adolescents with cerebral palsy and mental retardation with or without epilepsy. *Epilepsia* 2012; 53(12):2172–7.

29. Stephen LJ, McLellan AR, Harrison JH, et al. Bone density and antiepileptic drugs: a case-controlled study. *Seizure* 1999; 8(6):339–42.

30. Cummings SR, Nevitt MC, Browner WS, et al. Risk factors for hip fracture in white women. Study of osteoporotic fractures research group. *N Engl J Med* 1995; 332(12):767–73.

31. Ensrud KE, Walczak TS, Blackwell T, et al. Antiepileptic drug use increases rates of bone loss in older women: a prospective study. *Neurology* 2004; 62(11):2051–7.

32. Jette N, Lix LM, Metge CJ, et al. Association of antiepileptic drugs with nontraumatic fractures: a population-based analysis. *Arch Neurol* 2011; 68(1):107–12.

33. Sheth RD, Wesolowski CA, Jacob JC, et al. Effect of carbamazepine and valproate on bone mineral density. *J Pediatr* 1995; 127(2):256–62.

34. Kumandas S, Koklu E, Gumus H, et al. Effect of carbamezapine and valproic acid on bone mineral density, IGF-I and IGFBP-3. *J Pediatr Endocrinol Metab* 2006; 19(4):529–34.

35. Kim SH, Lee JW, Choi KG, et al. A 6-month longitudinal study of bone mineral density with antiepileptic drug monotherapy. *Epilepsy Behav* 2007; 10(2):291–5.

36. Hoikka V, Alhava EM, Karjalainen P, et al. Carbamazepine and bone mineral metabolism. *Acta Neurol Scand* 1984; 70(2):77–80.

37. Andress DL, Ozuna J, Tirschwell D, et al. Antiepileptic drug-induced bone loss in young male patients who have seizures. *Arch Neurol* 2002; 59(5):81–6.

38. El-Hajj Fuleihan G, Dib L, Yamout B, et al. Predictors of bone density in ambulatory patients on antiepileptic drugs. *Bone* 2008; 43(1):149–55.

39. Vestergaard P, Rejnmark L and Mosekilde L. Anxiolytics and sedatives and risk of fractures: effects of half-life. *Calcif Tissue Int* 2008; 82(1):34–43.

40. Guo CY, Ronen GM and Atkinson SA. Long-term valproate and lamotrigine treatment may be a marker for reduced growth and bone mass in children with epilepsy. *Epilepsia* 2001; 42(9): 1141–7.

41. Pack AM, Morrell MJ, Marcus R, et al. Bone mass and turnover in women with epilepsy on antiepileptic drug monotherapy. *Ann Neurol* 2005; 57(2): 252–7.

42. Pack AM, Morrell MJ, Randall A, et al. Bone health in young women with epilepsy after one year of antiepileptic drug monotherapy. *Neurology* 2008; 70(18):1586–93.

43. Nissen-Meyer LS, Svalheim S, Tauboll E, et al. Levetiracetam, phenytoin, and valproate act differently on rat bone mass, structure, and metabolism. *Epilepsia* 2007; 48(10):1850–60.

44. Koo DL, Joo EY, Kim D, et al. Effects of levetiracetam as a monotherapy on bone mineral density and biochemical markers of bone metabolism in patients with epilepsy. *Epilepsy Res* 2013; 104(1–2): 134–9.

45. Babayigit A, Dirik E, Bober E, et al. Adverse effects of antiepileptic drugs on bone mineral density. *Pediatr Neurol* 2006; 35(3):177–81.

46. Cansu A, Yesilkaya E, Serdaroglu A, et al. Evaluation of bone turnover in epileptic children using oxcarbazepine. *Pediatr Neurol* 2008; 39(4):266–71.

47. Cetinkaya Y, Kurtulmus YS, Tutkavul K, et al. The effect of oxcarbazepine on bone metabolism. *Acta Neurol Scand* 2009; 120(3):170–75.

48. Lado F, Spiegel R, Masur JH, et al. Value of routine screening for bone demineralization in an urban population of patients with epilepsy. *Epilepsy Res* 2008; 78(2–3):155–60.

49. Heo K, Rhee Y, Lee HW, et al. The effect of topiramate monotherapy on bone mineral density and markers of bone and mineral metabolism in premenopausal women with epilepsy. *Epilepsia* 2011; 52(10):1884–9.

50. Takahashi A, Onodera K, Kamei J, et al. Effects of chronic administration of zonisamide, an antiepileptic drug, on bone mineral density and their prevention with alfacalcidol in growing rats. *J Pharmacol Sci* 2003; 91(4):313–18.

51. Pascussi JM, Robert A, Nguyen M, et al. Possible involvement of pregnane X receptor-enhanced CYP24 expression in drug-induced osteomalacia. *J Clin Invest* 2005; 115(1):177–86.

52. Zhou C, Assem M, Tay JC, et al. Steroid and xenobiotic receptor and vitamin D receptor crosstalk mediates CYP24 expression and drug-induced osteomalacia. *J Clin Invest* 2006; 116(6):1703–12.

53. Cerveny L, Svecova L, Anzenbacherova E, et al. Valproic acid induces CYP3A4 and MDR1 gene expression by activation of constitutive androstane receptor and

pregnane X receptor pathways. *Drug Metab Dispos* 2007; 35(7):1032–41.

54. Vrzal R, Doricakova A, Novotna A, et al. Valproic acid augments vitamin D receptor-mediated induction of CYP24 by vitamin D3: a possible cause of valproic acid-induced osteomalacia? *Toxicol Lett* 2011; 200(3):146–53.

55. Kafali G, Erselcan T and Tanzer F. Effect of antiepileptic drugs on bone mineral density in children between ages 6 and 12 years. *Clin Pediatr (Phila)* 1999; 38(2):93–8.

56. Sato Y, Kondo I, Ishida S, et al. Decreased bone mass and increased bone turnover with valproate therapy in adults with epilepsy. *Neurology* 2001; 57(3):445–9.

57. Verrotti A, Agostinelli S, Coppola G, et al. A 12-month longitudinal study of calcium metabolism and bone turnover during valproate monotherapy. *Eur J Neurol* 2010; 17(2):232–7.

58. Verrotti A, Greco R, Morgese G, et al. Increased bone turnover in epileptic patients treated with carbamazepine. *Ann Neurol* 2000; 47(3):385–8.

59. Verrotti A, Greco R, Latini G, et al. Increased bone turnover in prepubertal, pubertal, and postpubertal patients receiving carbamazepine. *Epilepsia* 2002; 43(12):1488–92.

60. McCloskey E and Kanis JA. FRAX updates 2012. *Curr Opin Rheumatol* 2012; 24(5):554–60.

61. Mikati MA, Dib L, Yamout B, et al. Two randomized vitamin D trials in ambulatory patients on anticonvulsants: impact on bone. *Neurology* 2006; 67(11):2005–14.

62. IOM (Institute of Medicine). *Dietary reference intakes for calcium and vitamin D.* Washington, DC: The National Academies Press, 2011. www.iom.edu/vitamind.

Index

abortion
  induced, 116
  spontaneous, 11, 174
academic underachievement, 96
acetazolamide, 108
acetylcholine (ACh), 52
adolescent girls with epilepsy, 6–8
  adverse effects of AEDs, 93–4
  bone health, 95, 266–7
  contraception, 95
  endocrine effects of AEDs, 94–5
  psychosocial issues, 95–7
  reproductive endocrine dysfunction, 92–3
  seizure control, 95
  transition to adult care, 97
AEDs. See antiepileptic drugs
affective disorders. See mood disorders
agoraphobia, 5–6
Aicardi syndrome, 85–6
airway management, obstetric anesthesia, 207–8
alexithymia, 28
alfentanyl, 211–13
allopregnanolone
  catamenial epilepsy, 104–5
  mechanism of brain actions, 59–60, 62
  mediating progesterone actions, 58–60
amenorrhea, hypothalamic. See hypothalamic hypogonadism
androgenic neurosteroids, 53–60, 62
androstanediol, 61
anesthesia, obstetric. See obstetric anesthesia
anesthetic induction agents, 209–10
anovulatory cycles (inadequate luteal phase; ILP), 102–3, 106–7
antenatal management, 184–6
  AED therapy, 175, 184

anticholinesterases, 211
anticonvulsant drugs. See antiepileptic drugs
antidepressants, seizure risks, 28–9
antidiuretic hormone (ADH), 75–6
antiepileptic drugs (AEDs)
  adverse effects in children/adolescents, 93–4
  antenatal management, 175, 184
  assessing exposure of breastfed infants, 224–35
  bone health effects, 264–71
  breastfeeding and, 14, 149–50, 223–40
  childhood and adolescent epilepsy, 95
  contraceptive choice and, 135–6
  contraceptive interactions, 10, 128, 132–7
  cyclical use, catamenial epilepsy, 107–8
  domperidone interactions, 240
  endocrine effects in children/adolescents, 94–5
  enzyme-inducing. See enzyme-inducing antiepileptic drugs
  excretion into breast milk, 224–5
  fetal adverse effects, 11–12, 183–4, 252, 256–7
  fracture risk and, 266
  hormones and, 61–2, 65–76
  incidence of use in pregnancy, 251
  intrapartum therapy, 177, 186
  kinetics during pregnancy, 177–80
  metabolizing enzymes, 227–8
  neonatal withdrawal symptoms, 256
  obstetric anesthesia and, 208–9

osteoporosis risk, 15
  perimenstrual changes in metabolism, 105–6
  polytherapy. See polytherapy
  postpartum kinetics, 216–20
  preconception management, 138, 150–2, 175
  pregnancy outcomes and, 12–13
  and pregnancy registers, 144, 165–6
  in psychiatric comorbidities, 30
  psychiatric side effects, 28, 31
  psychotropic drug interactions, 30–2
  reproductive endocrine function and, 9, 65–71
  risks in pregnancy, 144–8, 157–67, 183–4
  role in infertility, 66, 120–2
  seizure control during pregnancy, 13–14
  selection for women of childbearing age, 123–5
  self-management in postpartum period, 245
  serum level monitoring. See therapeutic drug monitoring
  sleep effects, 38
  teratogenicity. See teratogenicity of AEDs
antipsychotic drugs, seizure risks, 28–9
anxiety, new mothers, 245
anxiety disorders, 5–6, 24
aortocaval compression, pregnant uterus, 208
Apgar scores, 184
aspiration pneumonitis, obstetric anesthesia, 207
atracurium, 210–11
attention deficit hyperactivity disorder (ADHD), 96
autism spectrum disorders, 163
autosomal dominant focal epilepsies, 143
awakening epilepsies, 36

barbiturates, induction of
anesthesia, 210, *See also*
phenobarbital
behavioral problems,
childhood, 94, 96
benzodiazepines (BZDs)
anesthesia induction, 209
catamenial epilepsy, 107–8
intrapartum therapy, 186
neonatal withdrawal
syndrome, 209, 236
postpartum seizure
management, 216
teratogenicity, 164, 212
bilateral periventricular
nodular heterotopia, 143
bipolar disorder, 24–5
bone, physiology, 265–6
bone health, 15, 264–71
bone mineral density (BMD),
265
adolescent girls, 95, 266–7
effects of AEDs, 266–70
factors associated with
reduced, 267
mechanisms of AED effects,
270
postmenopausal women, 268
screening, 270–1
treatment of reduced, 271
brain tumors, 197–200
brain-derived neurotrophic
factor (BDNF), 53
breast milk
factors influencing AED
excretion into, 224–5
indices of AED excretion
into, 226–7, 229
breastfeeding (lactation), 14,
223–40, 254, *See also*
postpartum period
assessing infant AED
exposure, 224–35
avoiding sleep deprivation,
247
benefits, 224
maternal adherence to, 235
neuroimaging with contrast
agents, 191–2, 202
preconception counseling,
149–50
psychotropic drugs, 30–1
specific AEDs, 236–40
treating refractory seizures,
220
bullying, 96

calcium homeostasis, 265
carbamazepine (CBZ)
bone health effects, 268,
270
breastfeeding mothers, 229,
236
cognitive effects of fetal
exposure, 147, 257
contraceptive interactions,
134
hyponatremic effects, 75
pharmacokinetics, 177, 225
postpartum period, 216
reproductive endocrine
effects, 66, 69–70, 121
teratogenicity, 146, 161
thyroid function effects, 74,
94
catamenial epilepsy, 8, 50,
101–11
animal models, 54
definition, 106
diagnosis, 107
hormonal influences, 55–6,
59, 61, 104–5
management, 107–11, 137–8
menopausal/perimenopausal
changes, 261
pathophysiology, 104–6
patterns, 102, 106–7
prevalence, 106
catheter angiography, 194–5
cavernous hemangioma, 199
CDKL5 gene mutations, 80–2
central nervous system
infections, 199
cerebral palsy, 118, 267
cerebral venous thrombosis,
194–6
cesarean section, 184, 186
childcare/parenting,
246–9
family involvement, 248–9
knowledge about, 242–3
safety, 152, 244–8
children of women with
epilepsy, *See also* infants;
neonates
cognitive outcomes.
See cognitive outcomes in
offspring
epilepsy risk, 6–7, 143–4,
183
follow-up, 256–7
maternal neuroimaging and,
190–2

children with epilepsy, female,
6–8
adverse effects of AEDs, 93–4
bone health, 95, 266–7
endocrine effects of AEDs,
94–5
psychosocial issues, 95–7
seizure control, 95
choriocarcinoma, metastatic,
199–200
clefts, oral/facial, 160, 162–3
clobazam
breastfeeding mothers, 229,
236
catamenial epilepsy, 107–8
contraceptive interactions,
135
intrapartum therapy, 177,
186
pharmacokinetics, 225
clomiphene citrate, 110, 124–5
clonazepam
breastfeeding mothers, 229,
236
pharmacokinetics, 225
cognitive adverse effects of
AEDs, 94
cognitive impairment (mental
retardation), 96
bone health and, 267
role in infertility, 116, 118
cognitive outcomes in offspring
breastfeeding and, 14, 149
fetal AED exposure, 12, 147,
162, 256–7
folic acid supplements and,
148
seizures during pregnancy
and, 149
combined hormonal
contraception, 131–2
combined oral contraceptive
pill (COC), 131, *See also*
oral contraceptives
comorbidities, 4–6
computed tomography (CT),
189–90, 201
pregnancy-related
conditions, 192, 195, 198
safety of unborn child, 190–1
congenital malformations,
159–67, *See also*
teratogenicity of AEDs
AED dose effects, 146
AED polytherapy vs.
monotherapy, 147

AED-related risks, 11–12,
    144–8, 159–67
antenatal screening, 185
folic acid supplements and,
    10–11, 148
late diagnosis, 256
major syndromes, 161
neonatal examination, 253–4
recurrence risks, 165
related to specific AEDs,
    255
worldwide registries, 144,
    165–6
contraception, 10, 127–38
adolescent girls, 95
AED interactions, 10, 128,
    132–7
clinical recommendations,
    135–6
dual method, 129
frequency of use, 128
methods, 128–32
preconception planning, 138
role in seizure control, 137–8
contraceptive implants, 129–30,
    137
contrast media
pregnant and lactating
    women, 201–2
safety of fetus/neonate,
    190–2
cooking safety, 247
copper intrauterine devices
    (IUDs), 129–30, 136
cosmetic adverse effects of
    AEDs, 93
curare, 210–11
cytochrome P450 enzymes, 227
cytokines, inflammatory, 266

danazol, 111
daytime sleepiness, excessive
    (EDS), 40–1, 47
DCX gene mutations, 84
dehydroepiandrosterone sulfate
    (DHEAS), 62, 70
depot-medroxyprogesterone
    acetate (DMPA) (Depo-
    Provera)
catamenial epilepsy, 109, 137
contraception, 130–1, 136
depression, 4–5, 20–3
childhood/adolescent
    epilepsy, 96
interictal, 21–2
postpartum (PPD), 5, 22–3

preictal, ictal, and postictal,
    21
role in infertility, 117
desflurane, 210
diabetes mellitus (DM), type 2,
    72–3
diazepam, 209, 216
diffuse epilepsies, 36
dihydrotestosterone, 61
domperidone, 240
driving, new mothers, 248
drowning risk, 172

eclampsia
difficult intubation, 207
neuroimaging, 192–4
postpartum, 220
electrolyte disturbances,
    obstetric patients, 208
endotracheal intubation,
    obstetric patients, 207
energy metabolism, effects of
    AEDs, 71–4
enflurane, 210
environmental safety, new
    mothers, 248
enzyme-inducing antiepileptic
    drugs (EIAEDs)
contraceptive interactions,
    10, 132–5
contraceptive selection,
    135–6
effects on bone health, 270
obstetric anesthesia and,
    208
psychotropic drug
    interactions, 30–2
reproductive endocrine
    effects, 61–2, 66, 69–70,
    121
thyroid function effects, 74–5
epidemiology, epilepsy, 1–4
epidural anesthesia, obstetric,
    177, 208
local anesthetic toxicity, 209
epilepsy and mental retardation
    limited to females
    (EFMR), 84–5
epilepsy surgery
mania after, 25
menstrual cycle changes
    after, 120
psychosis after, 26
epilepsy syndromes
hereditary, 8, 80–7
influencing fertility, 118

estrogen, 51–6
catamenial epilepsy and,
    55–6, 104
effects of AEDs, 61–2
effects on bone, 265
mechanisms of
    neuroexcitatory effects,
    51–3, 62, 260–1
neuroprotective effects, 53–5
perimenopausal changes,
    260
proconvulsant effects, 52–6
seizure susceptibility and,
    54–6
sleep effects, 38–9
testosterone conversion to,
    61
estrogen receptors (ER), 52
ethosuximide
breastfeeding mothers, 229,
    236–7
pharmacokinetics, 177, 225
etomidate, 210
excessive daytime sleepiness
    (EDS), 40–1, 47
Exposure Index, 228–35

falls, 266
family support, new mothers,
    248–9
felbamate
breastfeeding mothers, 229,
    237
contraceptive interactions,
    134
induced weight loss, 73
pharmacokinetics, 225
fentanyl, 211–13
fertility rates, 9, 114–15,
    See also infertility
fetal anticonvulsant syndrome,
    161
fetal growth restriction, 254
fetal hydantoin syndrome, 161
fetus, See also congenital
    malformations; infants
adverse effects of AEDs,
    11–12, 183–4, 252, 256–7
monitoring, 184–7
safety of maternal
    neuroimaging, 190–2
fluid intake, new mothers, 247
folic acid
supplementation, 10–11, 148,
    185
valproate interactions, 159

follicle-stimulating hormone (FSH), 67–8, 103
forced normalization, 26
FOXG1 gene mutations, 80, 82–3
fracture risk assessment tool (FRAX), 270–1
fractures, 15, 266

GABA (γ-aminobutyric acid), estrogen actions, 52–3
GABA-A receptors
neurosteroid interactions, 59–60
progesterone actions, 57–8, 60, 104
gabapentin
bone health effects, 268
breastfeeding mothers, 229, 237
induced weight gain, 72
pharmacokinetics, 177, 225
postpartum period, 217, 220
teratogenicity, 11–12, 163
gadolinium-based contrast media, 191–2, 201–2
ganaxolone, 110
gender differences
childhood/adolescent epilepsy, 7
epilepsy risk, 4
genetic causes of epilepsy in women, 8, 80–7
genetics, epilepsy, 6–7, 143–4
glioblastoma multiforme, 199
glucose metabolism, effects of AEDs, 71–4
glucuronosyltransferases (UGT), 228
glutamate, 52
glutamic acid decarboxylase (GAD), 53, 55
gonadotropin-releasing hormone (GnRH)
analogs, catamenial epilepsy, 111
pulsatile secretion, 67, 93, 103
goserelin, 111

halothane, 210
head growth, poor fetal, 254
HELLP syndrome, 194
hemorrhagic disease of newborn, 187, 253

heritability, epilepsy, 143–4, 183
hippocampus, estrogen actions, 52–4
home environment, safety, 248
hormonal contraceptives, 129–32
AED interactions, 10, 128, 132–7
catamenial epilepsy, 108–9, 137–8
hormonal therapy, catamenial epilepsy, 108–11
hormone replacement therapy (HRT), 14, 262
effects on sleep, 45–6
seizure frequency and, 262
hormones, 50–62
AEDs and, 61–2, 65–76
catamenial epilepsy and, 55–6, 59, 61, 104–5
effects on sleep problems, 38–40
epilepsy in adolescent girls and, 92–3
influences on brain activity, 51–61
perimenopausal changes, 260
household chores, 247
hydration, new mothers, 247
hydromorphone, 211–13
hyperandrogenism, 67–9
hypercarbia, obstetric patients, 208
hyperinsulinemia, 68–9, 72, 122
hyperparathyroidism, 270–1
hyperprolactinemia, 119
hyperventilation, obstetric patients, 208
hypoandrogenism, 69–70
hypocarbia, obstetric patients, 208, 210
hypoglycemia
neonatal, 256
obstetric patients, 208
hyponatremia, 75–6
hypothalamic hypogonadism (hypothalamic amenorrhea), 9, 70, 119
hypothalamic-pituitary-ovarian (or gonadal) axis, 103
effects of AEDs, 68, 121
effects of epileptic lesion, 67, 119–20
hypoxia, 207–8

implants, contraceptive, 129–30, 137
inadequate luteal phase (ILP) (anovulatory cycles), 102–3, 106–7
incidence, epilepsy, 2–3
infant dose, 226, 229
maternal weight-adjusted, 226, 229
infants, *See also* children of women with epilepsy; neonates
assessing AED exposure, 224–35
determinants of drug exposure levels, 226–35
drug clearance, 227–8
drug exposure indices, 226–7, 229
infertility, 113–25
epidemiology, 9, 114
etiology, 8–10, 116–22
evaluation, 122–4
management, 123–5
role of AEDs, 66, 120–2
inheritance, 6–7
insomnia, 41, 45
insulin resistance, 68–9, 72, 122
insulin-like growth factor-1 (IGF-1), 68
interictal discharges, sleep influences on, 37
interictal dysphoric disorder, 21–2
intracranial hemorrhage, neonates, 254
intrapartum management, 186
intrauterine devices (IUDs), 129–30
recommendations on use, 136
intrauterine growth restriction, 254
iodinated contrast media, 190–1, 201–2
iron deficiency, 42, 44
isoflurane, 210

juvenile absence epilepsy (JAE), 7
juvenile myoclonic epilepsy (JME), 7, 86
preconception planning, 150, 175

ketamine, 210

labor and delivery
  management, 186
  seizure management, 177
  seizures during, 173, 208
lactation. *See* breastfeeding
lamotrigine (LTG; LMT)
  adverse effects in children/
    adolescents, 93
  bone health effects, 268
  breastfeeding mothers, 229,
    237
  contraceptive interactions,
    135–6
  dose in pregnancy, 172
  kinetics during pregnancy,
    177, 179–80
  perimenstrual changes in
    serum levels, 105–6
  pharmacokinetics, 225
  postpartum period, 217
  reproductive endocrine
    effects, 69
  teratogenicity, 11–12, 146, 163
leptin, 265–6
levetiracetam (LEV)
  bone health effects, 269
  breastfeeding mothers, 229,
    238
  cognitive effects of fetal
    exposure, 147
  hyponatremia/SIADH due
    to, 76
  kinetics during pregnancy,
    177, 179
  pharmacokinetics, 225
  postpartum period, 217–18
  reproductive endocrine
    effects, 69
  teratogenicity, 11–12, 146,
    163–4
levonorgestrel-releasing
    intrauterine device (LNG
    IUD), 129–30, 136
libido, reduced. *See* sexual
    dysfunction
lithium, 30
local anesthetics, obstetric
    patients, 209
long-acting reversible
    contraception (LARC)
    methods, 129–31
lorazepam, 216
low birth weight infants, 174–5
luteinizing hormone (LH),
    67–8, 103
  pulsatile secretion, 119–20

magnesium sulfate, 177
magnetic resonance imaging
    (MRI), 200–1
  pregnancy-related
    conditions, 192–7,
    199–200
  pregnant and lactating
    women, 201–3
  safety of unborn child, 191–2
Mallampati classification, 207
mania
  post-epilepsy surgery, 25
  postictal, 25
marriage rates, 9–10, 116
maternal weight-adjusted
    infant dose, 226, 229
meal preparation, 247
MeCP2 gene, 80, 82
medroxyprogesterone acetate
    (MPA)
  catamenial epilepsy, 109, 137
  depot. *See* depot-
    medroxyprogesterone
    acetate
meningioma, 199
menopause, 14–15, 260–2,
    See also hormone
    replacement therapy
  age at, 260
  management, 262
  premature, 119, 262
  seizures at, 261
  sleep problems, 44–5
menstrual cycle, 101–4, *See also*
    catamenial epilepsy
  AED metabolism during,
    105–6
  after epilepsy surgery, 120
  effects on sleep, 39–40
menstrual disorders, 8–9
mental retardation.
    See cognitive impairment
meperidine, 211
metabolic syndrome, 71
midazolam, 209, 216
milk-to-plasma drug-
    concentration ratio
    (MP ratio), 226, 228,
    235
Mini International
    Neuropsychiatric
    Interview (MINI), 27
miscarriage (spontaneous
    abortion), 11, 174
mood changes, new mothers,
    246

mood disorders, 4–5, 20–5
morphine, 211–13
muscle relaxants.
    See neuromuscular
    blocking agents
myelomeningocele, 185–6
myopia, in offspring, 256

neonates, 251–7, *See also*
    infants
  AED withdrawal symptoms,
    256
  benzodiazepine withdrawal
    syndrome, 209, 236
  delivery room care, 253
  drug clearance, 227–8
  feeding, 247
  immediate care and pre-
    discharge assessment,
    254–6
  long-term follow-up, 256–7
  opioid withdrawal syndrome,
    212, 236
  parenting safety, 152, 244–9
  physical examination, 253–4
  potential complications,
    183–4, 253–6
  vitamin K supplements, 187,
    253
neuraxial anesthesia, obstetric,
    208–9
neurodevelopmental outcomes.
    See cognitive outcomes in
    offspring
neuroimaging in pregnancy,
    189–203
  brain tumors, 197–200
  cerebral venous thrombosis,
    194–6
  modalities, 189–90
  other conditions, 199–200
  postpartum cerebral
    angiopathy, 197–8
  pre-eclampsia and eclampsia,
    192–4
  recommended protocol,
    200–1
  safety of unborn child,
    190–2
neuromuscular blocking agents,
    208, 210–11
neuropeptide Y (NPY), 53, 55
neurosteroids
  endogenous, 53–60, 62
  therapy, catamenial epilepsy,
    110

non-rapid eye movement (NREM) sleep, 35, 37
norepinephrine, 265

obesity, 68, 121–2, *See also* weight gain
obstetric anesthesia, 206–13
  AED interactions, 208–9
  airway management, 207–8
  anesthetic induction agents, 209–10
  neuromuscular blocking agents, 208, 210–11
  opioid analgesics, 211–13
  volatile anesthetics, 210
obstetric monitoring, 184–7
obstructive sleep apnea (OSA), 6, 41–2, 44–5
offspring of women with epilepsy. *See* children of women with epilepsy
opioid analgesics, 211–13
opioid withdrawal syndrome, neonatal, 212, 236
oral contraceptives (OC), 10, 131–2
  adolescent girls, 95
  AED interactions, 132–6
  catamenial epilepsy, 109, 138
  recommendations on use, 135
oral/facial clefts, 160, 162–3
osmolarity, serum, effects of AEDs, 75–6
osteoporosis, 15, 268
ovulation, measuring, 107
oxcarbazepine (OXC)
  bone health effects, 269
  breastfeeding mothers, 229, 238
  contraceptive interactions, 134, 136
  hyponatremic effects, 75
  kinetics during pregnancy, 177, 179
  pharmacokinetics, 225
  postpartum period, 218, 220
  teratogenicity, 11–12, 164
  thyroid function effects, 74–5

pancuronium, 210–11
panic disorder, 5–6
parathyroid hormone (PTH), 265

parenting. *See* childcare/ parenting
PCDH19 gene mutations, 85
perimenopause, *See also* hormone replacement therapy
  hormonal changes, 260
  management, 262
  seizures at, 261
perinatal death, 184
periodic limb movement disorder (PLMD), 42–3
periodic limb movements of sleep (PLMS), 42, 44
pethidine (meperidine), 211
phenobarbital (PB)
  bone health effects, 269–70
  breastfeeding mothers, 229, 238
  contraceptive interactions, 133
  kinetics during pregnancy, 177
  metabolism in infants, 227
  pharmacokinetics, 225
  postpartum period, 218
  reproductive endocrine effects, 66, 69–70
  teratogenicity, 146, 162
phenytoin (PHT)
  bone health effects, 269–70
  breastfeeding mothers, 229, 239
  contraceptive interactions, 134
  cosmetic adverse effects, 93
  inhibition of ADH release, 75
  kinetics during pregnancy, 177
  metabolism in infants, 227
  perimenstrual changes in metabolism, 105
  pharmacokinetics, 225
  postpartum period, 219
  reproductive endocrine effects, 66, 69–70
  thyroid function effects, 74
polycystic ovary syndrome (PCOS), 9, 66–9, 92–3, 118
polysomnography (PSG), 42, 47
polytherapy
  congenital malformation risk, 147
  seizure risk in pregnancy, 171

post-epilepsy surgery mania, 25
post-epilepsy surgery psychosis, 26
posterior reversible encephalopathy syndrome (PRES), 192–4
postmenopausal women, bone health, 268
postpartum blues, 22
postpartum cerebral angiopathy, 197–8
postpartum depression (PPD), 5, 22–3
postpartum period, 215–21, *See also* breastfeeding; neonates
  kinetics of individual AEDs, 216–20
  problem of seizure control, 215
  recommendations for seizure control, 220
  safety considerations, 242–9
  status epilepticus, 220
  treating breakthrough seizures, 216
  treating refractory seizures, 220
  vitamin K supplements, 187, 253
postpartum psychosis (PPP), 22–3
pre-eclampsia, 12–13, 184
  difficult intubation, 207
  neuroimaging, 192–4
preconception counseling, 10–11, 141–53
  AED management, 138, 150–2, 175
  approach to, 141–2
  common questions asked, 143–50
  key elements, 141–2
  safety and social support, 152
pregabalin
  induced weight gain, 72
  kinetics during pregnancy, 177, 179
pregnancy, 12–14, 170–80, 182–7
  adverse effects of seizures, 149, 174–5
  adverse outcomes, 12–13, 183–4
  AED management, 175, 184

AED pharmacokinetics,
177–80
antenatal management, 184–6
incidence of AED use, 251
neuroimaging in, 189–203
obstetric and fetal
monitoring, 184–7
postnatal management, 14,
187
psychotropic drugs, 30–1
registers, 144, 165–6
risks of AEDs, 144–8,
157–67, 183–4
seizure frequency, 148–9,
170–2, 182–3
seizure management, 13–14,
177
sleep problems, 43–4
status epilepticus, 172–3
pregnenolone sulfate, 59–60
premature ovarian failure
(POF), 119, 262
premenstrual dysphoric
disorder (PMDD), 23–4
pre-term delivery, 12–13,
174–5, 253
prevalence, epilepsy, 1–2
primidone
breastfeeding mothers, 229,
239
contraceptive interactions,
134
pharmacokinetics, 225
progesterone, 56–9
mechanisms of
neuroinhibitory effects,
56–7, 60, 261
perimenopausal changes, 260
role in catamenial epilepsy,
59, 104–5
seizure susceptibility and,
58–9
sleep effects, 39
therapy, catamenial epilepsy,
109–10, 138
progesterone receptors (PR),
56–7, 60
progestin-only pill (POP), 131
prolactin, 118–19, 265
propofol, 210
psychiatric comorbidities, 4–6,
20–32
children and adolescents, 94,
96
psychogenic non-epileptic
seizures (PNES), 27–8

psychosis, 25–6
alternative, 26
interictal, 26
post-epilepsy surgery, 26
postpartum, 22–3
preictal, postictal, and ictal,
25–6
psychosocial issues, childhood/
adolescent epilepsy, 95–7
psychotropic drugs
AED interactions, 30–2
in pregnancy and lactation,
30–1
seizure risks, 28–9

quality of life, childhood/
adolescent epilepsy, 97

radiation exposure, fetus/
embryo, 190
rapid eye movement (REM)
sleep, 35–6
5α-reductase, 104
regional anesthesia, obstetric,
208–9
remifentanil, 211–13
reminders, medication, 245
renal function, neonates, 228
reproductive dysfunction,
8–10
adolescent girls, 92–3
AED selection and, 123–5
as cause of infertility, 118–19
regular monitoring, 124
role of AEDs, 9, 65–71
signs and evaluation, 122–4
respiratory distress, neonatal,
253
restless legs syndrome (RLS),
42–4
Rett syndrome, 80–3
risk-taking behavior, 96
rocuronium, 210–11
rufinamide, contraceptive
interactions, 135

safety considerations
childcare/parenting, 152, 244–8
neuroimaging in pregnancy,
190–2
schizophrenia, 26
seizures
adolescent girls with
epilepsy, 95
adverse effects in pregnancy,
149

estrogen effects, 54–6
fetal effects, 174–5
fracture risk, 266
frequency in pregnancy,
148–9, 170–2, 182–3
management in pregnancy,
13–14, 177
menopause/perimenopause,
261
neonatal, 254
peripartum, 173
postpartum management,
216, 220
postpartum triggers, 245–6
psychogenic non-epileptic
seizures (PNES), 27–8
self-management, 243–5
sleep disruption, 37–8
sleep-wake timing, 36–7
self-management, postpartum
period, 242–9
common needs, 243
defined, 243
medication management,
245
seizure management, 243–5
seizure triggers, 245–6
serotonin, 266
sevoflurane, 210
sex hormone-binding globulin
(SHBG), 66, 70
sex steroid hormones.
See estrogen;
progesterone; testosterone
sexual dysfunction, 8, 70
as cause of infertility, 117,
120
sexually transmitted infections,
132
sleep, 34–40
epilepsy interactions, 36–8
hormonal influences, 38–40
physiology of epilepsy
interactions, 35–6
stages, 35
sleep deprivation
EEG, 37
effects, 40–1
new mothers, 245–7
sleep epilepsies, 36
sleep-disordered breathing,
41–5
sleep-related comorbidities, 6,
40–7
small for gestational age (SGA),
13, 174–5, 183–4

social factors, leading to infertility, 116
social support, new mothers, 152, 245
sodium
   homeostasis, effects of AEDs, 75–6
   serum level monitoring, 76
spina bifida, 160, 162
   antenatal screening, 185–6
status epilepticus
   antenatal management, 177
   induction of anesthesia, 209–10
   postpartum, 220
   risk during pregnancy, 172–3
stigma, as cause of infertility, 116
stress, new mothers, 245–6
subcortical band heterotopia (SBH), 83–4, 144
sudden unexpected death in epilepsy (SUDEP), 36–7, 172
sufentanyl, 211–13
suicide, 26–7
   children and adolescents, 94, 96
syndrome of inappropriate antidiuretic hormone (SIADH), 76

temporal lobe epilepsy (TLE)
   catamenial epilepsy, 107
   hypothalamic hypogonadism, 9, 119
   infertility, 118
   PCOS association, 67
   reproductive disorders, 66
   sexual dysfunction, 8, 70
teratogenesis, principles, 158
teratogenicity of AEDs, 11–12, 157–67, See also congenital malformations
   categories of risk, 159–60
   dose effects, 146
   folic acid supplements and, 10–11, 148
   newer AEDs, 159
   older AEDs, 158–9
   polytherapy vs. monotherapy, 147
   preconception counseling, 144–8
teratology, 157–8
termination of pregnancy, 116

testosterone
   effects on sleep, 39
   mechanism of effects on brain, 53–60, 62
therapeutic drug monitoring (TDM)
   postpartum period, 216, 220
   preconception planning, 150–2
   pregnancy, 175, 180
thrombotic thrombocytopenic purpura (TTP), 194
thyroid hormones, effects of AEDs, 74–5, 94
tiagabine
   breastfeeding mothers, 229, 239
   pharmacokinetics, 177, 225
topiramate
   bone health effects, 269
   breastfeeding mothers, 229, 239
   cognitive adverse effects, 94
   contraceptive interactions, 134
   induced weight loss, 72–3
   kinetics during pregnancy, 177, 179
   pharmacokinetics, 225
   postpartum period, 219–20
   teratogenicity, 11–12, 146, 162
transition to adult care, 97
trimethadione syndrome, 161
triptorelin, 111

ultrasonography, antenatal, 185

vagus nerve stimulator (VNS), 220
valproic acid (VPA)
   adverse effects in children/ adolescents, 93
   bone health effects, 269–70
   breastfeeding mothers, 229, 239–40
   cognitive effects of fetal exposure, 12, 147, 162, 257
   contraceptive interactions, 136
   during pregnancy, 184
   fertility effects, 121–2
   hyponatremia/SIADH due to, 76
   hypothalamic hypogonadism due to, 70

induced weight gain, 68–9, 71–4
   kinetics during pregnancy, 177–9
   mechanism of teratogenesis, 159
   PCOS association, 9, 66–9, 93
   perimenstrual changes in serum levels, 105–6
   pharmacokinetics, 225
   postpartum period, 219
   preconception planning, 150
   sexual dysfunction due to, 71
   teratogenicity, 11, 146–7, 162–3
   use in women of reproductive age, 69
vecuronium, 210–11
vigabatrin
   breastfeeding mothers, 229, 240
   induced weight gain, 72
   kinetics during pregnancy, 177, 179
   pharmacokinetics, 225
vitamin D, 265, 270–1
vitamin K, 187, 253
volatile anesthetic agents, 210

water balance
   catamenial epilepsy and, 105
   effects of AEDs, 75–6
weight gain
   AEDs inducing, 71–2, 94–5, 121–2
   pregnancy-related, difficult airway, 207
   valproate-induced, 68–9, 71–4
weight loss, AEDs inducing, 72–3

zonisamide
   bone health effects, 269
   breastfeeding mothers, 229, 240
   induced weight loss, 73
   kinetics during pregnancy, 177, 179
   pharmacokinetics, 225
   teratogenicity, 164